Treatments for Squamous Cell Cancer

Treatments for Squamous Cell Cancer

Editor

Charbel Darido

MDPI • Basel • Beijing • Wuhan • Barcelona • Belgrade • Manchester • Tokyo • Cluj • Tianjin

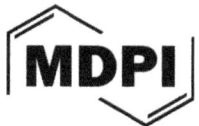

Editor
Charbel Darido
The Sir Peter MacCallum
Department of Oncology
University of Melbourne
Melbourne
Australia

Editorial Office
MDPI
St. Alban-Anlage 66
4052 Basel, Switzerland

This is a reprint of articles from the Special Issue published online in the open access journal *Cancers* (ISSN 2072-6694) (available at: www.mdpi.com/journal/cancers/special_issues/Squamous_Cell_Cancer).

For citation purposes, cite each article independently as indicated on the article page online and as indicated below:

LastName, A.A.; LastName, B.B.; LastName, C.C. Article Title. *Journal Name* **Year**, *Volume Number*, Page Range.

ISBN 978-3-0365-4758-9 (Hbk)
ISBN 978-3-0365-4757-2 (PDF)

© 2022 by the authors. Articles in this book are Open Access and distributed under the Creative Commons Attribution (CC BY) license, which allows users to download, copy and build upon published articles, as long as the author and publisher are properly credited, which ensures maximum dissemination and a wider impact of our publications.

The book as a whole is distributed by MDPI under the terms and conditions of the Creative Commons license CC BY-NC-ND.

Contents

About the Editor vii

Preface to "Treatments for Squamous Cell Cancer" ix

Imran Khan and Charbel Darido
Squamous Cell Carcinoma—A Summary of Novel Advances in Pathogenesis and Therapies
Reprinted from: *Cancers* **2022**, *14*, 2523, doi:10.3390/cancers14102523 1

Alesha A. Thai, Annette M. Lim, Benjamin J. Solomon and Danny Rischin
Biology and Treatment Advances in Cutaneous Squamous Cell Carcinoma
Reprinted from: *Cancers* **2021**, *13*, 5645, doi:10.3390/cancers13225645 5

Alexandre Bozec, Dorian Culié, Gilles Poissonnet, François Demard and Olivier Dassonville
Current Therapeutic Strategies in Patients with Oropharyngeal Squamous Cell Carcinoma:
Impact of the Tumor HPV Status
Reprinted from: *Cancers* **2021**, *13*, 5456, doi:10.3390/cancers13215456 25

Linda Kessler, Shivani Malik, Mollie Leoni and Francis Burrows
Potential of Farnesyl Transferase Inhibitors in Combination Regimens in Squamous Cell
Carcinomas
Reprinted from: *Cancers* **2021**, *13*, 5310, doi:10.3390/cancers13215310 43

Yuchen Bai, Jarryd Boath, Gabrielle R. White, Uluvitike G. I. U. Kariyawasam, Camile S. Farah and Charbel Darido
The Balance between Differentiation and Terminal Differentiation Maintains Oral Epithelial
Homeostasis
Reprinted from: *Cancers* **2021**, *13*, 5123, doi:10.3390/cancers13205123 57

Natalia García-Sancha, Roberto Corchado-Cobos, Lorena Bellido-Hernández, Concepción Román-Curto, Esther Cardeñoso-Álvarez and Jesús Pérez-Losada et al.
Overcoming Resistance to Immunotherapy in Advanced Cutaneous Squamous Cell Carcinoma
Reprinted from: *Cancers* **2021**, *13*, 5134, doi:10.3390/cancers13205134 75

Nguyen Huu Tu, Kenji Inoue, Elyssa Chen, Bethany M. Anderson, Caroline M. Sawicki and Nicole N. Scheff et al.
Cathepsin S Evokes PAR_2-Dependent Pain in Oral Squamous Cell Carcinoma Patients and
Preclinical Mouse Models
Reprinted from: *Cancers* **2021**, *13*, 4697, doi:10.3390/cancers13184697 101

Eric Miller and Jose Bazan
De-Escalation of Therapy for Patients with Early-Stage Squamous Cell Carcinoma of the Anus
Reprinted from: *Cancers* **2021**, *13*, 2099, doi:10.3390/cancers13092099 123

Kendrick Koo, Dmitri Mouradov, Christopher M. Angel, Tim A. Iseli, David Wiesenfeld and Michael J. McCullough et al.
Genomic Signature of Oral Squamous Cell Carcinomas from Non-Smoking Non-Drinking
Patients
Reprinted from: *Cancers* **2021**, *13*, 1029, doi:10.3390/cancers13051029 137

Darido Charbel
Treatments of Squamous Cell Cancer
Reprinted from: *Cancers* **2020**, *12*, 3229, doi:10.3390/cancers12113229 155

About the Editor

Charbel Darido

Dr Charbel Darido graduated with a Master's in Endocrinology and a Master's in Physiology before completing his PhD studies on colon cancer at the University of Montpellier in France. He then conducted post-doctoral studies at the Royal Melbourne Hospital and the University of Melbourne in Australia. He initiated a cancer project that led to the identification of a critical tumour-suppressor gene against squamous cell carcinoma (SCC) of skin and head and neck tissues. Following his first postdoc, he relocated to Monash University to lead the cancer program in the "epidermal development laboratory"at the Central Clinical School (The Alfred Centre). More recently, Dr Darido was appointed to a Group Leader position within the Cancer Therapeutic Program at Peter Mac to establish a vibrant research program on head and neck cancer. The main focus of his lab is to develop model systems for the investigation of head and neck SCC with an emphasis on studying the initiating lesions and identifying the cells of origin of these cancers. His research group studies the molecular basis of cancer, with emphasis on the basic mechanisms of tumour suppression and signal transduction and their dysregulation in skin and head and neck squamous cell carcinogenesis. He is recognised for his pioneering research aimed at unravelling the complexity of the intracellular signalling circuitries by which the loss of transcription factors promotes oncogenic addiction, thereby leading to malignant transformation and cancer cell proliferation. Dr Darido's current investigations are made possible through the use of genetically engineered mouse models and carcinogenic protocols, orthotopic SCC xenografts and cultured cancer-derived cell lines. His ultimate goal is to translate molecular insights into new strategies of preventing and treating this disease, which causes significant mortality and morbidity worldwide.

Preface to "Treatments for Squamous Cell Cancer"

Squamous cell cancer (SCC) is the most frequent solid cancer. SCC is a malignant tumor of epidermal keratinocytes and consists of a disease spectrum ranging from hyperplasia, dysplasia, and carcinoma in situ to locally invasive and, finally, metastatic disease. The common risk factors for SCC initiation and progression include environmental insults such as UV irradiation; tobacco smoke and frequent alcohol use; poor hygiene; human papillomavirus (HPV) infections; lack of dietary nutrients; and immunosuppression and genetic predisposition. Considering these differing etiologies, it is not surprising that SCC is a highly heterogeneous disease.

This reprint presents our current understanding of predisposing factors and biological mechanisms that underlie heterogeneous SCC development and highlight recent preclinical and clinical advances for the effective prevention and treatment of the disease.

Charbel Darido
Editor

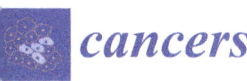

Editorial

Squamous Cell Carcinoma—A Summary of Novel Advances in Pathogenesis and Therapies

Imran Khan [1,2] and Charbel Darido [1,2,*]

1. Peter MacCallum Cancer Centre, 305 Grattan St., Melbourne, VIC 3000, Australia; imran.i.khan@petermac.org
2. The Sir Peter MacCallum Department of Oncology, The University of Melbourne, Parkville, VIC 3010, Australia
* Correspondence: charbel.darido@petermac.org; Tel.: +61-3-8559-7111; Fax: +61-3-8559-5489

Citation: Khan, I.; Darido, C. Squamous Cell Carcinoma—A Summary of Novel Advances in Pathogenesis and Therapies. *Cancers* 2022, 14, 2523. https://doi.org/10.3390/cancers14102523

Received: 5 May 2022
Accepted: 12 May 2022
Published: 20 May 2022

Publisher's Note: MDPI stays neutral with regard to jurisdictional claims in published maps and institutional affiliations.

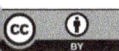

Copyright: © 2022 by the authors. Licensee MDPI, Basel, Switzerland. This article is an open access article distributed under the terms and conditions of the Creative Commons Attribution (CC BY) license (https://creativecommons.org/licenses/by/4.0/).

Squamous cell carcinomas (SCCs) are cancers of epithelial cells lining the aerodigestive and genitourinary tract [1]. SCCs are known to occur in the skin, head and neck, oesophagus, lung, cervix, pancreas, thyroid, bladder, and prostate [2]. SCCs are the leading causes of cancer worldwide [3], and their incidence is on the rise due to an increase in exposure to carcinogens such as tobacco, alcohol consumption, sunlight, and human papilloma virus (HPV) infection.

In this Special Issue, experts in the field describe the cellular and molecular events in SCC development, recurrence, and metastasis. They provide an updated snapshot on our understanding of the heterogeneity of SCC pathogenesis with novel opportunities in precision therapeutics to achieve better clinical outcomes. In addition, the researchers highlight the current advances in therapy development, outcome-predicting biomarkers, and molecular mechanisms of therapy resistance along with possible remedial measures.

Bai et al. [4] describe the molecular mechanisms of oral epithelium (OE) formation, repair, and homeostasis. They focus on key molecular mechanisms involved in OE terminal differentiation that go awry during oral SCC development. The authors also describe current therapeutics available to treat oral SCC and propose targeted approaches to restore OE differentiation as a novel oral SCC treatment strategy.

Thai et al. [5] describe the risk factors and molecular mechanisms involved in the development of cutaneous SCC. They explain how chronic exposure to ultraviolet radiation or immunosuppressive and kinase inhibiting drugs used to treat other ailments are *bona fide* risk factors for the development of cutaneous SCC. In addition, they discuss the risk for people suffering from chronic lymphocytic leukaemia, Marjolijn's ulcers, inherited bone marrow failure syndrome, and human papilloma virus (HPV) infection. The authors define common genetic aberrations involved in the development of cutaneous SCCs including the dysregulation of Notch signalling and inactivation of *TP53* and *CKN2A* tumour-suppressor genes. Finally, the authors describe current therapeutics available to treat cutaneous SCC including tumour-resection surgery and chemotherapy to treat localised cancers and the benefit of immunotherapy and kinase inhibitors in the treatment of advanced metastatic disease.

Garcia-Sancha et al. [6] describe mechanisms of immunotherapy resistance in cutaneous SCC. Similarly to Thai et al. [5], they highlight the immune-checkpoint inhibitors in cutaneous SCC treatment. In addition, the authors describe predictors of immunotherapy outcomes as well as primary and acquired mechanisms of immunotherapy resistance. Finally, the authors demonstrate how therapy can be improved by the combination of immunotherapy, radiotherapy and chemotherapies, immunotherapy with oncolytic viruses, cancer vaccines, and other therapies in treating cutaneous SCC.

SCC of the anus is a rare malignancy with an increasing incidence and mortality rates attributed to an aging population. Currently, chemoradiation therapy (CRT) is the standard of care treatment for early-stage disease; however, CRT involves a pronounced level of toxicity. It is not clear whether CRT is appropriate for early-stage anal SCC. Meill and Bazan [7] summarise the clinical trials and retrospective studies comparing radiation therapy (RT) to CRT, local excision versus CRT, and RT versus systemic treatment of early-stage anal SCC. In addition, the authors describe the utility of novel radiotherapy techniques to treat anal SCC. Overall, the authors propose investigations into the de-escalation of therapy to ameliorate therapy-induced toxicities and improve the prognosis in patients with early-stage anal SCC.

Oropharyngeal SCC incidence rates have been increasing. Oropharyngeal SCC is a highly heterogenous disease with distinct viral (HPV) and non-viral (alcohol, tobacco, etc.) aetiologies with differing clinical presentation, pathogenesis, and prognosis. HPV-positive oropharyngeal SCC have a higher propensity to metastasise to distant organs with frequent lymph-node involvement. Nevertheless, the prognosis of HPV-positive oropharyngeal SCC is generally better than non-viral oropharyngeal SCC. However, current therapeutics do not take the tumour HPV status into account. Bozec et al. [8] describe the impact of HPV status on oropharyngeal SCC treatment outcomes. The authors indicate that early-stage or locally advanced resectable HPV-positive oropharyngeal SCC can be treated with surgery or RT with favourable clinical outcomes. In contrast, at similar disease stages, the surgical interventions to treat non-viral oropharyngeal SCC lead to better clinical outcomes. The authors conclude that the overall surgical interventions lead to better oncologic outcomes; however, further consideration of the viral status needs to be incorporated in future therapeutic interventions.

Koo et al. [9] describe the mutational landscape of oral SCC with a special emphasis on non-smoking and non-drinking (NSND) patients. They used targeted gene-panel sequencing to identify frequent mutations in the tumour-suppressor gene *CDKN2A*, amplification of *EGFR*, and deletion of *BRCA2* in NSND oral SCC compared to smoking and drinking (SD) oral SCC patients. Overall, this study excluded HPV as a major driver of oral SCC development in NSND patients and identified critical differences in mutational landscapes of NSND and SD oral SCC patients driving oncogenic events.

Cathepsin S is a lysosomal cysteine protease and is upregulated in several human cancers including oral SCC [10]. Tu et al. [10] used a combination of animal and in vitro studies to identify Cathepsin-S-activated neuronal PAR_2 (protease-activated receptor-2), which induces cancer pain in oral SCC patients. This research opens new avenues in cancer-related pain management in oral SCC.

Finally, Kessler et al. [11] describe a novel treatment of head-and-neck SCC with RAS mutations. The RAS family of proto-oncogenes (KRAS, NRAS, and HRAS), which regulates the PI3K signalling pathway, is highly mutated in SCC [11]. Hyperactivation of RAS has been observed in head-and-neck, lung, and urinary-tract SCC. The authors describe the utility of Tipifarnib, an inhibitor of HRAS activity as mono or combination therapy in head-and-neck SCC. Using patient-derived xenograft mouse models, the researchers demonstrated that Tipifarnib sensitises head-and-neck SCC tumours to cetuximab (EGFR inhibitor), cisplatin (chemotherapy), Palbociclib (CDK4 and CDK6 inhibitor), and INK-128 (mTOR inhibitor).

In summary, this Special Issue describes the recent advances in SCC development and summarises the state-of-the-art therapeutics to treat primary and metastatic SCC. As Guest Editor, I thank all of the authors for their contribution to the challenging landscape of SCC biology and treatment.

Author Contributions: Conceptualization, C.D.; writing—original draft preparation, I.K.; writing—review and editing, C.D.; supervision, C.D. All authors have read and agreed to the published version of the manuscript.

Funding: This research received no external funding.

Conflicts of Interest: The authors declare no conflict of interest.

References

1. Campbell, J.D.; Yau, C.; Bowlby, R.; Liu, Y.; Brennan, K.; Fan, H.; Taylor, A.M.; Wang, C.; Walter, V.; Akbani, R.; et al. Genomic, Pathway Network, and Immunologic Features Distinguishing Squamous Carcinomas. *Cell Rep.* **2018**, *23*, 194–212.e196. [CrossRef] [PubMed]
2. Sanchez-Danes, A.; Blanpain, C. Deciphering the cells of origin of squamous cell carcinomas. *Nat. Rev. Cancer* **2018**, *18*, 549–561. [CrossRef]
3. Dotto, G.P.; Rustgi, A.K. Squamous Cell Cancers: A Unified Perspective on Biology and Genetics. *Cancer Cell* **2016**, *29*, 622–637. [CrossRef] [PubMed]
4. Bai, Y.; Boath, J.; White, G.R.; Kariyawasam, U.G.; Farah, C.S.; Darido, C. The Balance between Differentiation and Terminal Differentiation Maintains Oral Epithelial Homeostasis. *Cancers* **2021**, *13*, 5123. [CrossRef] [PubMed]
5. Thai, A.A.; Lim, A.M.; Solomon, B.J.; Rischin, D. Biology and Treatment Advances in Cutaneous Squamous Cell Carcinoma. *Cancers* **2021**, *13*, 5645. [CrossRef] [PubMed]
6. García-Sancha, N.; Corchado-Cobos, R.; Bellido-Hernández, L.; Román-Curto, C.; Cardeñoso-Álvarez, E.; Pérez-Losada, J.; Orfao, A.; Cañueto, J. Overcoming Resistance to Immunotherapy in Advanced Cutaneous Squamous Cell Carcinoma. *Cancers* **2021**, *13*, 5134. [CrossRef] [PubMed]
7. Miller, E.; Bazan, J. De-Escalation of Therapy for Patients with Early-Stage Squamous Cell Carcinoma of the Anus. *Cancers* **2021**, *13*, 2099. [CrossRef] [PubMed]
8. Bozec, A.; Culie, D.; Poissonnet, G.; Demard, F.; Dassonville, O. Current Therapeutic Strategies in Patients with Oropharyngeal Squamous Cell Carcinoma: Impact of the Tumor HPV Status. *Cancers* **2021**, *13*, 5456. [CrossRef] [PubMed]
9. Koo, K.; Mouradov, D.; Angel, C.M.; Iseli, T.A.; Wiesenfeld, D.; McCullough, M.J.; Burgess, A.W.; Sieber, O.M. Genomic Signature of Oral Squamous Cell Carcinomas from Non-Smoking Non-Drinking Patients. *Cancers* **2021**, *13*, 1029. [CrossRef] [PubMed]
10. Tu, N.H.; Inoue, K.; Chen, E.; Anderson, B.M.; Sawicki, C.M.; Scheff, N.N.; Tran, H.D.; Kim, D.H.; Alemu, R.G.; Yang, L.; et al. Cathepsin S Evokes PAR2-Dependent Pain in Oral Squamous Cell Carcinoma Patients and Preclinical Mouse Models. *Cancers* **2021**, *13*, 4697. [CrossRef] [PubMed]
11. Kessler, L.; Malik, S.; Leoni, M.; Burrows, F. Potential of Farnesyl Transferase Inhibitors in Combination Regimens in Squamous Cell Carcinomas. *Cancers* **2021**, *13*, 5310. [CrossRef] [PubMed]

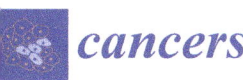

Review

Biology and Treatment Advances in Cutaneous Squamous Cell Carcinoma

Alesha A. Thai [1,2,*], Annette M. Lim [1,2], Benjamin J. Solomon [1,2] and Danny Rischin [1,2]

1   Department of Medical Oncology, Peter MacCallum Cancer Centre, 305 Grattan St., Parkville, Melbourne, VIC 3000, Australia; annette.lim@petermac.org (A.M.L.); ben.solomon@petermac.org (B.J.S.); danny.rischin@petermac.org (D.R.)
2   The Sir Peter MacCallum Department of Oncology, University of Melbourne, Melbourne, VIC 3000, Australia
*   Correspondence: alesha.thai@petermac.org

Simple Summary: Skin cancers are the most diagnosed type of cancer worldwide. Cutaneous squamous cell carcinoma—a type of skin cancer—usually affects older people who have chronic sun exposure, as well as people with weakened immune systems. There has been significant recent progress in the treatment of this type of cancer with immune checkpoint inhibitors that utilize the immune system to target cancer. In concert with advances in treatment, our understanding of the biology of skin cancer has also deepened. The authors have reviewed the risk factors, biology, and advances in treatment in this publication.

Abstract: Cutaneous squamous cell carcinoma (CSCC) is the second most common skin cancer diagnosed worldwide. CSCC is generally localized and managed with local therapies such as excision and/or radiotherapy. For patients with unresectable or metastatic disease, recent improvements in our understanding of the underlying biology have led to significant advancements in treatment approaches—including the use of immune checkpoint inhibition (ICI)—which have resulted in substantial gains in response and survival compared to traditional cytotoxic approaches. However, there is a lack of understanding of the biology underpinning CSCC in immunocompromised patients, in whom the risk of developing CSCC is hundreds of times higher compared to immunocompetent patients. Furthermore, current ICI approaches are associated with significant risk of graft rejection in organ transplant recipients who make up a significant proportion of immunocompromised patients. Ongoing scientific and clinical research efforts are needed in order to maintain momentum to increase our understanding and refine our therapeutic approaches for patients with CSCC.

Keywords: cutaneous squamous cell carcinoma; CSCC; treatment; advances; biology; immunocompromised; immune checkpoint inhibition; immunotherapy

1. Introduction

CSCC is the second most common skin cancer diagnosed worldwide [1]. Important risk factors for CSCC include ultraviolet (UV) radiation and immunosuppression. Most patients have curable, localized disease, but a small proportion (2–5%) develop unresectable locally advanced or metastatic disease [2,3]. Historically, systemic therapy options for these patients were limited; however, there have been advances in our understanding of the biology of CSCC—particularly, an appreciation of the high tumor mutational burden (TMB) observed in most cases of CSCC, and the role of the immune system in tumor prevention and control. This led to a pivotal study of an immune checkpoint inhibitor (ICI) in patients with metastatic or locally advanced, unresectable CSCC, and changed the treatment paradigm for these patients. Efforts are now underway to assess the benefit of ICI in patients with high-risk localized disease, where the chance for cure with improved neoadjuvant or adjuvant approaches is greater. This review discusses the epidemiology, risk factors, and genomic alterations underlying CSCC, and summarizes treatment advances for CSCC.

2. Epidemiology

Non-melanoma skin cancers (NMSCs) comprise of basal-cell carcinomas (BCCs; ~80%), CSCC (~20%), and rarer skin cancers. The incidence of CSCC is likely underestimated, as accurate figures are difficult to ascertain, with significant variation in cancer registry practices between countries as a result of the high incidence, relatively low mortality, and multiplicity of CSCC [4,5]. However, it is clear that NMSCs are the most common types of cancer diagnosed in many regions—including Australia, North America, and Europe—and their associated public health burden is significantly underestimated [4–8]. The incidence of CSCC in patients aged 75 years or older is 5–10 times higher than in their younger counterparts. Men are at higher risk of CSCC than women, which was traditionally hypothesized to be a reflection of higher occupational exposure, but there is some suggestion that differences in sexual biology may be a factor in the observed disparity [9–13]. As UV exposure is the strongest risk factor for CSCC, most cases arise in the head and neck region, where UV exposure is highest.

3. Risk Factors

The pathogenesis of CSCC is multifactorial. Chronic UV exposure plays an important role, but other risk factors include immunosuppression, environmental exposures, chronic inflammation, and drugs (Figure 1).

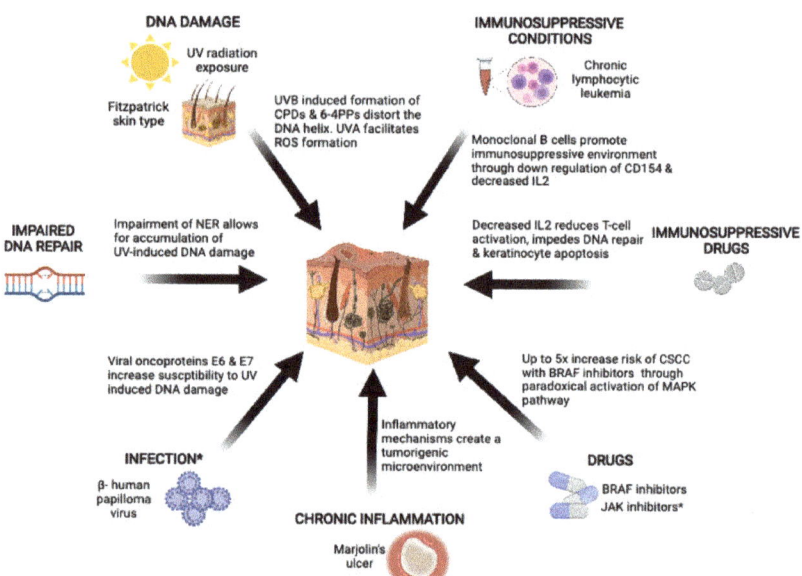

Figure 1. Risk factors for CSCC include UV radiation exposure, immunosuppressive conditions and drugs, inflammations such as those from chronic wounds, and impaired DNA repair. * Infection with β-human papillomavirus and JAK inhibitors are also thought to increase the risk of CSCC, but clear evidence and the underlying biology are not as well established. Created using biorender.com (accessed on 1 September 2021).

3.1. Ultraviolet Radiation

Chronic UV exposure is the most important risk factor for CSCC [14]. Sunlight produces three main types of UV radiation: UVA, UVB, and UVC. UVA radiation exposure increases the risk of CSCC, but is less mutagenic than UVB. UVA radiation causes indirect

DNA damage by facilitating the formation of reactive oxygen species, which can interact with DNA, lipids, and proteins to form pre-mutagenic adducts [15]. UVB radiation directly damages DNA and RNA by causing the formation of cyclobutane-pyrimidine dimers (CPDs) and 6-4 photoproducts (6-4PPs), which distort the DNA helix, impeding transcription and replication [15]. Particular genomic positions, as a result of their structure, are more vulnerable to UVB-induced DNA damage—for instance, the *TP53* gene, which is the most frequently mutated gene in CSCC [16]. In vivo studies show that mice exposed to chronic UV radiation develop inactivating *TP53* mutations as early as 1 week post-exposure [17]. UVC has the shortest wavelength, and is completely absorbed by the Earth's ozone layer.

There is marked global variation in CSCC incidence, reflecting not only varying levels of UV exposure, but also genetic propensity to UV damage. The amount of melanin pigment in the skin can be categorized using the Fitzpatrick skin type scale, and is correlated with UV susceptibility and skin cancer risk [18]. Pale or white skin that burns easily and does not tan, classified as Fitzpatrick type 1, has a higher risk of developing skin cancers compared to people with Fitzpatrick type 6 skin, who have very pigmented skin that rarely or never burns [18]. As such, Australia, as a consequence of its location, relative lack of ozone, and high proportion of Anglo-Saxon population, has one of the highest incidences of NMSCs, including CSCC [4,19].

3.2. Immunosuppression

The role of the immune system in the development of CSCC has long been recognized from the significantly increased risk of CSCC observed in immunosuppressed patients [20]. Furthermore, the success of ICI (discussed in detail below) highlights the anticancer potency of an intact immune system.

Immunosuppression can be a result of host factors—such as chronic lymphocytic leukemia (CLL) or HIV—or extrinsic factors, such as drugs. This review will address the most common causes of immunosuppression, such as CLL and immunosuppressive drugs.

3.2.1. Chronic Lymphocytic Leukemia

CLL is a low-grade lymphoproliferative malignancy characterized by clonal proliferation of functionally incompetent B cells; it is the most common leukemia in developed countries, accounting for up to 35% of all leukemias [21]. CLL was the most common cause of immunosuppression (34%, $n = 20/59$) in a multicenter retrospective study of patients with CSCC receiving immune checkpoint inhibition [22]. Patients with CLL are 5–8 times more likely to develop CSCC compared to patients without CLL [23–25]. Furthermore, the risk of recurrence and CSCC-specific mortality is increased in patients with CLL [26,27]. The risk of metastasis at 5 years has been reported to be 18%, with a standardized mortality ratio of 17.0 (95% CI 14.4–19.8) [27].

CLL is typically diagnosed in older people, with a median age of 70 years. Older age, a higher incidence in men, and the associated immunosuppressive effects of CLL all contribute to the higher risk of CSCC. The strongest risk factor for developing CSCC in the setting of CLL is prior history of any skin cancer, but other CLL risk factors associated with a higher risk of developing CSCC include CLL international prognostic index, Rai stage, and lymphocyte doubling time [28].

The biology underlying the increased risk of CSCC is not fully understood. B cells are traditionally known for antigen presentation, antibody production, and the release of effector cytokines that modulate T-cell responses. There is growing evidence, however, that a newly identified, heterogeneous group of B cells—called regulatory B cells—can modulate the immune response to tumors [29]. In the setting of CLL, monoclonal B cells have been shown to promote an immunosuppressive environment via the downregulation of CD154 in activated T cells in preclinical models. CD154 plays a critical role in stimulating B cells, monocytes, and dendritic cells to differentiate and proliferate [30]. Additionally, in clinical tumor samples, higher levels of interleukin-2 (IL-2) receptors have been detected in patients with CLL compared to patients without CLL. IL-2 receptors are thought to be secreted from T-regulatory cells, and bind free IL-2, thus decreasing its availability [31]. Suppression of IL-2 has been shown to induce CD8+ T-cell anergy [32]. Other immune deficits have been identified in patients with CLL, such as impaired phagocytosis and functional defects in helper B cells [33]. It has also been hypothesized that in addition to the immunosuppressive effects of CLL, shared genetic risk factors between CLL and NMSC can contribute to the association between the two diseases [28,34].

3.2.2. Drugs

A number of drugs are associated with an increased risk of CSCC via different mechanisms, ranging from immunosuppression, to the paradoxical activation of pathways that lead to keratinocyte proliferation and loss of apoptosis.

Immunosuppressive Drugs

Long-term immunosuppressive drug regimens are most commonly utilized in organ transplant recipients (OTRs), and involve multiple classes of drugs to minimize graft rejection. As a result, their immunosuppressive effects can be profound, and increase the risk of CSCC by hundreds-fold. In one long-term observational study, approximately 30% of OTRs developed NMSCs, the majority of which were CSCC. The mean time from transplant to first CSCC was 9.9 years, and overall cumulative incidence increased over time to 10.6%, 24.8%, 53.9%, and 73.9% at 5, 10, 20, and 30 years post-transplant, respectively [20]. Patients who have undergone heart or lung transplantations are more susceptible to CSCC formation than renal transplant recipients, likely reflecting the more potent immunosuppressive regimens required for those organs [35,36]. CSCCs developing in OTRs have a higher risk of recurrence, metastases, and cancer-specific death compared to non-transplant patients [37].

Calcineurin inhibitors such as cyclosporine and tacrolimus are a commonly used class of immunosuppressive drugs. They reduce IL-2 production and IL-2 receptor expression, leading to reduced T-cell activation. Cyclosporine, however, also impedes the UV-induced DNA repair mechanisms and keratinocyte apoptosis, by counteracting p53 through ATF3 [38,39]. Furthermore, there is in vitro evidence that cyclosporine can induce epithelial–mesenchymal transition via the upregulation of TGF-β, thus altering the phenotype to a more invasive and aggressive tumor type [40].

Tacrolimus is a more modern calcineurin inhibitor, which has been increasingly used since the 1990s [41]. Interestingly, studies have shown that tacrolimus is not associated with an increased risk of CSCC [42,43], and does not confer resistance to UV-induced apoptosis in keratinocytes—unlike cyclosporine [44].

Since the early 2000s, there has been increasing use of mechanistic target of rapamycin (mTOR) inhibitors—such as rapamycin and sirolimus—as immunosuppressants. mTOR is a protein kinase that plays a role in cell proliferation and survival, as well as modulation of the innate and adaptive immune system [45,46]. Interestingly, however, in vivo studies of mice show that sirolimus—an mTOR inhibitor—significantly delays CSCC development and reduces its multiplicity, even if co-administered with cyclosporine, through inhibition of the transcription factor ATF3 [47–49]. ATF3 downregulates expression of *TP53*, which is one of the most commonly mutated genes in CSCC [38,50]. Furthermore, randomized controlled trials (RCTs) also show a significantly reduced incidence of CSCC in patients receiving mTOR inhibitors compared to cyclosporine [51], as well as in patients who were prescribed sirolimus after three months of treatment with cyclosporine (1.2% vs. 4.3%, $p < 0.001$) [43,52].

Oral glucocorticoids are a frequently used immunosuppressant, but data regarding the risk associated with the development of CSCC are inconsistent. Two studies—a case–control study, and a planned sub-study of an RCT—found no association between oral steroid use and risk of CSCC [53,54]. In contrast, a cohort study found that patients on prolonged courses of oral glucocorticoids were at higher risk of developing CSCC (standardized incidence ratio 2.45; 95% CI 1.37–4.04) [55]. Another study of OTRs found that higher cumulative immunosuppression from a combination of cyclosporine, azathioprine, and oral prednisolone increased the risk of CSCC by fourfold compared to lower cumulative doses [56]. However, there was no association between the cumulative doses of each drug alone and risk of CSCC. This highlights the possibility that the overall level and duration of immunosuppression, regardless of agent, is a factor impacting the risk of developing CSCC. Ultimately, it will be difficult to ascertain the true risk of CSCC arising in patients taking a commonly used drug such as oral glucocorticoids. There are many indications for oral glucocorticoids, thus increasing potential confounders and biases. Furthermore, accurate information regarding duration of therapy—which can vary widely, from a few days, to many months or years—is difficult to gather at a population-based level.

BRAF Inhibitors

A number of targeted therapies are associated with cutaneous side effects. Squamoproliferative lesions such as actinic keratoses and CSCC are most commonly seen with BRAF inhibitors such as vemurafenib, dabrafenib, and encorafenib, which can be used as monotherapies for patients with metastatic melanoma harboring *BRAF* V600E mutations. A meta-analysis of seven randomized trials found that 18% (95% CI 0.12–0.26) of patients on vemurafenib develop CSCC [57]. In patients taking dabrafenib, CSCC develops in 6–26% of patients [58,59]. BRAF-inhibitor-associated abnormal squamous proliferation is thought to be induced by the paradoxical activation of the mitogen-activated protein kinase (MAPK) pathway, and subsequent ERK-mediated transcription in wild-type BRAF keratinocytes—particularly in the presence of oncogenic RAS mutations [60–63]. CSCC arising from BRAF inhibition typically occurs within the first 3 months of treatment, and age has been identified as an independent risk factor [64]. Following the establishment of efficacy of BRAF inhibition in metastatic melanoma, overall survival and response with the combination of BRAF with MEK inhibition was found to be superior compared to BRAF monotherapy. Dual blockade of BRAF and MEK is now the standard of care for patients with metastatic *BRAF* V600E mutations. Fortunately, the risk of squamoproliferative lesions—including CSCC—significantly decreased with the addition of MEK inhibition, with a reported incidence of 0–2% [65–67].

JAK1/2 Inhibitors

Janus kinase (JAK)1/2 inhibitors such as ruxolitinib are used to treat myelofibrosis or polycythemia vera. A number of cases have been reported wherein the initiation of JAK1/2 inhibitors is associated with the development of multiple, rapidly progressing CSCCs [68–70]. The incidence of newly diagnosed non-melanoma skin cancer was 17.1% in patients receiving ruxolitinib compared to 2.1% in those receiving best available therapy for myelofibrosis in the long-term follow-up of a phase III RCT [71]. The exact mechanism of tumorigenesis is unknown, but JAK1/2 aberrant hyperactivation has been associated with tumor proliferation and survival in different cancer types [72]. Interestingly, ruxolitinib was shown to reduce tumor progression in in vitro experiments of cyclosporine-induced CSCC cell lines [73].

3.3. Marjolin's Ulcers

Marjolin's ulcers describe a rare form of CSCC that arises from areas of chronic inflammation such as burn scars, venous stasis ulcers, and pressure sores [74]. Marjolin's ulcers are more aggressive than spontaneous CSCC, with the risk of recurrence or metastases reported to be approximately 30% in case series [75,76]. There is a long latency period from initial injury to the development of CSCC, with an average time of 30 years reported [74,77,78]. The relationship between inflammation and tumorigenesis has long been appreciated, with examples of cancers arising from patients' inflammatory bowel disease and *Helicobacter*-induced gastritis [79]. Inflammatory mechanisms ensure appropriate responses to infections, and promote wound healing, but can also create a microenvironment that promotes tumorigenesis via the recruitment of immune cells and subsequent release of cytokines and growth factors [80].

3.4. Environmental Exposure

Other environmental risk factors include chronic arsenic exposure, which most commonly occurs from contaminated drinking water [81]. Arsenic-induced CSCC can develop even in non-sun-exposed sites. Ionizing radiation via environmental, therapeutic, or diagnostic exposure is also a known risk factor, although the risk of BCC is higher than that of CSCC, as the basal layer of the epidermis is more affected than more superficial layers [82–84]. Occupational exposure to aromatic hydrocarbons such as benzene and mineral oil have also been identified as risk factors for the development of CSCC, and are of particular importance in occupations such as firefighting and petroleum work [85,86].

3.5. Inherited Bone Marrow Failure Sydromes (IBMFSs)

IBMFSs comprise of rare diseases typically characterized by genetic mutations resulting in bone marrow failure. These syndromes include Fanconi anemia and dyskeratosis congenita as the most common disorders, which are associated with defects in DNA repair and telomere function, respectively. Patients with these conditions are at increased risk of hematological and solid malignancies due to multiple factors that arise from the genetic disruption, resulting in genomic instability and bone marrow failure. The risk of CSCC is more notable in patients with Fanconi anemia and dyskeratosis congenita. Skin cancers make up approximately 10–20% of cancer cases in patients with Fanconi anemia and dyskeratosis congenita, and typically occur at a median age of approximately 30 years [87–89].

3.6. Beta Human Papillomavirus

HPV comprises several heterogeneous subgroups; α-papillomavirus (α-HPV) subtypes are associated with mucosal SCCs, such as cervical and oropharyngeal cancer, but it is the β-papillomavirus (β-HPV) subtypes that are hypothesized to be a risk factor for CSCCs. β-HPV was first discovered in the context of patients with a rare skin disorder—epidermodysplasia verruciformis. Patients develop pre-cancerous wart-like lesions that progress to CSCC in UV-exposed areas. Multiple β-HPV types were found in these lesions, thus raising the possibility of the carcinogenic role of β-HPV. Complicating matters, however, is the relative ubiquitousness of β-HPV in the skin. β-HPV DNA is detected in the skin of 39–91% of immunocompetent patients—particularly in hair follicles, which are considered to be a natural reservoir [90,91]. There are, however, multiple factors that suggest that β-HPV may be a risk factor for the development of CSCC.

Firstly, immunocompromised patients have an increased risk of CSCC, and have significantly higher rates of β-HPV infection and higher viral loads, suggesting a potential causal relationship between β-HPV and CSCC [92]. Second, observational studies have shown an association between β-HPV DNA and/or serum antibodies and CSCC in both immunocompromised and immunocompetent patients [93]. A meta-analysis of over 3000 immunocompetent patients found an overall association of β-HPV and CSCC (OR 1.42; 95% CI 1.18–1.72) [94]. Notably, some of these studies incorporated BCC cases, and no associations were observed between β-HPV and BCC [95–97]. Thirdly, there are increasing preclinical data supporting the role of β-HPV in tumor initiation, but not necessarily in tumor maintenance [98]. β-HPV DNA is detected at high levels in pre-cancerous lesions such as actinic keratoses, whereas lower levels are detected in CSCC lesions [99,100]. In vitro and in vivo studies have shown that the HPV oncoproteins E6 and/or E7 from HPV types 5, 8, and 38 can increase susceptibility to UV-induced oncogenesis via alterations in p53 and Notch1 signaling [101–108]. β-HPV is also thought to infect and expand adult tissue stem cells, thus enabling cells to persist and accumulate mutations [109]. It is hypothesized that once cells have accumulated mutations such as *TP53* and *Notch*, which allow for ongoing cell proliferation, expression of viral oncogenes becomes redundant, and they are no longer positively selected.

4. Biology and Pathogenesis

There have been significant advances in our understanding of the biological pathways in CSCC development, with multiple genes identified as playing a critical role in tumor initiation and persistence. CSCC, however, has one of the highest median TMBs of any tumor type; thus, hundreds of mutations can be found per megabase [110]. One of the challenges in understanding the biological pathways involved in CSCC is separating true oncogenic mutations from passenger mutations. Here, we discuss the oncogenic roles of selected commonly mutated genes such as *TP53*, *Notch*, and *CDKN2A*. No specific oncogenic drivers of CSCC have been identified.

p53 functions predominantly as a transcription factor, and can activate or repress a large number of target genes. In particular, p53 plays an important role in modulating nucleotide excision repair (NER) and other DNA repair pathways that are essential in the repair of UV-induced DNA damage [111]. Mutations in *TP53* allow for ongoing, unrepaired UV-induced DNA damage. As an example, the risk of CSCCs is significantly higher if there are genetically impaired DNA repair mechanisms, such as in patients with xeroderma pigmentosum who develop NMSCs during childhood [112].

Mutations in *TP53* occur early in CSCC development, and are often found in normal keratinocytes [113–115] and pre-malignant lesions [116]. Whole-exome sequencing of CSCC has identified bi-allelic *TP53* mutations in nearly all tumors, again suggesting that the loss of wild-type *TP53* is an early step in carcinogenesis [117–119]. This is in contrast to other solid malignancies, where *TP53* gene mutations occur later in tumor evolution [120–122]. Further evidence of the oncogenic role of *TP53* in CSCC has been shown in in vivo studies, where homozygous p53-knockout mice rapidly developed CSCC after UV exposure [123,124]. p53-mutant cells are more resistant to UV-induced apoptosis, and have a proliferative advantage over wild-type keratinocytes [125].

The Notch signaling pathway is commonly affected, and *Notch* mutations are found in 60–80% of CSCCs [118,119,126]. Notch is a highly conserved intercellular signaling mechanism that plays a critical role in the development and maintenance of tissue homeostasis [127]. Genes of the *Notch* family encode four transmembrane receptors (Notch1–4). In the epidermis, Notch signaling is involved in the terminal differentiation of keratinocytes [128]. Interestingly, *Notch* can have oncogenic or tumor-suppressive functions depending on the cell context [129]. Constitutive Notch1 signaling as a result of activating mutations is the initiating step in almost all T-cell acute lymphoblastic leukemia (T-ALL) cases [130,131]. In contrast, loss of Notch signaling—particularly Notch1 and Notch2—is associated with carcinogenesis in keratinocytes [118,132,133]. Preclinical studies have shown that Notch1 is a downstream positive target of p53 in keratinocytes; thus, inactivating *TP53* mutations can further lead to reduced Notch1 expression [134]. Several in vivo experiments have shown Notch1 deficiency or Notch1 inhibition in mice can result in the spontaneous development of CSCC [135]. A possible mechanism is via upregulation of the Wnt/β-catenin pathway [132]. Intriguingly, Notch deficiency or loss does not purely exert its effect autonomously on cells, but can also create a pro-tumorigenic microenvironment. Loss of Notch signaling disrupts skin barrier function, creating a chronic wound-like environment [136]. As a result, mesenchymal components are recruited for repair, which also stimulates a vascularized and growth-factor-rich stroma, providing an ideal environment for tumor formation [136]. There is also clinical evidence of Notch inactivation resulting in increased CSCC risk. Semagacestat, a γ-secretase inhibitor, was developed as a drug for Alzheimer's disease. A phase III RCT of semagacestat was halted early due to lack of efficacy as well as an increased risk of CSCC. γ-Secretase, in addition to converting amyloid precursor protein to amyloid-β is also responsible for cleaving and activating Notch1; thus, its inhibition indirectly inactivates Notch1 [137].

The cyclin-dependent kinase inhibitor 2A *(CDKN2A)* gene encodes two tumor-suppressor genes: $p16^{INK4a}$ and $p14^{ARF}$. Both genes regulate cell cycling: $p16^{INK4A}$ binds to CDK4 and CDK6, thus preventing Rb protein phosphorylation and G1-S phase progression, while $p14^{ARF}$ binds to MDM2, preventing p53 degradation and Rb inactivation, causing cell arrest. Methylation of the promoter region is the most common mechanism of p16 and p14 inactivation in CSCC, followed by point mutations and loss of heterozygosity [138]. Alterations in *CDKN2A* are found in up to 80% of CSCCs [119]. Inactivating mutations of *CDKN2A* result in uncontrolled cell cycling and proliferation. A recent analysis, however, consistently found upregulation of *CDKN2A* in gene expression profiles and cell lines, in contrast to the pre-existing literature; the authors hypothesized that ERK signaling in CSCC may upregulate *CDKN2A* as a stress response to induce senescence rather than stimulating cell cycling [139].

RAS gene mutations are among the most common activating mutations found in human cancers, and also present a significant therapeutic challenge due to their molecular characteristics. The *RAS* gene encodes four RAS proteins: HRAS, NRAS, and two splice variants of KRAS. RAS proteins belong to a family of small GTPases that cycle between "off" and "on" states [140]. Activating *RAS* mutations can result in oncogenic constitutive activation of the RAF-MEK-ERK and PI3K-AKT pathways, leading to cell proliferation [141]. In CSCC, *HRAS* mutations are most common, and are found in 3–20% of CSCCs [118,133]. In keratinocytes, upregulated expression of RAS alone is not sufficient to induce tumorigenesis [142]. Concomitant *Notch1* deletion, IκBα co-expression, or CDK4-mediated bypass of Rb cell cycle restraints increase CSCC formation in the presence of activated RAS [132,143,144].

5. Tumor Mutation Burden

As a result of the chronic nature of UV exposure and the mechanism of DNA damage, there are cumulative DNA aberrations in CSCCs. In a study examining TMB in over 100,000 tumor samples, CSCC had the highest median TMB (45.2 mutations/Mb) compared to other tumor types [110]. High TMB is predictive of response to ICI, although prospective validation is lacking [145]. The impressive and durable responses observed with ICI in CSCC are thought to be due to high TMB representing a large number of immunostimulatory neoantigens.

6. Tumor Mutational Signatures

Somatic mutations in cancer cells can create a characteristic mutational signature, which reflects the mutational process involved in carcinogenesis. The UV mutation signature—the first characterized signature—is found in the great majority of CSCCs, and even in immunocompromised hosts. UV radiation damage most commonly results in cytosine to thymine or cytosine–cytosine to thymine–thymine changes—i.e., C > T or CC > TT—at dipyrimidine sites [146,147]. Recent studies have also identified signatures in CSCC associated with azathioprine exposure [139] and hyperactivity of endogenous cytidine deaminases (APOBEC)—specifically in patients with epidermolysis bullosa [148].

7. Treatment Advances

7.1. Localized Resectable High-Risk Disease

Most CSCCs are small, indolent, and surgically resectable, and adjuvant therapy is often not required. Post-operative radiotherapy, however, is considered for patients with resected high-risk localized disease—usually defined as tumors showing involved resection margins, depth of invasion of more than 2–6 mm, extensive perineural invasion, or large nerve involvement [2,149]. Other indications include lymph node involvement and large primary tumors [150,151].

7.1.1. Post-Operative Chemoradiotherapy

Platinum chemotherapy agents such as cisplatin and carboplatin are often used concurrently with postoperative radiotherapy in patients with mucosal head and neck squamous cell carcinoma (HNSCC), as several studies have shown a survival benefit [152–155]. The results of these trials have been extrapolated and applied to patients with cutaneous SCC. Until recently, there was no definitive prospective study supporting its use in this population.

A phase III trial randomized patients with high-risk resected CSCC to postoperative radiotherapy alone, or with concurrent weekly carboplatin chemotherapy [156]. Concurrent cisplatin is considered the gold standard in HNSCC, but its significant toxicity profile often precludes its use in patients with CSCC who are generally older, and with significant comorbidities. Thus, carboplatin is more frequently used. High-risk disease was defined as patients with primary tumors > 5 cm or T4 disease, resected intra-parotid nodal disease, two or more cervical nodal diseases, or with a node $\geq$ 3 cm or extranodal extension. Contrary to the results of mucosal HNSCC, no benefit was observed in freedom from locoregional relapse, nor in disease-free or overall survival, in patients with CSCC receiving concurrent chemotherapy. Based on the results of this trial, and the lack of evidence with other regimens, concurrent chemotherapy is generally not recommended in the adjuvant treatment of CSCC outside of clinical trials [151].

7.1.2. Neo/Adjuvant Immunotherapy

The success of ICI in patients with advanced disease has driven efforts to incorporate treatment into earlier stages of disease in order to reduce (a) the morbidity associated with resections of large tumors, and (b) the risk of locoregional relapse or metastasis.

Neoadjuvant immunotherapy is particularly appealing for clinical and translational purposes. Immune activation may be potentiated by the presence of neoantigens and intratumoral immune cells within the unresected cancer, and changes in the tumor and stroma can be compared between pretreatment biopsies and the resection specimen [157–159]. Furthermore, neoadjuvant studies allow for earlier assessment, using pathologic response, compared to adjuvant studies, where survival data can take many years to mature. A pilot phase II study of two doses of neoadjuvant cemiplimab for patients with locally advanced, curable CSCC resulted in 14/20 patients (70%; 95% CI 45.7–88.1) with a pathological complete response (n = 11) or major pathological response (n = 3) [160]; this was despite only 30% (95% CI 11.9–54.3) showing a partial response by RECIST, highlighting the challenges of assessing ICI response using current radiological criteria. Neoadjuvant studies of other ICIs, as well as combination neoadjuvant treatment with dual anti-PD(L)1 with anti-cytotoxic T-lymphocyte-associated protein 4 (CTLA-4) blockade, are ongoing [NCT04154943] [161,162]. Furthermore, there are two large phase III adjuvant studies of pembrolizumab or cemiplimab [163,164].

7.2. Unresectable Locally Advanced or Metastatic Disease

Historically, no standard of care for systemic therapies existed for patients with unresectable or metastatic CSCC. Cytotoxic chemotherapies such as platinums, fluoropyrimidines, and taxanes have shown activity in retrospective analyses. Response rates are generally low, and the toxicity profiles of therapies often preclude their use in elderly patients with CSCC [165]. ICI with monoclonal antibodies against PD1 and PD-L1 has transformed the treatment landscape for many solid tumors, including CSCC. Other treatment approaches include targeting the epidermal growth factor receptor (EGFR) pathway.

7.2.1. Immunotherapy

A practice-changing phase II study demonstrated the efficacy of cemiplimab—an anti-PD-1 monoclonal antibody—in patients with unresectable or metastatic CSCC [166,167]. Responses were observed in 54.4% (95% CI 47.1–61.6) of patients (both previously treated and untreated) [167]. In patients with initial response, 76% (95% CI 64.1–84.4%) had ongoing response at 24 months, demonstrating the excellent durability of disease response; estimated overall survival at 24 months was 73.3% (95% CI 66.1–79.2) [167–169]. As a result of this study, cemiplimab was approved by the FDA, and became the standard treatment for patients with locally advanced or metastatic CSCC who are not candidates for curative surgery or radiation.

Other ICIs, such as pembrolizumab, have shown comparable activity. Two studies—CARSKIN, and KEYNOTE-629—assessed the efficacy of pembrolizumab in advanced

CSCC. The objective response rate was 34.3% (95% CI 25.3–44.2%) in KEYNOTE-629 in a heavily pretreated population, and median overall survival has not been ascertained [170]. Based on KEYNOTE-629, pembrolizumab has also been approved by the FDA for advanced CSCC.

The CARKSIN study enrolled treatment-naïve patients with unresectable or metastatic CSCC to receive pembrolizumab [171]. Response rate (RR) at 15 weeks was the primary objective of the study, and was 41% (95% CI 26–58%), including 13 partial and 3 complete responses. Similarly, nivolumab has shown robust results in a phase II first-line study of patients with advanced CSCC [172]. Recently, real-world data regarding the use of ICIs in 245 patients—including immunocompromised patients—were reported to be comparable to trial data [22]. The estimated 12-month OS was 63% (95% CI 51–70); 50% of patients achieved a complete response or partial response (95% CI 44–57), and there were no unexpected toxicities. In univariate and multivariate analysis, ECOG score > 2 was the only clinical factor that was significantly associated with poor OS and PS in the first 6 months.

More aggressive approaches are also being considered for select patients with unresectable localized disease where cure may be possible. A phase II study of neoadjuvant avelumab, followed by curative-dose radiotherapy with concurrent avelumab, is ongoing [173].

Combination strategies of ICIs with cetuximab and oncolytic viruses are being investigated in order to address the challenges of resistance and improve durability of response. CSCC and melanoma share similar features, such as chronic UV exposure and high TMB. Studies of immunotherapy have been established longer in melanoma than in CSCC; thus, approaches that are efficacious or promising in melanoma are being tested in patients with CSCC. Talimogene laherparepvec (T-VEC) is a modified attenuated oncolytic herpes simplex virus containing the granulocyte macrophage colony-stimulating factor (GM-CSF) gene. Production of intratumoral GM-CSF can induce cellular immunity, and the direct oncolytic effect from viral infection of tumor cells can cause an antitumor response. Early-phase studies in metastatic melanoma show that intralesional injections of T-VEC combined with immune checkpoint blockade resulted in an objective response rate of 39% and 50% with concurrent ipilimumab and pembrolizumab, respectively [174–176]. Currently, there are studies in CSCC combining oncolytic viruses such as T-VEC and RP1 with ICI or EGFR antibodies [177,178]. EGFR antibodies, which are discussed in more detail below, are also being investigated in combination with anti-PD(L)1 antibodies. A phase II trial will randomize immunocompetent patients with unresectable/metastatic CSCC to avelumab alone, or in combination with cetuximab [179].

7.2.2. EGFR Pathway Inhibition

EGFR is a transmembrane glycoprotein with an extracellular binding domain, along with an intracellular tyrosine kinase domain that regulates cell proliferation via pathways such as MAPK and PI3K. The EGFR protein is highly expressed in CSCC [180–182]. EGFR monoclonal antibodies such as cetuximab and panitumumab have shown activity in CSCC in small phase II trials. In a phase II trial of cetuximab in patients with locally advanced unresectable or metastatic CSCC, 28% achieved a response, while 41% had stable disease [183]. An ORR of 31% was observed in a study of panitumumab [184].

Cetuximab has also been used in the neoadjuvant setting. Five out of nine patients receiving neoadjuvant cetuximab alone had a response that allowed for surgical resection and, of these, three had a complete pathological response [185].

Oral tyrosine inhibitors such as gefitinib and dacomitinib, which target the intracellular tyrosine kinase domain, are typically used in patients with EGFR-driven non-small-cell lung cancer, where responses are seen in approximately 75% of patients. These agents have activity in CSCC, with overall response rates of 16% and 28% observed in early phase trials of gefitinib and dacomitinib, respectively [186–188].

Combination therapies with drugs known to target common EGFR resistance mechanisms such as fibroblast growth factor receptor (FGFR) signaling are also being investigated.

A phase I study of cetuximab with lenvatinib—a multitarget tyrosine kinase inhibitor that has activity against FGFR—in patients with metastatic CSCC or HNSCC is underway [189].

7.2.3. Other Approaches

The risk of BRAF-induced CSCC is abrogated with the addition of MEK inhibition, forming the rationale for investigating the potential role of MEK inhibition in the treatment of CSCC. In vivo studies have shown that MEK induces CSCC cell senescence, but not apoptosis. Interestingly, MEK inhibition also significantly delayed or prevented CSCC development in murine models [190]. Currently, there is a phase II study investigating the efficacy of cobimetinib—an MEK inhibitor—with atezolizumab [191].

Future therapeutic approaches may include novel small molecule inhibitors of both PI3K and mTOR. The oral dual PI3K/mTOR inhibitors—GDC-0084 and LY3023414—have been shown to inhibit proliferation and promote apoptosis in CSCC cell lines [192,193]. GDC-0084 and LY3023414 have been shown to be safe and tolerable in early-phase studies in patients with solid tumors, and there were promising signals of activity [194,195].

8. Therapeutic Options for Immunocompromised Patients

Immunocompromised patients have historically been excluded from clinical trials, but with the success of ICI for immunocompetent patients with CSCC, it became apparent that high-level data to guide treatment for immunocompromised patients were lacking. There are several ongoing studies investigating approaches in different groups of immunocompromised patients. A major concern with the use of ICIs in solid organ transplant patents is graft rejection. Case reports and case series have reported up to a 40% risk of graft rejection with the use of anti-PD(L)1 antibodies [196,197]. To potentially ameliorate that risk, two studies are investigating the combination of tacrolimus—an immunosuppressant—with ipilimumab plus nivolumab, and sirolimus with cemiplimab [198]. Tacrolimus and sirolimus—both mTOR inhibitors—may reduce the risk of CSCC development, as discussed earlier in the review. Cemiplimab is also being investigated in patients with CLL, HIV, or allogenic hematopoietic stem cell transplants [199,200].

Recently, real-world data of patients with CSCC receiving cemiplimab included a cohort of immunocompromised patients. Somewhat surprisingly, given the poor prognosis of immunocompromised patients with CSCC compared to immunocompetent patients, ORR and OS did not differ between immunocompetent and immunocompromised patients. Several patients experienced graft rejection as expected. The causes of immunosuppression in this cohort were heterogeneous, ranging from CLL to OTRs and patients with HIV.

Given the increased risk of developing CSCC and its increased lethality in immunocompromised patients, there is an urgent need to better understand the underlying biology driving this disparity, and to identify potential novel treatment approaches for this cohort.

9. Conclusions

Our understanding of the underlying biology of CSCC—such as the mechanisms and sequelae of UV-induced DNA damage—has resulted in significant advances in the management of patients with CSCC. ICI is established as the first-line management of advanced CSCC, but focus has now shifted to more challenging questions. Can we reduce the risk of patients with localized disease developing recurrent or metastatic disease? How can we improve current treatment paradigms, particularly in immunocompromised patients, where the risk of treatment-related adverse events—particularly graft rejection in OTRs—is high? Finally, what do we do for patients who do not respond to—or have progressed despite—immunotherapy? Current and future scientific research efforts towards identifying predictive biomarkers and understanding the biology behind clinically disparate groups will hopefully address these clinical challenges.

Author Contributions: All authors were involved in the conceptualization, writing, and review of the published manuscript. All authors have read and agreed to the published version of the manuscript.

Funding: This research received no external funding.

Conflicts of Interest: A.A.T. has no conflict of interest to declare. A.M.L. has served on uncompensated advisory boards for Merck Sharp & Dohme and Bristol-Myers Squibb, with travel and accommodation expenses; and uncompensated consultancy for Eisai. B.S. has served on advisory boards for AstraZeneca, Roche-Genentech, Sanofi-Regeneron, Pfizer, Novartis, Merck, Bristol Myers Squibb, Lilly, and Amgen, and received institutional research funding from Sanofi/Regeneron. D.R. has received institutional research grants and funding from Regeneron Pharmaceuticals, Inc., Roche, Merck Sharp & Dohme, Bristol-Myers Squibb, GlaxoSmithKline, Sanofi, Replimune, and Kura Oncology, and has served on uncompensated scientific committees and advisory boards for Merck Sharp & Dohme, Regeneron Pharmaceuticals, Inc., Sanofi, GlaxoSmithKline, and Bristol-Myers Squibb.

References

1. Bray, F.; Ferlay, J.; Soerjomataram, I.; Siegel, R.L.; Torre, L.A.; Jemal, A. Global cancer statistics 2018: GLOBOCAN estimates of incidence and mortality worldwide for 36 cancers in 185 countries. *CA A Cancer J. Clin.* **2018**, *68*, 394–424. [CrossRef]
2. Brantsch, K.D.; Meisner, C.; Schönfisch, B.; Trilling, B.; Wehner-Caroli, J.; Röcken, M.; Breuninger, H. Analysis of risk factors determining prognosis of cutaneous squamous cell carcinoma: A prospective study. *Lancet Oncol.* **2008**, *9*, 713–720. [CrossRef]
3. Brougham, N.D.; Dennett, E.R.; Cameron, R.; Tan, S.T. The incidence of metastasis from cutaneous squamous cell carcinoma and the impact of its risk factors. *J. Surg. Oncol.* **2012**, *106*, 811–815. [CrossRef] [PubMed]
4. Lomas, A.; Leonardi-Bee, J.; Bath-Hextall, F. A systematic review of worldwide incidence of nonmelanoma skin cancer. *Br. J. Dermatol.* **2012**, *166*, 1069–1080. [CrossRef]
5. Pandeya, N.; Olsen, C.M.; Whiteman, D.C. The incidence and multiplicity rates of keratinocyte cancers in Australia. *Med. J. Aust.* **2017**, *207*, 339–343. [CrossRef]
6. Goon, P.K.C.; Greenberg, D.C.; Igali, L.; Levell, N.J. Predicted cases of U.K. skin squamous cell carcinoma and basal cell carcinoma in 2020 and 2025: Horizon planning for National Health Service dermatology and dermatopathology. *Br. J. Dermatol.* **2017**, *176*, 1351–1353. [CrossRef] [PubMed]
7. Karia, P.S.; Han, J.; Schmults, C.D. Cutaneous squamous cell carcinoma: Estimated incidence of disease, nodal metastasis, and deaths from disease in the United States, 2012. *J. Am. Acad. Dermatol.* **2013**, *68*, 957–966. [CrossRef] [PubMed]
8. Ronconi, G.; Piccinni, C.; Dondi, L.; Calabria, S.; Pedrini, A.; Esposito, I.; Ascierto, P.A.; Naldi, L.; Martini, N. Identification of cases and estimate of direct costs of unresectable and advanced cutaneous squamous cell carcinoma: Real-world data from a large Italian database. *Br. J. Dermatol.* **2020**, *183*, 172–174. [CrossRef]
9. Foote, J.A.; Harris, R.B.; Giuliano, A.R.; Roe, D.J.; Moon, T.E.; Cartmel, B.; Alberts, D.S. Predictors for cutaneous basal-and squamous cell carcinoma among actinically damaged adults. *Int. J. Cancer* **2001**, *95*, 7–11. [CrossRef]
10. Armstrong, B.K.; Kricker, A. The epidemiology of UV induced skin cancer. *J. Photochem. Photobiol. B Biol.* **2001**, *63*, 8–18. [CrossRef]
11. Hall, H.I.; May, D.S.; Lew, R.A.; Koh, H.K.; Nadel, M. Sun protection behaviors of the US white population. *Prev. Med.* **1997**, *26*, 401–407. [CrossRef]
12. McCarthy, E.M.; Ethridge, K.P.; Wagner Jr, R. Beach holiday sunburn: The sunscreen paradox and gender differences. *Cutis* **1999**, *64*, 37–42.
13. Thomas-Ahner, J.M.; Wulff, B.C.; Tober, K.L.; Kusewitt, D.F.; Riggenbach, J.A.; Oberyszyn, T.M. Gender Differences in UVB-Induced Skin Carcinogenesis, Inflammation, and DNA Damage. *Cancer Res.* **2007**, *67*, 3468–3474. [CrossRef]
14. Rosso, S.; Zanetti, R.; Martinez, C.; Tormo, M.J.; Schraub, S.; Sancho-Garnier, H.; Franceschi, S.; Gafà, L.; Perea, E.; Navarro, C.; et al. The multicentre south European study 'Helios'. II: Different sun exposure patterns in the aetiology of basal cell and squamous cell carcinomas of the skin. *Br. J. Cancer* **1996**, *73*, 1447–1454. [CrossRef]
15. Sinha, R.P.; Häder, D.P. UV-induced DNA damage and repair: A review. *Photochem. Photobiol. Sci.* **2002**, *1*, 225–236. [CrossRef]
16. Benjamin, C.L.; Ananthaswamy, H.N. p53 and the pathogenesis of skin cancer. *Toxicol. Appl. Pharm.* **2007**, *224*, 241–248. [CrossRef] [PubMed]
17. Benavides, F.; Oberyszyn, T.M.; VanBuskirk, A.M.; Reeve, V.E.; Kusewitt, D.F. The hairless mouse in skin research. *J. Dermatol. Sci.* **2009**, *53*, 10–18. [CrossRef] [PubMed]
18. Fitzpatrick, T.B. The validity and practicality of sun-reactive skin types I through VI. *Arch. Dermatol.* **1988**, *124*, 869–871. [CrossRef] [PubMed]
19. Staples, M.P.; Elwood, M.; Burton, R.C.; Williams, J.L.; Marks, R.; Giles, G.G. Non-melanoma skin cancer in Australia: The 2002 national survey and trends since 1985. *Med. J. Aust.* **2006**, *184*, 6–10. [CrossRef] [PubMed]
20. Harwood, C.A.; Mesher, D.; McGregor, J.M.; Mitchell, L.; Leedham-Green, M.; Raftery, M.; Cerio, R.; Leigh, I.M.; Sasieni, P.; Proby, C.M. A Surveillance Model for Skin Cancer in Organ Transplant Recipients: A 22-Year Prospective Study in an Ethnically Diverse Population. *Am. J. Transplant.* **2013**, *13*, 119–129. [CrossRef]
21. Chiorazzi, N.; Rai, K.R.; Ferrarini, M. Chronic lymphocytic leukemia. *N. Engl. J. Med.* **2005**, *352*, 804–815. [CrossRef]

22. Hober, C.; Fredeau, L.; Pham-Ledard, A.; Boubaya, M.; Herms, F.; Celerier, P.; Aubin, F.; Beneton, N.; Dinulescu, M.; Jannic, A.; et al. Cemiplimab for Locally Advanced and Metastatic Cutaneous Squamous Cell Carcinomas: Real-Life Experience from the French CAREPI Study Group. *Cancers* **2021**, *13*, 3547. [CrossRef]
23. Brewer, J.D.; Shanafelt, T.D.; Khezri, F.; Seda, I.M.S.; Zubair, A.S.; Baum, C.L.; Arpey, C.J.; Cerhan, J.R.; Call, T.G.; Roenigk, R.K. Increased incidence and recurrence rates of nonmelanoma skin cancer in patients with non-Hodgkin lymphoma: A Rochester Epidemiology Project population-based study in Minnesota. *J. Am. Acad. Dermatol.* **2015**, *72*, 302–309. [CrossRef]
24. Levi, F.; Randimbison, L.; Te, V.C.; La Vecchia, C. Non-Hodgkin's lymphomas, chronic lymphocytic leukaemias and skin cancers. *Br. J. Cancer* **1996**, *74*, 1847–1850. [CrossRef]
25. Que, S.K.T.; Zwald, F.O.; Schmults, C.D. Cutaneous squamous cell carcinoma: Incidence, risk factors, diagnosis, and staging. *J. Am. Acad. Dermatol.* **2018**, *78*, 237–247. [CrossRef] [PubMed]
26. Mehrany, K.; Weenig, R.H.; Lee, K.K.; Pittelkow, M.R.; Otley, C.C. Increased metastasis and mortality from cutaneous squamous cell carcinoma in patients with chronic lymphocytic leukemia. *J. Am. Acad. Dermatol.* **2005**, *53*, 1067–1071. [CrossRef] [PubMed]
27. Royle, J.A.; Baade, P.D.; Joske, D.; Girschik, J.; Fritschi, L. Second cancer incidence and cancer mortality among chronic lymphocytic leukaemia patients: A population-based study. *Br. J. Cancer* **2011**, *105*, 1076–1081. [CrossRef] [PubMed]
28. Kleinstern, G.; Rishi, A.; Achenbach, S.J.; Rabe, K.G.; Kay, N.E.; Shanafelt, T.D.; Ding, W.; Leis, J.F.; Norman, A.D.; Call, T.G.; et al. Delineation of clinical and biological factors associated with cutaneous squamous cell carcinoma among patients with chronic lymphocytic leukemia. *J. Am. Acad. Dermatol.* **2020**, *83*, 1581–1589. [CrossRef]
29. Sarvaria, A.; Madrigal, J.A.; Saudemont, A. B cell regulation in cancer and anti-tumor immunity. *Cell. Mol. Immunol.* **2017**, *14*, 662–674. [CrossRef] [PubMed]
30. Cantwell, M.; Hua, T.; Pappas, J.; Kipps, T.J. Acquired CD40-ligand deficiency in chronic lymphocytic leukemia. *Nat. Med.* **1997**, *3*, 984–989. [CrossRef]
31. Lindqvist, C.A.; Christiansson, L.H.; Simonsson, B.; Enblad, G.; Olsson-Strömberg, U.; Loskog, A.S.I. T regulatory cells control T-cell proliferation partly by the release of soluble CD25 in patients with B-cell malignancies. *Immunology* **2010**, *131*, 371–376. [CrossRef] [PubMed]
32. Chikuma, S.; Terawaki, S.; Hayashi, T.; Nabeshima, R.; Yoshida, T.; Shibayama, S.; Okazaki, T.; Honjo, T. PD-1-mediated suppression of IL-2 production induces CD8+ T cell anergy in vivo. *J. Immunol.* **2009**, *182*, 6682–6689. [CrossRef] [PubMed]
33. Riches, J.C.; Ramsay, A.G.; Gribben, J.G. Immune reconstitution in chronic lymphocytic leukemia. *Curr. Hematol. Malig. Rep.* **2012**, *7*, 13–20. [CrossRef]
34. Besson, C.; Moore, A.; Wu, W.; Camp, N.J.; Vajdic, C.; Morton, L.M.; Smedby, K.E.; de Sanjose, S.; Shanafelt, T.D.; Brewer, J.; et al. Common Genetic Polymorphisms Contribute to the Association between Non-Melanoma Skin Cancer and Chronic Lymphocytic Leukemia. *Blood* **2017**, *130*, 1454. [CrossRef]
35. Veness, M.J.; Quinn, D.I.; Ong, C.S.; Keogh, A.M.; Macdonald, P.S.; Cooper, S.G.; Morgan, G.W. Aggressive cutaneous malignancies following cardiothoracic transplantation: The Australian experience. *Cancer Interdiscip. Int. J. Am. Cancer Soc.* **1999**, *85*, 1758–1764. [CrossRef]
36. Jensen, P.; Hansen, S.; Møller, B.; Leivestad, T.; Pfeffer, P.; Geiran, O.; Fauchald, P.; Simonsen, S. Skin cancer in kidney and heart transplant recipients and different long-term immunosuppressive therapy regimens. *J. Am. Acad. Dermatol.* **1999**, *40*, 177–186. [CrossRef]
37. Garrett, G.L.; Lowenstein, S.E.; Singer, J.P.; He, S.Y.; Arron, S.T. Trends of skin cancer mortality after transplantation in the United States: 1987 to 2013. *J. Am. Acad. Dermatol.* **2016**, *75*, 106–112. [CrossRef]
38. Wu, X.; Nguyen, B.-C.; Dziunycz, P.; Chang, S.; Brooks, Y.; Lefort, K.; Hofbauer, G.F.L.; Dotto, G.P. Opposing roles for calcineurin and ATF3 in squamous skin cancer. *Nature* **2010**, *465*, 368–372. [CrossRef]
39. Yarosh, D.B.; Pena, A.V.; Nay, S.L.; Canning, M.T.; Brown, D.A. Calcineurin Inhibitors Decrease DNA Repair and Apoptosis in Human Keratinocytes Following Ultraviolet B Irradiation. *J. Investig. Dermatol.* **2005**, *125*, 1020–1025. [CrossRef]
40. Walsh, S.B.; Xu, J.; Xu, H.; Kurundkar, A.R.; Maheshwari, A.; Grizzle, W.E.; Timares, L.; Huang, C.C.; Kopelovich, L.; Elmets, C.A.; et al. Cyclosporine a mediates pathogenesis of aggressive cutaneous squamous cell carcinoma by augmenting epithelial-mesenchymal transition: Role of TGFβ signaling pathway. *Mol. Carcinog.* **2011**, *50*, 516–527. [CrossRef]
41. Hong, J.C.; Kahan, B.D. Immunosuppressive agents in organ transplantation: Past, present, and future. *Semin. Nephrol.* **2000**, *20*, 108–125. [PubMed]
42. Coghill, A.E.; Johnson, L.G.; Berg, D.; Resler, A.J.; Leca, N.; Madeleine, M.M. Immunosuppressive Medications and Squamous Cell Skin Carcinoma: Nested Case-Control Study Within the Skin Cancer after Organ Transplant (SCOT) Cohort. *Am. J. Transplant.* **2016**, *16*, 565–573. [CrossRef]
43. Salgo, R.; Gossmann, J.; Schöfer, H.; Kachel, H.; Kuck, J.; Geiger, H.; Kaufmann, R.; Scheuermann, E. Switch to a sirolimus-based immunosuppression in long-term renal transplant recipients: Reduced rate of (pre-) malignancies and nonmelanoma skin cancer in a prospective, randomized, assessor-blinded, controlled clinical trial. *Am. J. Transplant.* **2010**, *10*, 1385–1393. [CrossRef] [PubMed]
44. Norman, K.G.; Canter, J.A.; Shi, M.; Milne, G.L.; Morrow, J.D.; Sligh, J.E. Cyclosporine A suppresses keratinocyte cell death through MPTP inhibition in a model for skin cancer in organ transplant recipients. *Mitochondrion* **2010**, *10*, 94–101. [CrossRef]
45. Thomson, A.W.; Turnquist, H.R.; Raimondi, G. Immunoregulatory functions of mTOR inhibition. *Nat. Rev. Immunol.* **2009**, *9*, 324–337. [CrossRef]

46. Hackstein, H.; Taner, T.; Zahorchak, A.F.; Morelli, A.E.; Logar, A.J.; Gessner, A.; Thomson, A.W. Rapamycin inhibits IL-4—Induced dendritic cell maturation in vitro and dendritic cell mobilization and function in vivo. *Blood* **2003**, *101*, 4457–4463. [CrossRef]
47. de Gruijl, F.R.; Koehl, G.E.; Voskamp, P.; Strik, A.; Rebel, H.G.; Gaumann, A.; de Fijter, J.W.; Tensen, C.P.; Bavinck, J.N.B.; Geissler, E.K. Early and late effects of the immunosuppressants rapamycin and mycophenolate mofetil on UV carcinogenesis. *Int. J. Cancer* **2010**, *127*, 796–804. [CrossRef]
48. Wulff, B.C.; Kusewitt, D.F.; VanBuskirk, A.M.; Thomas-Ahner, J.M.; Duncan, F.J.; Oberyszyn, T.M. Sirolimus reduces the incidence and progression of UVB-induced skin cancer in SKH mice even with co-administration of cyclosporine A. *J. Investig. Dermatol.* **2008**, *128*, 2467–2473. [CrossRef]
49. Schaper-Gerhardt, K.; Walter, A.; Schmitz-Rode, C.; Satzger, I.; Gutzmer, R. The mTOR-inhibitor Sirolimus decreases the cyclosporine-induced expression of the oncogene ATF3 in human keratinocytes. *J. Dermatol. Sci.* **2018**, *92*, 172–180. [CrossRef]
50. Kim, M.S.; In, S.G.; Park, O.J.; Won, C.H.; Lee, M.W.; Choi, J.H.; Kim, C.W.; Kim, S.E.; Moon, K.C.; Chang, S. Increased expression of activating transcription factor 3 is related to the biologic behavior of cutaneous squamous cell carcinomas. *Hum. Pathol.* **2011**, *42*, 954–959. [CrossRef] [PubMed]
51. Euvrard, S.; Kanitakis, J.; Decullier, E.; Butnaru, A.C.; Lefrançois, N.; Boissonnat, P.; Sebbag, L.; Garnier, J.-L.; Pouteil-Noble, C.; Cahen, R. Subsequent skin cancers in kidney and heart transplant recipients after the first squamous cell carcinoma. *Transplantation* **2006**, *81*, 1093–1100. [CrossRef] [PubMed]
52. Alberú, J.; Pascoe, M.D.; Campistol, J.M.; Schena, F.P.; del Carmen Rial, M.; Polinsky, M.; Neylan, J.F.; Korth-Bradley, J.; Goldberg-Alberts, R.; Maller, E.S. Lower malignancy rates in renal allograft recipients converted to sirolimus-based, calcineurin inhibitor-free immunotherapy: 24-month results from the CONVERT trial. *Transplantation* **2011**, *92*, 303–310. [CrossRef] [PubMed]
53. Jensen, A.; Thomsen, H.F.; Engebjerg, M.C.; Olesen, A.B.; Friis, S.; Karagas, M.R.; Sørensen, H.T. Use of oral glucocorticoids and risk of skin cancer and non-Hodgkin's lymphoma: A population-based case–control study. *Br. J. Cancer* **2009**, *100*, 200–205. [CrossRef]
54. Baibergenova, A.T.; Weinstock, M.A.; Group, V.T. Oral prednisone use and risk of keratinocyte carcinoma in non-transplant population. The VATTC trial. *J. Eur. Acad. Dermatol. Venereol.* **2012**, *26*, 1109–1115. [CrossRef]
55. Sørensen, H.T.; Mellemkjær, L.; Nielsen, G.L.; Baron, J.A.; Olsen, J.H.; Karagas, M.R. Skin Cancers and Non-Hodgkin Lymphoma Among Users of Systemic Glucocorticoids: A Population-Based Cohort Study. *JNCI J. Natl. Cancer Inst.* **2004**, *96*, 709–711. [CrossRef] [PubMed]
56. Fortina, A.B.; Piaserico, S.; Caforio, A.L.P.; Abeni, D.; Alaibac, M.; Angelini, A.; Iliceto, S.; Peserico, A. Immunosuppressive Level and Other Risk Factors for Basal Cell Carcinoma and Squamous Cell Carcinoma in Heart Transplant Recipients. *Arch. Dermatol.* **2004**, *140*, 1079–1085. [CrossRef]
57. Chen, P.; Chen, F.; Zhou, B. Systematic review and meta-analysis of prevalence of dermatological toxicities associated with vemurafenib treatment in patients with melanoma. *Clin. Exp. Dermatol.* **2019**, *44*, 243–251. [CrossRef]
58. Anforth, R.; Fernandez-Peñas, P.; Long, G.V. Cutaneous toxicities of RAF inhibitors. *Lancet. Oncol.* **2013**, *14*, e11–e18. [CrossRef]
59. Ascierto, P.A.; Minor, D.; Ribas, A.; Lebbe, C.; O'Hagan, A.; Arya, N.; Guckert, M.; Schadendorf, D.; Kefford, R.F.; Grob, J.J.; et al. Phase II trial (BREAK-2) of the BRAF inhibitor dabrafenib (GSK2118436) in patients with metastatic melanoma. *J. Clin. Oncol.* **2013**, *31*, 3205–3211. [CrossRef]
60. Gibney, G.T.; Messina, J.L.; Fedorenko, I.V.; Sondak, V.K.; Smalley, K.S.M. Paradoxical oncogenesis—The long-term effects of BRAF inhibition in melanoma. *Nat. Rev. Clin. Oncol.* **2013**, *10*, 390–399. [CrossRef]
61. Heidorn, S.J.; Milagre, C.; Whittaker, S.; Nourry, A.; Niculescu-Duvas, I.; Dhomen, N.; Hussain, J.; Reis-Filho, J.S.; Springer, C.J.; Pritchard, C. Kinase-dead BRAF and oncogenic RAS cooperate to drive tumor progression through CRAF. *Cell* **2010**, *140*, 209–221. [CrossRef]
62. Poulikakos, P.I.; Zhang, C.; Bollag, G.; Shokat, K.M.; Rosen, N. RAF inhibitors transactivate RAF dimers and ERK signalling in cells with wild-type BRAF. *Nature* **2010**, *464*, 427–430. [CrossRef]
63. Su, F.; Viros, A.; Milagre, C.; Trunzer, K.; Bollag, G.; Spleiss, O.; Reis-Filho, J.S.; Kong, X.; Koya, R.C.; Flaherty, K.T. RAS mutations in cutaneous squamous-cell carcinomas in patients treated with BRAF inhibitors. *N. Engl. J. Med.* **2012**, *366*, 207–215. [CrossRef] [PubMed]
64. Anforth, R.; Menzies, A.; Byth, K.; Carlos, G.; Chou, S.; Sharma, R.; Scolyer, R.A.; Kefford, R.; Long, G.V.; Fernandez-Peñas, P. Factors influencing the development of cutaneous squamous cell carcinoma in patients on BRAF inhibitor therapy. *J. Am. Acad. Dermatol.* **2015**, *72*, 809–815.e801. [CrossRef] [PubMed]
65. Robert, C.; Karaszewska, B.; Schachter, J.; Rutkowski, P.; Mackiewicz, A.; Stroiakovski, D.; Lichinitser, M.; Dummer, R.; Grange, F.; Mortier, L.; et al. Improved overall survival in melanoma with combined dabrafenib and trametinib. *N. Engl. J. Med.* **2015**, *372*, 30–39. [CrossRef]
66. Long, G.V.; Flaherty, K.T.; Stroyakovskiy, D.; Gogas, H.; Levchenko, E.; de Braud, F.; Larkin, J.; Garbe, C.; Jouary, T.; Hauschild, A.; et al. Dabrafenib plus trametinib versus dabrafenib monotherapy in patients with metastatic BRAF V600E/K-mutant melanoma: Long-term survival and safety analysis of a phase 3 study. *Ann. Oncol.* **2017**, *28*, 1631–1639. [CrossRef] [PubMed]
67. Carlos, G.; Anforth, R.; Clements, A.; Menzies, A.M.; Carlino, M.S.; Chou, S.; Fernandez-Peñas, P. Cutaneous Toxic Effects of BRAF Inhibitors Alone and in Combination with MEK Inhibitors for Metastatic Melanoma. *JAMA Derm.* **2015**, *151*, 1103–1109. [CrossRef] [PubMed]

68. March-Rodriguez, Á.; Bellosillo, B.; Álvarez-Larrán, A.; Besses, C.; Pujol, R.M.; Toll, A. Rapidly Growing and Aggressive Cutaneous Squamous Cell Carcinomas in a Patient Treated with Ruxolitinib. *Ann. Derm.* **2019**, *31*, 204–208. [CrossRef]
69. Aboul-Fettouh, N.; Nijhawan, R.I. Aggressive squamous cell carcinoma in a patient on the Janus kinase inhibitor ruxolitinib. *JAAD Case Rep.* **2018**, *4*, 455–457. [CrossRef]
70. Aleisa, A.I.; Plante, J.G.; Hsia, L.-L.B. A case of aggressive squamous cell carcinoma with lymphovascular invasion during treatment with the Janus kinase inhibitor tofacitinib. *JAAD Case Rep.* **2020**, *6*, 727–730. [CrossRef]
71. Harrison, C.N.; Vannucchi, A.M.; Kiladjian, J.J.; Al-Ali, H.K.; Gisslinger, H.; Knoops, L.; Cervantes, F.; Jones, M.M.; Sun, K.; McQuitty, M.; et al. Long-term findings from COMFORT-II, a phase 3 study of ruxolitinib vs best available therapy for myelofibrosis. *Leukemia* **2016**, *30*, 1701–1707. [CrossRef]
72. Johnson, D.E.; O'Keefe, R.A.; Grandis, J.R. Targeting the IL-6/JAK/STAT3 signalling axis in cancer. *Nat. Rev. Clin. Oncol.* **2018**, *15*, 234–248. [CrossRef] [PubMed]
73. Abikhair Burgo, M.; Roudiani, N.; Chen, J.; Santana, A.L.; Doudican, N.; Proby, C.; Felsen, D.; Carucci, J.A. Ruxolitinib inhibits cyclosporine-induced proliferation of cutaneous squamous cell carcinoma. *JCI Insight* **2020**, *3*, e120750. [CrossRef] [PubMed]
74. Kerr-Valentic, M.A.; Samimi, K.; Rohlen, B.H.; Agarwal, J.P.; Rockwell, W.B. Marjolin's Ulcer: Modern Analysis of an Ancient Problem. *Plast. Reconstr. Surg.* **2009**, *123*, 184–191. [CrossRef] [PubMed]
75. Xiang, F.; Song, H.-P.; Huang, Y.-S. Clinical features and treatment of 140 cases of Marjolin's ulcer at a major burn center in southwest China. *Exp. Med.* **2019**, *17*, 3403–3410. [CrossRef] [PubMed]
76. Kadir, A.R. Burn scar neoplasm. *Ann. Burn. Fire Disasters* **2007**, *20*, 185–188.
77. Das, K.K.; Chakaraborty, A.; Rahman, A.; Khandkar, S. Incidences of malignancy in chronic burn scar ulcers: Experience from Bangladesh. *Burns* **2015**, *41*, 1315–1321. [CrossRef]
78. Yu, N.; Long, X.; Lujan-Hernandez, J.R.; Hassan, K.Z.; Bai, M.; Wang, Y.; Wang, X.; Zhao, R. Marjolin's ulcer: A preventable malignancy arising from scars. *World J. Surg. Oncol.* **2013**, *11*, 313. [CrossRef]
79. Grivennikov, S.I.; Greten, F.R.; Karin, M. Immunity, Inflammation, and Cancer. *Cell* **2010**, *140*, 883–899. [CrossRef]
80. Greten, F.R.; Grivennikov, S.I. Inflammation and Cancer: Triggers, Mechanisms, and Consequences. *Immunity* **2019**, *51*, 27–41. [CrossRef]
81. Yu, H.S.; Liao, W.T.; Chai, C.Y. Arsenic carcinogenesis in the skin. *J. Biomed. Sci.* **2006**, *13*, 657–666. [CrossRef] [PubMed]
82. Kishikawa, M.; Koyama, K.; Iseki, M.; Kobuke, T.; Yonehara, S.; Soda, M.; Ron, E.; Tokunaga, M.; Preston, D.L.; Mabuchi, K.; et al. Histologic characteristics of skin cancer in Hiroshima and Nagasaki: Background incidence and radiation effects. *Int. J. Cancer* **2005**, *117*, 363–369. [CrossRef]
83. Yoshinaga, S.; Hauptmann, M.; Sigurdson, A.J.; Doody, M.M.; Freedman, D.M.; Alexander, B.H.; Linet, M.S.; Ron, E.; Mabuchi, K. Nonmelanoma skin cancer in relation to ionizing radiation exposure among U.S. radiologic technologists. *Int. J. Cancer* **2005**, *115*, 828–834. [CrossRef]
84. Lichter, M.D.; Karagas, M.R.; Mott, L.A.; Spencer, S.K.; Stukel, T.A.; Greenberg, E.R. Therapeutic ionizing radiation and the incidence of basal cell carcinoma and squamous cell carcinoma. The New Hampshire Skin Cancer Study Group. *Arch. Dermatol.* **2000**, *136*, 1007–1011. [CrossRef] [PubMed]
85. Stenehjem, J.S.; Robsahm, T.E.; Bråtveit, M.; Samuelsen, S.O.; Kirkeleit, J.; Grimsrud, T.K. Aromatic hydrocarbons and risk of skin cancer by anatomical site in 25 000 male offshore petroleum workers. *Am. J. Ind. Med.* **2017**, *60*, 679–688. [CrossRef]
86. Pukkala, E.; Martinsen, J.I.; Weiderpass, E.; Kjaerheim, K.; Lynge, E.; Tryggvadottir, L.; Sparén, P.; Demers, P.A. Cancer incidence among firefighters: 45 years of follow-up in five Nordic countries. *Occup. Environ. Med.* **2014**, *71*, 398–404. [CrossRef]
87. Alter, B.P.; Giri, N.; Savage, S.A.; Rosenberg, P.S. Cancer in dyskeratosis congenita. *Blood* **2009**, *113*, 6549–6557. [CrossRef]
88. Alter, B.P.; Giri, N.; Savage, S.A.; Peters, J.A.; Loud, J.T.; Leathwood, L.; Carr, A.G.; Greene, M.H.; Rosenberg, P.S. Malignancies and survival patterns in the National Cancer Institute inherited bone marrow failure syndromes cohort study. *Br. J. Haematol.* **2010**, *150*, 179–188. [CrossRef]
89. Risitano, A.M.; Marotta, S.; Calzone, R.; Grimaldi, F.; Zatterale, A. Twenty years of the Italian Fanconi Anemia Registry: Where we stand and what remains to be learned. *Haematologica* **2016**, *101*, 319–327. [CrossRef]
90. de Koning, M.N.C.; Weissenborn, S.J.; Abeni, D.; Bouwes Bavinck, J.N.; Euvrard, S.; Green, A.C.; Harwood, C.A.; Naldi, L.; Neale, R.; Nindl, I.; et al. Prevalence and associated factors of betapapillomavirus infections in individuals without cutaneous squamous cell carcinoma. *J. Gen. Virol.* **2009**, *90*, 1611–1621. [CrossRef] [PubMed]
91. Antonsson, A.; Forslund, O.; Ekberg, H.; Sterner, G.; Hansson, B.G. The ubiquity and impressive genomic diversity of human skin papillomaviruses suggest a commensalic nature of these viruses. *J. Virol.* **2000**, *74*, 11636–11641. [CrossRef] [PubMed]
92. Neale, R.E.; Weissenborn, S.; Abeni, D.; Bavinck, J.N.B.; Euvrard, S.; Feltkamp, M.C.W.; Green, A.C.; Harwood, C.; de Koning, M.; Naldi, L.; et al. Human Papillomavirus Load in Eyebrow Hair Follicles and Risk of Cutaneous Squamous Cell Carcinoma. *Cancer Epidemiol. Biomark. Prev.* **2013**, *22*, 719–727. [CrossRef]
93. Bouwes Bavinck, J.N.; Feltkamp, M.C.W.; Green, A.C.; Fiocco, M.; Euvrard, S.; Harwood, C.A.; Nasir, S.; Thomson, J.; Proby, C.M.; Naldi, L.; et al. Human papillomavirus and posttransplantation cutaneous squamous cell carcinoma: A multicenter, prospective cohort study. *Am. J. Transplant.* **2018**, *18*, 1220–1230. [CrossRef]
94. Chahoud, J.; Semaan, A.; Chen, Y.; Cao, M.; Rieber, A.G.; Rady, P.; Tyring, S.K. Association Between β-Genus Human Papillomavirus and Cutaneous Squamous Cell Carcinoma in Immunocompetent Individuals—A Meta-analysis. *JAMA Dermatol.* **2016**, *152*, 1354–1364. [CrossRef] [PubMed]

95. Karagas, M.R.; Nelson, H.H.; Sehr, P.; Waterboer, T.; Stukel, T.A.; Andrew, A.; Green, A.C.; Bouwes Bavinck, J.N.; Perry, A.; Spencer, S.; et al. Human Papillomavirus Infection and Incidence of Squamous Cell and Basal Cell Carcinomas of the Skin. *JNCI J. Natl. Cancer Inst.* **2006**, *98*, 389–395. [CrossRef]
96. Andersson, K.; Waterboer, T.; Kirnbauer, R.; Slupetzky, K.; Iftner, T.; de Villiers, E.-M.; Forslund, O.; Pawlita, M.; Dillner, J. Seroreactivity to Cutaneous Human Papillomaviruses among Patients with Nonmelanoma Skin Cancer or Benign Skin Lesions. *Cancer Epidemiol. Biomark. Prev.* **2008**, *17*, 189–195. [CrossRef] [PubMed]
97. Iannacone, M.R.; Gheit, T.; Waterboer, T.; Giuliano, A.R.; Messina, J.L.; Fenske, N.A.; Cherpelis, B.S.; Sondak, V.K.; Roetzheim, R.G.; Ferrer-Gil, S.; et al. Case–Control Study of Cutaneous Human Papillomavirus Infection in Basal Cell Carcinoma of the Skin. *J. Investig. Dermatol.* **2013**, *133*, 1512–1520. [CrossRef]
98. Howley, P.M.; Pfister, H.J. Beta genus papillomaviruses and skin cancer. *Virology* **2015**, *479–480*, 290–296. [CrossRef]
99. Weissenborn, S.J.; Nindl, I.; Purdie, K.; Harwood, C.; Proby, C.; Breuer, J.; Majewski, S.; Pfister, H.; Wieland, U. Human papillomavirus-DNA loads in actinic keratoses exceed those in non-melanoma skin cancers. *J. Investig. Dermatol.* **2005**, *125*, 93–97. [CrossRef]
100. Conforti, C.; Paolini, F.; Venuti, A.; Dianzani, C.; Zalaudek, I. The detection rate of human papillomavirus in well-differentiated squamous cell carcinoma and keratoacanthoma: Is there new evidence for a viral pathogenesis of keratoacanthoma? *Br. J. Dermatol.* **2019**, *181*, 1309–1311. [CrossRef]
101. Viarisio, D.; Decker, K.M.; Aengeneyndt, B.; Flechtenmacher, C.; Gissmann, L.; Tommasino, M. Human papillomavirus type 38 E6 and E7 act as tumour promoters during chemically induced skin carcinogenesis. *J. Gen. Virol.* **2013**, *94*, 749–752. [CrossRef] [PubMed]
102. Wallace, N.A.; Robinson, K.; Howie, H.L.; Galloway, D.A. HPV 5 and 8 E6 abrogate ATR activity resulting in increased persistence of UVB induced DNA damage. *PLoS Pathog.* **2012**, *8*, e1002807. [CrossRef]
103. Cornet, I.; Bouvard, V.; Campo, M.S.; Thomas, M.; Banks, L.; Gissmann, L.; Lamartine, J.; Sylla, B.S.; Accardi, R.; Tommasino, M. Comparative Analysis of Transforming Properties of E6 and E7 from Different Beta Human Papillomavirus Types. *J. Virol.* **2012**, *86*, 2366–2370. [CrossRef]
104. Caldeira, S.; Zehbe, I.; Accardi, R.; Malanchi, I.; Dong, W.; Giarrè, M.; de Villiers, E.-M.; Filotico, R.; Boukamp, P.; Tommasino, M. The E6 and E7 Proteins of the Cutaneous Human Papillomavirus Type 38 Display Transforming Properties. *J. Virol.* **2003**, *77*, 2195–2206. [CrossRef]
105. Brimer, N.; Lyons, C.; Wallberg, A.E.; Vande Pol, S.B. Cutaneous papillomavirus E6 oncoproteins associate with MAML1 to repress transactivation and NOTCH signaling. *Oncogene* **2012**, *31*, 4639–4646. [CrossRef]
106. Meyers, J.M.; Uberoi, A.; Grace, M.; Lambert, P.F.; Munger, K. Cutaneous HPV8 and MmuPV1 E6 Proteins Target the NOTCH and TGF-β Tumor Suppressors to Inhibit Differentiation and Sustain Keratinocyte Proliferation. *PLoS Pathog.* **2017**, *13*, e1006171. [CrossRef] [PubMed]
107. Tan, M.J.A.; White, E.A.; Sowa, M.E.; Harper, J.W.; Aster, J.C.; Howley, P.M. Cutaneous β-human papillomavirus E6 proteins bind Mastermind-like coactivators and repress Notch signaling. *Proc. Natl. Acad. Sci. USA* **2012**, *109*, E1473–E1480. [CrossRef]
108. Rozenblatt-Rosen, O.; Deo, R.C.; Padi, M.; Adelmant, G.; Calderwood, M.A.; Rolland, T.; Grace, M.; Dricot, A.; Askenazi, M.; Tavares, M.; et al. Interpreting cancer genomes using systematic host network perturbations by tumour virus proteins. *Nature* **2012**, *487*, 491–495. [CrossRef]
109. Olivero, C.; Lanfredini, S.; Borgogna, C.; Gariglio, M.; Patel, G.K. HPV-Induced Field Cancerisation: Transformation of Adult Tissue Stem Cell Into Cancer Stem Cell. *Front. Microbiol.* **2018**, *9*, 546. [CrossRef]
110. Chalmers, Z.R.; Connelly, C.F.; Fabrizio, D.; Gay, L.; Ali, S.M.; Ennis, R.; Schrock, A.; Campbell, B.; Shlien, A.; Chmielecki, J.; et al. Analysis of 100,000 human cancer genomes reveals the landscape of tumor mutational burden. *Genome Med.* **2017**, *9*, 34. [CrossRef] [PubMed]
111. Sengupta, S.; Harris, C.C. p53: Traffic cop at the crossroads of DNA repair and recombination. *Nat. Rev. Mol. Cell Biol.* **2005**, *6*, 44–55. [CrossRef]
112. Kraemer, K.H.; Tamura, D.; Khan, S.G.; Digiovanna, J.J. Burning issues in the diagnosis of xeroderma pigmentosum. *Br. J. Dermatol.* **2013**, *169*, 1176. [CrossRef] [PubMed]
113. Nakazawa, H.; English, D.; Randell, P.L.; Nakazawa, K.; Martel, N.; Armstrong, B.K.; Yamasaki, H. UV and skin cancer: Specific p53 gene mutation in normal skin as a biologically relevant exposure measurement. *Proc. Natl. Acad. Sci. USA* **1994**, *91*, 360–364. [CrossRef]
114. Jonason, A.S.; Kunala, S.; Price, G.J.; Restifo, R.J.; Spinelli, H.M.; Persing, J.A.; Leffell, D.J.; Tarone, R.E.; Brash, D.E. Frequent clones of p53-mutated keratinocytes in normal human skin. *Proc. Natl. Acad. Sci. USA* **1996**, *93*, 14025–14029. [CrossRef]
115. Ren, Z.P.; Hedrum, A.; Pontén, F.; Nistér, M.; Ahmadian, A.; Lundeberg, J.; Uhlén, M.; Pontén, J. Human epidermal cancer and accompanying precursors have identical p53 mutations different from p53 mutations in adjacent areas of clonally expanded non-neoplastic keratinocytes. *Oncogene* **1996**, *12*, 765–773.
116. Ziegler, A.; Jonason, A.S.; Leffell, D.J.; Simon, J.A.; Sharma, H.W.; Kimmelman, J.; Remington, L.; Jacks, T.; Brash, D.E. Sunburn and p53 in the onset of skin cancer. *Nature* **1994**, *372*, 773–776. [CrossRef] [PubMed]
117. Durinck, S.; Ho, C.; Wang, N.J.; Liao, W.; Jakkula, L.R.; Collisson, E.A.; Pons, J.; Chan, S.-W.; Lam, E.T.; Chu, C.; et al. Temporal Dissection of Tumorigenesis in Primary Cancers. *Cancer Discov.* **2011**, *1*, 137–143. [CrossRef] [PubMed]

118. South, A.P.; Purdie, K.J.; Watt, S.A.; Haldenby, S.; den Breems, N.Y.; Dimon, M.; Arron, S.T.; Kluk, M.J.; Aster, J.C.; McHugh, A.; et al. NOTCH1 Mutations Occur Early during Cutaneous Squamous Cell Carcinogenesis. *J. Investig. Dermatol.* **2014**, *134*, 2630–2638. [CrossRef]
119. Di Nardo, L.; Pellegrini, C.; Di Stefani, A.; Del Regno, L.; Sollena, P.; Piccerillo, A.; Longo, C.; Garbe, C.; Fargnoli, M.C.; Peris, K. Molecular genetics of cutaneous squamous cell carcinoma: Perspective for treatment strategies. *J. Eur. Acad. Dermatol. Venereol.* **2020**, *34*, 932–941. [CrossRef]
120. Fearon, E.R.; Vogelstein, B. A genetic model for colorectal tumorigenesis. *Cell* **1990**, *61*, 759–767. [CrossRef]
121. Hruban, R.H.; Goggins, M.; Parsons, J.; Kern, S.E. Progression model for pancreatic cancer. *Clin. Cancer Res.* **2000**, *6*, 2969–2972. [PubMed]
122. Olivier, M.; Langerød, A.; Carrieri, P.; Bergh, J.; Klaar, S.; Eyfjord, J.; Theillet, C.; Rodriguez, C.; Lidereau, R.; Bièche, I.; et al. The clinical value of somatic TP53 gene mutations in 1794 patients with breast cancer. *Clin. Cancer Res.* **2006**, *12*, 1157–1167. [CrossRef]
123. Berg, R.J.; van Kranen, H.J.; Rebel, H.G.; de Vries, A.; van Vloten, W.A.; Van Kreijl, C.F.; van der Leun, J.C.; de Gruijl, F.R. Early p53 alterations in mouse skin carcinogenesis by UVB radiation: Immunohistochemical detection of mutant p53 protein in clusters of preneoplastic epidermal cells. *Proc. Natl. Acad. Sci. USA* **1996**, *93*, 274–278. [CrossRef] [PubMed]
124. Li, G.; Tron, V.; Ho, V. Induction of squamous cell carcinoma in p53-deficient mice after ultraviolet irradiation. *J. Investig. Dermatol.* **1998**, *110*, 72–75. [CrossRef]
125. Mudgil, A.V.; Segal, N.; Andriani, F.; Wang, Y.; Fusenig, N.E.; Garlick, J.A. Ultraviolet B irradiation induces expansion of intraepithelial tumor cells in a tissue model of early cancer progression. *J. Investig. Dermatol.* **2003**, *121*, 191–197. [CrossRef]
126. Li, Y.Y.; Hanna, G.J.; Laga, A.C.; Haddad, R.I.; Lorch, J.H.; Hammerman, P.S. Genomic analysis of metastatic cutaneous squamous cell carcinoma. *Clin. Cancer Res.* **2015**, *21*, 1447–1456. [CrossRef]
127. Artavanis-Tsakonas, S.; Rand, M.D.; Lake, R.J. Notch Signaling: Cell Fate Control and Signal Integration in Development. *Science* **1999**, *284*, 770–776. [CrossRef] [PubMed]
128. Watt, F.M.; Estrach, S.; Ambler, C.A. Epidermal Notch signalling: Differentiation, cancer and adhesion. *Curr. Opin. Cell Biol.* **2008**, *20*, 171–179. [CrossRef]
129. Nowell, C.S.; Radtke, F. Notch as a tumour suppressor. *Nat. Rev. Cancer* **2017**, *17*, 145–159. [CrossRef]
130. Balint, K.; Xiao, M.; Pinnix, C.C.; Soma, A.; Veres, I.; Juhasz, I.; Brown, E.J.; Capobianco, A.J.; Herlyn, M.; Liu, Z.J. Activation of Notch1 signaling is required for beta-catenin-mediated human primary melanoma progression. *J. Clin. Investig.* **2005**, *115*, 3166–3176. [CrossRef]
131. Weng, A.P.; Ferrando, A.A.; Lee, W.; Morris, J.P.t.; Silverman, L.B.; Sanchez-Irizarry, C.; Blacklow, S.C.; Look, A.T.; Aster, J.C. Activating mutations of NOTCH1 in human T cell acute lymphoblastic leukemia. *Science* **2004**, *306*, 269–271. [CrossRef] [PubMed]
132. Nicolas, M.; Wolfer, A.; Raj, K.; Kummer, J.A.; Mill, P.; van Noort, M.; Hui, C.-c.; Clevers, H.; Dotto, G.P.; Radtke, F. Notch1 functions as a tumor suppressor in mouse skin. *Nat. Genet.* **2003**, *33*, 416–421. [CrossRef] [PubMed]
133. Pickering, C.R.; Zhou, J.H.; Lee, J.J.; Drummond, J.A.; Peng, S.A.; Saade, R.E.; Tsai, K.Y.; Curry, J.L.; Tetzlaff, M.T.; Lai, S.Y. Mutational landscape of aggressive cutaneous squamous cell carcinoma. *Clin. Cancer Res.* **2014**, *20*, 6582–6592. [CrossRef] [PubMed]
134. Lefort, K.; Mandinova, A.; Ostano, P.; Kolev, V.; Calpini, V.; Kolfschoten, I.; Devgan, V.; Lieb, J.; Raffoul, W.; Hohl, D.; et al. Notch1 is a p53 target gene involved in human keratinocyte tumor suppression through negative regulation of ROCK1/2 and MRCKalpha kinases. *Genes Dev* **2007**, *21*, 562–577. [CrossRef]
135. Proweller, A.; Tu, L.; Lepore, J.J.; Cheng, L.; Lu, M.M.; Seykora, J.; Millar, S.E.; Pear, W.S.; Parmacek, M.S. Impaired Notch Signaling Promotes De novo Squamous Cell Carcinoma Formation. *Cancer Res.* **2006**, *66*, 7438–7444. [CrossRef]
136. Demehri, S.; Turkoz, A.; Kopan, R. Epidermal Notch1 Loss Promotes Skin Tumorigenesis by Impacting the Stromal Microenvironment. *Cancer Cell* **2009**, *16*, 55–66. [CrossRef]
137. Extance, A. Alzheimer's failure raises questions about disease-modifying strategies. *Nat. Rev. Drug Discov.* **2010**, *9*, 749–751. [CrossRef]
138. Brown, V.L.; Harwood, C.A.; Crook, T.; Cronin, J.G.; Kelsell, D.P.; Proby, C.M. p16INK4a and p14ARF Tumor Suppressor Genes Are Commonly Inactivated in Cutaneous Squamous Cell Carcinoma. *J. Investig. Dermatol.* **2004**, *122*, 1284–1292. [CrossRef]
139. Inman, G.J.; Wang, J.; Nagano, A.; Alexandrov, L.B.; Purdie, K.J.; Taylor, R.G.; Sherwood, V.; Thomson, J.; Hogan, S.; Spender, L.C.; et al. The genomic landscape of cutaneous SCC reveals drivers and a novel azathioprine associated mutational signature. *Nat. Commun.* **2018**, *9*, 3667. [CrossRef]
140. Ryan, M.B.; Corcoran, R.B. Therapeutic strategies to target RAS-mutant cancers. *Nat. Rev. Clin. Oncol.* **2018**, *15*, 709–720. [CrossRef]
141. Fruman, D.A.; Chiu, H.; Hopkins, B.D.; Bagrodia, S.; Cantley, L.C.; Abraham, R.T. The PI3K pathway in human disease. *Cell* **2017**, *170*, 605–635. [CrossRef] [PubMed]
142. D'Arcy, M.E.; Pfeiffer, R.M.; Rivera, D.R.; Hess, G.P.; Cahoon, E.K.; Arron, S.T.; Brownell, I.; Cowen, E.W.; Israni, A.K.; Triplette, M.A.; et al. Voriconazole and the Risk of Keratinocyte Carcinomas among Lung Transplant Recipients in the United States. *JAMA Dermatol.* **2020**, *156*, 772–779. [CrossRef] [PubMed]
143. Dajee, M.; Lazarov, M.; Zhang, J.Y.; Cai, T.; Green, C.L.; Russell, A.J.; Marinkovich, M.P.; Tao, S.; Lin, Q.; Kubo, Y.; et al. NF-κB blockade and oncogenic Ras trigger invasive human epidermal neoplasia. *Nature* **2003**, *421*, 639–643. [CrossRef] [PubMed]

144. Ridky, T.W.; Chow, J.M.; Wong, D.J.; Khavari, P.A. Invasive three-dimensional organotypic neoplasia from multiple normal human epithelia. *Nat. Med.* **2010**, *16*, 1450–1455. [CrossRef]
145. Rizvi, N.A.; Hellmann, M.D.; Snyder, A.; Kvistborg, P.; Makarov, V.; Havel, J.J.; Lee, W.; Yuan, J.; Wong, P.; Ho, T.S.; et al. Cancer immunology. Mutational landscape determines sensitivity to PD-1 blockade in non-small cell lung cancer. *Science* **2015**, *348*, 124–128. [CrossRef] [PubMed]
146. Howard, B.D.; Tessman, I. Identification of the altered bases in mutated single-stranded DNA: II. In vivo mutagenesis by 5-bromodeoxyuridine and 2-aminopurine. *J. Mol. Biol.* **1964**, *9*, 364–371. [CrossRef]
147. Setlow, R.; Carrier, W. Pyrimidine dimers in ultraviolet-irradiated DNA's. *J. Mol. Biol.* **1966**, *17*, 237–254. [CrossRef]
148. Cho, R.J.; Alexandrov, L.B.; den Breems, N.Y.; Atanasova, V.S.; Farshchian, M.; Purdom, E.; Nguyen, T.N.; Coarfa, C.; Rajapakshe, K.; Prisco, M.; et al. APOBEC mutation drives early-onset squamous cell carcinomas in recessive dystrophic epidermolysis bullosa. *Sci. Transl. Med.* **2018**, *10*, eaas9668. [CrossRef]
149. Haisma, M.S.; Plaat, B.E.C.; Bijl, H.P.; Roodenburg, J.L.N.; Diercks, G.F.H.; Romeijn, T.R.; Terra, J.B. Multivariate analysis of potential risk factors for lymph node metastasis in patients with cutaneous squamous cell carcinoma of the head and neck. *J. Am. Acad. Dermatol.* **2016**, *75*, 722–730. [CrossRef]
150. Koyfman, S.A.; Cooper, J.S.; Beitler, J.J.; Busse, P.M.; Jones, C.U.; McDonald, M.W.; Quon, H.; Ridge, J.A.; Saba, N.F.; Salama, J.K.; et al. ACR Appropriateness Criteria(®) Aggressive Nonmelanomatous Skin Cancer of the Head and Neck. *Head Neck* **2016**, *38*, 175–182. [CrossRef]
151. National Comprehensive Cancer Network. Squamous Cell Skin Cancer. (Version 1). 2021. Available online: https://www.nccn.org/professionals/physician_gls/pdf/squamous.pdf (accessed on 5 April 2021).
152. Cooper, J.S.; Pajak, T.F.; Forastiere, A.A.; Jacobs, J.; Campbell, B.H.; Saxman, S.B.; Kish, J.A.; Kim, H.E.; Cmelak, A.J.; Rotman, M. Postoperative concurrent radiotherapy and chemotherapy for high-risk squamous-cell carcinoma of the head and neck. *N. Engl. J. Med.* **2004**, *350*, 1937–1944. [CrossRef]
153. Bernier, J.; Domenge, C.; Ozsahin, M.; Matuszewska, K.; Lefèbvre, J.-L.; Greiner, R.H.; Giralt, J.; Maingon, P.; Rolland, F.; Bolla, M. Postoperative irradiation with or without concomitant chemotherapy for locally advanced head and neck cancer. *N. Engl. J. Med.* **2004**, *350*, 1945–1952. [CrossRef]
154. Denis, F.; Garaud, P.; Bardet, E.; Alfonsi, M.; Sire, C.; Germain, T.; Bergerot, P.; Rhein, B.; Tortochaux, J.; Calais, G. Final results of the 94-01 French Head and Neck Oncology and Radiotherapy Group randomized trial comparing radiotherapy alone with concomitant radiochemotherapy in advanced-stage oropharynx carcinoma. *J. Clin. Oncol.* **2004**, *22*, 69–76. [CrossRef] [PubMed]
155. Bourhis, J.; Sire, C.; Graff, P.; Grégoire, V.; Maingon, P.; Calais, G.; Gery, B.; Martin, L.; Alfonsi, M.; Desprez, P.; et al. Concomitant chemoradiotherapy versus acceleration of radiotherapy with or without concomitant chemotherapy in locally advanced head and neck carcinoma (GORTEC 99-02): An open-label phase 3 randomised trial. *Lancet Oncol.* **2012**, *13*, 145–153. [CrossRef]
156. Porceddu, S.V.; Bressel, M.; Poulsen, M.G.; Stoneley, A.; Veness, M.J.; Kenny, L.M.; Wratten, C.; Corry, J.; Cooper, S.; Fogarty, G.B.; et al. Postoperative Concurrent Chemoradiotherapy Versus Postoperative Radiotherapy in High-Risk Cutaneous Squamous Cell Carcinoma of the Head and Neck: The Randomized Phase III TROG 05.01 Trial. *J. Clin. Oncol.* **2018**, *36*, 1275–1283. [CrossRef]
157. Jamal-Hanjani, M.; Wilson, G.A.; McGranahan, N.; Birkbak, N.J.; Watkins, T.B.K.; Veeriah, S.; Shafi, S.; Johnson, D.H.; Mitter, R.; Rosenthal, R.; et al. Tracking the Evolution of Non–Small-Cell Lung Cancer. *N. Engl. J. Med.* **2017**, *376*, 2109–2121. [CrossRef]
158. McGranahan, N.; Furness, A.J.; Rosenthal, R.; Ramskov, S.; Lyngaa, R.; Saini, S.K.; Jamal-Hanjani, M.; Wilson, G.A.; Birkbak, N.J.; Hiley, C.T.; et al. Clonal neoantigens elicit T cell immunoreactivity and sensitivity to immune checkpoint blockade. *Science* **2016**, *351*, 1463–1469. [CrossRef]
159. Liu, J.; Blake, S.J.; Yong, M.C.; Harjunpää, H.; Ngiow, S.F.; Takeda, K.; Young, A.; O'Donnell, J.S.; Allen, S.; Smyth, M.J.; et al. Improved Efficacy of Neoadjuvant Compared to Adjuvant Immunotherapy to Eradicate Metastatic Disease. *Cancer Discov* **2016**, *6*, 1382–1399. [CrossRef]
160. Ferrarotto, R.; Amit, M.; Nagarajan, P.; Rubin, M.L.; Yuan, Y.; Bell, D.; El-Naggar, A.K.; Johnson, J.M.; Morrison, W.H.; Rosenthal, D.I.; et al. Pilot Phase II Trial of Neoadjuvant Immunotherapy in Locoregionally Advanced, Resectable Cutaneous Squamous Cell Carcinoma of the Head and Neck. *Clin. Cancer Res.* **2021**. [CrossRef] [PubMed]
161. Neoadjuvant Atezolizumab in Surgically Resectable Advanced Cutaneous Squamous Cell Carcinoma. U.S. National Library of Medicine. 2020. Available online: https://clinicaltrials.gov/ct2/show/NCT04710498 (accessed on 15 June 2021).
162. Neo-adjuvant Nivolumab or Nivolumab With Ipilimumab in Advanced Cutaneous Squamous Cell Carcinoma Prior to Surgery (MATISSE)—NCT04620200. U.S. National Library of Medicine. 2020. Available online: https://clinicaltrials.gov/ct2/show/NCT04620200 (accessed on 1 August 2021).
163. Rischin, D.; Fury, M.G.; Lowy, I.; Stankevich, E.; Han, H.; Porceddu, S. A phase III, randomized, double-blind study of adjuvant cemiplimab versus placebo post-surgery and radiation therapy (RT) in patients (pts) with high-risk cutaneous squamous cell carcinoma (CSCC). *J. Clin. Oncol.* **2020**, *38*, TPS10084. [CrossRef]
164. Geiger, J.L.; Daniels, G.A.; Cohen, E.E.W.; Ge, J.Y.; Gumuscu, B.; Swaby, R.F.; Chang, A.L.S. KEYNOTE-630: Phase 3 study of adjuvant pembrolizumab versus placebo in patients with high-risk, locally advanced cutaneous squamous cell carcinoma. *J. Clin. Oncol.* **2019**, *37*, TPS9597. [CrossRef]
165. Jarkowski, A., 3rd; Hare, R.; Loud, P.; Skitzki, J.J.; Kane, J.M., 3rd; May, K.S.; Zeitouni, N.C.; Nestico, J.; Vona, K.L.; Groman, A.; et al. Systemic Therapy in Advanced Cutaneous Squamous Cell Carcinoma (CSCC): The Roswell Park Experience and a Review of the Literature. *Am. J. Clin. Oncol.* **2016**, *39*, 545–548. [CrossRef]

166. Migden, M.R.; Rischin, D.; Schmults, C.D.; Guminski, A.; Hauschild, A.; Lewis, K.D.; Chung, C.H.; Hernandez-Aya, L.; Lim, A.M.; Chang, A.L.S.; et al. PD-1 Blockade with Cemiplimab in Advanced Cutaneous Squamous-Cell Carcinoma. *N. Engl. J. Med.* **2018**, *379*, 341–351. [CrossRef]
167. Rischin, D.; Khushalani, N.I.; Schmults, C.D.; Guminski, A.D.; Chang, A.L.S.; Lewis, K.D.; Lim, A.M.L.; Hernandez-Aya, L.F.; Hughes, B.G.M.; Schadendorf, D.; et al. Phase II study of cemiplimab in patients (pts) with advanced cutaneous squamous cell carcinoma (CSCC): Longer follow-up. *J. Clin. Oncol.* **2020**, *38*, 10018. [CrossRef]
168. Rischin, D.; Migden, M.R.; Lim, A.M.; Schmults, C.D.; Khushalani, N.I.; Hughes, B.G.M.; Schadendorf, D.; Dunn, L.A.; Hernandez-Aya, L.; Chang, A.L.S.; et al. Phase 2 study of cemiplimab in patients with metastatic cutaneous squamous cell carcinoma: Primary analysis of fixed-dosing, long-term outcome of weight-based dosing. *J. Immunother. Cancer* **2020**, *8*, e000775. [CrossRef]
169. Rischin, D.; Khushalani, N.I.; Schmults, C.D.; Guminski, A.; Chang, A.L.S.; Lewis, K.D.; Lim, A.M.; Hernandez-Aya, L.; Hughes, B.G.M.; Schadendorf, D.; et al. Integrated analysis of a phase 2 study of cemiplimab in advanced cutaneous squamous cell carcinoma: Extended follow-up of outcomes and quality of life analysis. *J. Immunother. Cancer* **2021**, *9*, e002757. [CrossRef] [PubMed]
170. Grob, J.J.; Gonzalez, R.; Basset-Seguin, N.; Vornicova, O.; Schachter, J.; Joshi, A.; Meyer, N.; Grange, F.; Piulats, J.M.; Bauman, J.R.; et al. Pembrolizumab Monotherapy for Recurrent or Metastatic Cutaneous Squamous Cell Carcinoma: A Single-Arm Phase II Trial (KEYNOTE-629). *J. Clin. Oncol.* **2020**, *38*, 2916–2925. [CrossRef] [PubMed]
171. Maubec, E.; Boubaya, M.; Petrow, P.; Beylot-Barry, M.; Basset-Seguin, N.; Deschamps, L.; Grob, J.-J.; Dréno, B.; Scheer-Senyarich, I.; Bloch-Queyrat, C.; et al. Phase II Study of Pembrolizumab As First-Line, Single-Drug Therapy for Patients With Unresectable Cutaneous Squamous Cell Carcinomas. *J. Clin. Oncol.* **2020**, *38*, 3051–3061. [CrossRef] [PubMed]
172. Munhoz, R.R.; Camargo, V.P.D.; Marta, G.N.; Martins, J.C.; Nardo, M.; Barbosa, C.C.; Souza, C.E.d.; Barbosa, I.; Ricci, H.; Mattos, M.R.d.; et al. CA209-9JC: A phase II study of first-line nivolumab (NIVO) in patients (pts) with locally advanced or metastatic cutaneous squamous cell carcinoma. *J. Clin. Oncol.* **2020**, *38*, 10044. [CrossRef]
173. The UNSCARRed Study: UNresectable Squamous Cell Carcinoma Treated With Avelumab and Radical Radiotherapy (UN-SCARRed). U.S. National Library of Medicine. 2020. Available online: https://clinicaltrials.gov/ct2/show/NCT03737721 (accessed on 14 July 2021).
174. Andtbacka, R.H.; Kaufman, H.L.; Collichio, F.; Amatruda, T.; Senzer, N.; Chesney, J.; Delman, K.A.; Spitler, L.E.; Puzanov, I.; Agarwala, S.S.; et al. Talimogene Laherparepvec Improves Durable Response Rate in Patients with Advanced Melanoma. *J. Clin. Oncol.* **2015**, *33*, 2780–2788. [CrossRef]
175. Puzanov, I.; Milhem, M.M.; Minor, D.; Hamid, O.; Li, A.; Chen, L.; Chastain, M.; Gorski, K.S.; Anderson, A.; Chou, J.; et al. Talimogene Laherparepvec in Combination with Ipilimumab in Previously Untreated, Unresectable Stage IIIB-IV Melanoma. *J. Clin. Oncol.* **2016**, *34*, 2619–2626. [CrossRef]
176. Long, G.; Dummer, R.; Johnson, D.; Michielin, O.; Martin-Algarra, S.; Treichel, S.; Chan, E.; Diede, S.; Ribas, A. 429 Long-term analysis of MASTERKEY-265 phase 1b trial of talimogene laherparepvec (T-VEC) plus pembrolizumab in patients with unresectable stage IIIB-IVM1c melanoma. *J. Immunother. Cancer* **2020**, *8*, A261. [CrossRef]
177. Study Evaluating Cemiplimab Alone and Combined With RP1 in Treating Advanced Squamous Skin Cancer (CERPASS) U.S National Library of Medicine. 2020. Available online: https://clinicaltrials.gov/ct2/show/NCT04050436 (accessed on 2 September 2021).
178. Talimogene Laherparepvec and Panitumumab for the Treatment of Locally Advanced or Metastatic Squamous Cell Carcinoma of the Skin U.S National Library of Medicine. 2021. Available online: https://clinicaltrials.gov/ct2/show/NCT04163952 (accessed on 2 September 2021).
179. Avelumab with or without Cetuximab in Treating Patients with Advanced Skin Squamous Cell Cancer. U.S. National Library of Medicine. 2020. Available online: https://clinicaltrials.gov/ct2/show/NCT03944941 (accessed on 14 July 2021).
180. Salomon, D.S.; Brandt, R.; Ciardiello, F.; Normanno, N. Epidermal growth factor-related peptides and their receptors in human malignancies. *Crit. Rev. Oncol. Hematol.* **1995**, *19*, 183–232. [CrossRef]
181. Maubec, E.; Duvillard, P.; Velasco, V.; Crickx, B.; Avril, M.F. Immunohistochemical analysis of EGFR and HER-2 in patients with metastatic squamous cell carcinoma of the skin. *Anticancer Res.* **2005**, *25*, 1205–1210.
182. Shimizu, T.; Izumi, H.; Oga, A.; Furumoto, H.; Murakami, T.; Ofuji, R.; Muto, M.; Sasaki, K. Epidermal Growth Factor Receptor Overexpression and Genetic Aberrations in Metastatic Squamous-Cell Carcinoma of the Skin. *Dermatology* **2001**, *202*, 203–206. [CrossRef]
183. Maubec, E.; Petrow, P.; Scheer-Senyarich, I.; Duvillard, P.; Lacroix, L.; Gelly, J.; Certain, A.; Duval, X.; Crickx, B.; Buffard, V.; et al. Phase II study of cetuximab as first-line single-drug therapy in patients with unresectable squamous cell carcinoma of the skin. *J. Clin. Oncol.* **2011**, *29*, 3419–3426. [CrossRef]
184. Foote, M.C.; McGrath, M.; Guminski, A.; Hughes, B.G.M.; Meakin, J.; Thomson, D.; Zarate, D.; Simpson, F.; Porceddu, S.V. Phase II study of single-agent panitumumab in patients with incurable cutaneous squamous cell carcinoma. *Ann. Oncol.* **2014**, *25*, 2047–2052. [CrossRef] [PubMed]
185. Reigneau, M.; Robert, C.; Routier, E.; Mamelle, G.; Moya-Plana, A.; Tomasic, G.; Mateus, C. Efficacy of neoadjuvant cetuximab alone or with platinum salt for the treatment of unresectable advanced nonmetastatic cutaneous squamous cell carcinomas. *Br. J. Dermatol.* **2015**, *173*, 527–534. [CrossRef]

186. William, W.N., Jr.; Feng, L.; Ferrarotto, R.; Ginsberg, L.; Kies, M.; Lippman, S.; Glisson, B.; Kim, E.S. Gefitinib for patients with incurable cutaneous squamous cell carcinoma: A single-arm phase II clinical trial. *J. Am. Acad. Dermatol.* **2017**, *77*, 1110–1113.e1112. [CrossRef]
187. Gold, K.A.; Kies, M.S.; William, W.N.; Johnson, F.M.; Lee, J.J.; Glisson, B.S. Erlotinib in the treatment of recurrent or metastatic cutaneous squamous cell carcinoma: A single-arm phase 2 clinical trial. *Cancer* **2018**, *124*, 2169–2173. [CrossRef] [PubMed]
188. Cavalieri, S.; Perrone, F.; Miceli, R.; Ascierto, P.A.; Locati, L.D.; Bergamini, C.; Granata, R.; Alfieri, S.; Resteghini, C.; Galbiati, D.; et al. Efficacy and safety of single-agent pan-human epidermal growth factor receptor (HER) inhibitor dacomitinib in locally advanced unresectable or metastatic skin squamous cell cancer. *Eur. J. Cancer* **2018**, *97*, 7–15. [CrossRef]
189. Dunn, L.; Ho, A.L.; Eng, J.; Michel, L.S.; Fetten, J.V.; Warner, E.; Kriplani, A.; Zhi, W.I.; Ng, K.K.; Haque, S.; et al. A phase I/Ib study of lenvatinib and cetuximab in patients with recurrent/metastatic (R/M) head and neck squamous cell carcinoma (HNSCC). *J. Clin. Oncol.* **2020**, *38*, 6541. [CrossRef]
190. Adelmann, C.H.; Truong, K.A.; Liang, R.J.; Bansal, V.; Gandee, L.; Saporito, R.C.; Lee, W.; Du, L.; Nicholas, C.; Napoli, M.; et al. MEK Is a Therapeutic and Chemopreventative Target in Squamous Cell Carcinoma. *J. Investig. Dermatol.* **2016**, *136*, 1920–1924. [CrossRef] [PubMed]
191. Cobimetinib and Atezolizumab in Treating Participants with Advanced or Refractory Rare Tumors. U.S. National Library of Medicine. 2021. Available online: https://clinicaltrials.gov/ct2/show/NCT03108131 (accessed on 2 September 2021).
192. Ding, L.T.; Zhao, P.; Yang, M.L.; Lv, G.Z.; Zhao, T.L. GDC-0084 inhibits cutaneous squamous cell carcinoma cell growth. *Biochem. Biophys. Res. Commun.* **2018**, *503*, 1941–1948. [CrossRef]
193. Zou, Y.; Ge, M.; Wang, X. Targeting PI3K-AKT-mTOR by LY3023414 inhibits human skin squamous cell carcinoma cell growth in vitro and in vivo. *Biochem. Biophys. Res. Commun.* **2017**, *490*, 385–392. [CrossRef] [PubMed]
194. Bendell, J.C.; Varghese, A.M.; Hyman, D.M.; Bauer, T.M.; Pant, S.; Callies, S.; Lin, J.; Martinez, R.; Wickremsinhe, E.; Fink, A.; et al. A First-in-Human Phase 1 Study of LY3023414, an Oral PI3K/mTOR Dual Inhibitor, in Patients with Advanced Cancer. *Clin. Cancer Res.* **2018**, *24*, 3253–3262. [CrossRef]
195. Wen, P.Y.; De Groot, J.F.; Battiste, J.D.; Goldlust, S.A.; Garner, J.S.; Simpson, J.A.; Kijlstra, J.; Olivero, A.; Cloughesy, T.F. Escalation portion of phase II study to evaluate the safety, pharmacokinetics, and clinical activity of the PI3K/mTOR inhibitor paxalisib (GDC-0084) in glioblastoma (GBM) with unmethylated O6-methylguanine-methyltransferase (MGMT) promotor status. *J. Clin. Oncol.* **2020**, *38*, 2550. [CrossRef]
196. Manohar, S.; Thongprayoon, C.; Cheungpasitporn, W.; Markovic, S.N.; Herrmann, S.M. Systematic Review of the Safety of Immune Checkpoint Inhibitors among Kidney Transplant Patients. *Kidney Int. Rep.* **2019**, *5*, 149–158. [CrossRef]
197. Lai, H.-C.; Lin, J.-F.; Hwang, T.I.S.; Liu, Y.-F.; Yang, A.-H.; Wu, C.-K. Programmed Cell Death 1 (PD-1) Inhibitors in Renal Transplant Patients with Advanced Cancer: A Double-Edged Sword? *Int. J. Mol. Sci.* **2019**, *20*, 2194. [CrossRef] [PubMed]
198. Tacrolimus, Nivolumab, and Ipilimumab in Treating Kidney Transplant Recipients with Selected Unresectable or Metastatic Cancers. U.S National Library of Medicine. 2020. Available online: https://clinicaltrials.gov/ct2/show/NCT03816332 (accessed on 2 July 2021).
199. Cemiplimab in AlloSCT/SOT Recipients with CSCC (CONTRAC) U.S. National Library of Medicine. 2020. Available online: https://clinicaltrials.gov/ct2/show/NCT04339062 (accessed on 2 July 2021).
200. Cemiplimab-rwlc for Unresectable Locally Recurrent and/or Metastatic CSCC U.S National Library of Medicine. 2020. Available online: https://clinicaltrials.gov/ct2/show/NCT04242173 (accessed on 2 July 2021).

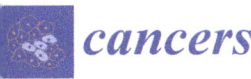

Review

Current Therapeutic Strategies in Patients with Oropharyngeal Squamous Cell Carcinoma: Impact of the Tumor HPV Status

Alexandre Bozec *, Dorian Culié, Gilles Poissonnet, François Demard and Olivier Dassonville

Institut Universitaire de la Face et du Cou, Centre Antoine Lacassagne, Université Côte d'Azur, 06100 Nice, France; dorian.culie@nice.unicancer.fr (D.C.); gilles.poissonnet@nice.unicancer.fr (G.P.); francois.demard@nice.unicancer.fr (F.D.); olivier.dassonville@nice.unicancer.fr (O.D.)
* Correspondence: alexandre.bozec@nice.unicancer.fr

Simple Summary: Contrary to other head and neck subsites, oropharyngeal squamous cell carcinoma (OPSCC) has shown a considerable increase in incidence over the past 20 years. This growing incidence is largely due to the increasing place of human papillomavirus (HPV)-related tumors. HPV-positive and HPV-negative OPSCC are two distinct entities with considerable differences in terms of treatment response and prognosis. However, there are no specific recommendations yet in the therapeutic management of OPSCC patients according to their tumor HPV-status. The aim of this review is therefore to discuss the therapeutic management of patients with OPSCC and the impact of HPV status on treatment selection.

Abstract: Since there is no published randomized study comparing surgical and non-surgical therapeutic strategies in patients with oropharyngeal squamous cell carcinoma (OPSCC), the therapeutic management of these patients remains highly controversial. While human papillomavirus (HPV)-positive and HPV-negative OPSCC are now recognized as two distinct diseases with different epidemiological, biological, and clinical characteristics, the impact of HPV status on the management of OPSCC patients is still unclear. In this review, we analyze the current therapeutic options in patients with OPSCC, highlighting the most recent advances in surgical and non-surgical therapies, and we discuss the impact of HPV status on the therapeutic strategy.

Keywords: oropharynx; neoplasm; squamous cell carcinoma; human papillomavirus; therapeutic management; treatment selection

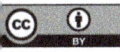

1. Introduction

Head and neck squamous cell carcinoma (HNSCC) accounts for more than 600,000 new cases each year worldwide and represents the 6th cause of cancer deaths [1–3]. In western countries, about 25% of all HNSCC arise from the oropharynx [2]. Beside alcohol and tobacco consumption, which are well-known risk factors, human papillomavirus (HPV) has been also implicated in the carcinogenesis of oropharyngeal squamous cell carcinoma (OPSCC) [1]. Contrary to other head and neck subsites, OPSCC incidence has considerably increased in the past 20 years [2,4]. This growing incidence is largely due to the increasing place of HPV-related OPSCC [2,4]. Indeed, to date, HPV-positive OPSCC represents up to 80% of OPSCC in North America and Northern Europe, and 30 to 60% in Western Europe [5,6]. HPV-positive and HPV-negative OPSCC are two distinct entities with molecular, histological, epidemiological, and prognostic differences [7]. However, there are no specific recommendations yet in the therapeutic management of patients with OPSCC according to their tumor HPV-status [8,9].

There has been considerable debate over the last three decades regarding the initial therapeutic management of OPSCC [10,11]. To date, there is no published prospective randomized clinical trial comparing surgical and non-surgical approaches for OPSCC patients. It is therefore widely acknowledged that the therapeutic decision has to be made by a tumor board, where the cases of individual cancer patients are thoroughly reviewed by a team of physicians and other health professionals from different specialties (surgeons, medical and radiation oncologists, radiologists, and pathologists). This results in great variability in the therapeutic management of patients with OPSCC between medical teams, according to their particular experience and skills [11].

In the light of the results of larynx preservation programs, the 1990s saw an increased use of non-surgical treatments, for OPSCC, combining radiotherapy (RT) with chemotherapy (CT), commonly referred to as an organ-sparing therapy protocol [10,12]. This switch from primary conventional open surgery to definitive (chemo)-RT ((C)RT) was made in many centers despite the lack of high-quality evidence from randomized controlled trials in patients with OPSCC. In the meantime, HPV-positive OPSCC has been identified as a unique disease, with improved radiosensitivity and survival [13]. Thus, the favorable outcomes reported with non-surgical therapeutic strategies in previous North American and European studies could be explained by a high yet unknown proportion of HPV-related OPSCC [14]. Recently, the presumed equivalence in terms of oncological results between surgical and non-surgical therapeutic strategies in patients with HPV-negative OPSCC was rediscussed, because the HPV status of OPSCC patients was not determined before 2010 and could be a major bias in earlier studies [15]. Simultaneously, the development of minimally-invasive surgical procedures and the progress in microvascular reconstructive surgery have considerably reduced the classic sequelae of oropharyngeal oncologic surgery [16,17]. Altogether, these data explain why the role of upfront surgery and the impact of tumor HPV status in the initial management of OPSCC remain largely debated.

The aim of this review article is therefore to discuss current therapeutic strategies in patients with OPSCC and the potential impact of tumor HPV status.

2. HPV-Positive and HPV-Negative OPSCC Are Two Distinct Diseases

HPV-positive OPSCC is a unique entity both clinically and demographically [2,7]. HPV-positive OPSCC patients displayed less comorbidity, less alcohol and tobacco consumption, higher educational level and socio-economic status, lower T stage, higher N stage, and more frequent involvement of the tongue base and tonsillar fossa than HPV-negative OPSCC patients [11,18]. Moreover, recent studies showed that the risk of synchronous or metachronous second primary neoplasia was significantly reduced in HPV-negative OPSCC patients [19–21].

At the molecular level, HPV-induced carcinogenesis leads to functional abrogation of p53 and pRb pathways, mediated by the expression of the viral oncoproteins E6 and E7 [22]. E6 binds wild-type p53 and induces its degradation, leading to impaired apoptosis. E7 binds pRb, causing the release of the transcriptional factor E2F that activates cellular proliferation [22]. Independently of pRb inhibition, the transcriptional induction of KDM6B by E7 accounts for expression of the p16 protein, an inhibitor of cyclin-dependent kinases (CDK) 4 and 6 [23]. Consequently, contrary to their HPV-negative counterparts, HPV-positive OPSCC bear high p16 levels, and the overexpression of p16 is used in routine clinical practice as a surrogate marker of tumor HPV status [24]. However, although p16 overexpression is a cost-effective and practical marker of HPV-positive OPSCC, the link between p16 overexpression and HPV-induced carcinogenesis is not totally specific, and 5 to 20% of p16-positive OPSCC are not HPV-related [24,25].

In a comprehensive genomic characterization of HNSCC, the Cancer Genome Atlas Network showed that HPV-associated tumors are dominated by helical domain mutations of the oncogene PIK3CA, novel alterations involving loss of TRAF3, and amplification of the cell cycle gene E2F1 [26]. By contrast, smoking-related HNSCCs demonstrate near universal loss-of-function TP53 mutations and CDKN2A inactivation with frequent copy number alterations including amplification of 3q26/28 and 11q13/22 [26].

Regarding clinical presentation, HPV-positive OPSCC are characterized by a frequent discordance between small primary tumor size and significant lymph node involvement [27]. This explains that an isolated neck mass (carcinoma of unknown primary: "CUP" syndrome) is a common initial presentation of HPV-positive OPSCC. Neck metastases are often cystic and, therefore, solitary cystic metastatic lymph node of occult HPV-positive OPSCC can mimic a second branchial cleft cyst [28]. Moreover, the primary tumor can be difficult to see and to delineate in the lymphoepithelial tissue of the tongue base or tonsillar fossa.

Multiple studies demonstrated that HPV tumor status was the main prognostic factor in OPSCC patients [6,7,29]. The improved prognosis for HPV-positive OPSCC can be explained by several factors. Firstly, due to lower alcohol/tobacco consumption, patients with an HPV-positive OPSCC display a lower level of comorbidity than patients with an HPV-negative OPSCC. This better general health status makes HPV-positive OPSCC patients more likely to benefit from the treatment at any stage of the disease [27].

Secondly, HPV-positive OPSCC are characterized by an improved chemo- and radiosensitivity compared to HPV-negative OPSCC [29,30]. Complete response rates after CRT are considerably higher for HPV-positive than for HPV-negative patients [29]. Moreover, the risk of locoregional or distant recurrence is significantly lower for HPV-positive than for HPV-negative patients irrespective of the therapeutic strategy (surgical or nonsurgical treatment) [31,32]. The pattern of recurrence is also different according to the HPV tumor status. Indeed, a recent multicentric study showed that locoregional recurrence was the most frequent type of treatment failure in HPV-negative patients, whereas distant metastasis was the main type of recurrence in HPV-positive patients [31]. In HPV-positive OPSCC, the risk of locoregional recurrence is inferior to 15% and most locoregional recurrences correspond to nodal persistent/recurrent disease frequently amenable to salvage neck dissection [31]. At the opposite, locoregional failures in HPV-negative OPSCC patients are most often local recurrence or combine local with nodal recurrences and are rarely amenable to successful surgical salvage [31,33].

Thirdly, HPV-positive OPSCC patients display a lower risk of second primary neoplasia than HPV negative OPSCC patients [19,20]. The significant risk of second cancer in HPV-negative patients is mainly explained by their alcohol/tobacco consumption with the concept of field cancerization and affects mostly the head and neck, the lung, and the esophagus [19,34]. It is considered to be one of the leading causes of death in patients that have been cured from their primary OPSCC [19]. The HPV oncogenic properties at other cancer sites and in particular the anogenital organs are well demonstrated [35,36]. In this regard, in a recent study investigating sequential acquisition of HPV infection between genital and oral anatomic sites in males, Dickey et al. showed that the Hazard ratio of a sequential genital to oral HPV infection was 2.3 (95% CI: 1.7–3.1) and 3.5 (95% CI: 1.9–6.4) for oral to genital infection [35]. However, the risk of a second HPV-induced primary malignancy seems relatively low and does not represent an important cause of death in HPV-positive OPSCC patients [19,21].

All these differences and particularly the considerable discrepancy in terms of prognosis have led to the creation of two distinct TNM classifications, in the 8th UICC/AJCC staging system, according to the p16 tumor status of OPSCC patients [13,37]. The most important change for p16-positive OPSCC concerns nodal staging where clinically involved lymph nodes, whether one or multiple, as long as they are ipsilateral and less than 6 cm in size, are included in the same N category—N1—since there is no significant impact on survival. Survival with clinically palpable and/or radiographically evident, bilateral, or contralateral lymph nodes was distinguishable, with a worse outcome than N1. Therefore, contralateral or bilateral lymph nodes are classified as N2, without, conversely to p16-negative OPSCC, the classical three N2 sub-stages (N2a, b, or c) [13]. Of note, extranodal extension is not considered as a staging criterion for p16-positive OPSCC. Finally, the 8th edition staging of p16-positive OPSCC gives a much more accurate and reasonable prediction of survival [13]. For example, a patient that presents with a 2 cm p16-positive tonsil cancer and 2 metastatic neck lymph nodes in the same side was stage IV in the 7th edition staging manual but is stage I in the 8th edition. The psychological benefit of having stage I vs. stage IV cancer is significant and means that clinicians can much more readily reassure patients that they have a good prognosis. However, currently, this new classification should not be used to modify the therapeutic strategy, and, in particular, the de-escalation of treatment intensity for p16-positive patients should only be tested in clinical trials [38].

Interestingly, several studies demonstrated that, besides p16 tumor status, tobacco consumption was an important prognostic factor in OPSCC patients [39,40]. Indeed, p16-positive OPSCC occurring in smokers (>10 pack-years) exhibit an intermediate prognosis between p16-positive tumors in non-smokers, which are associated with the best prognosis, and p16-negative tumors, which are associated with the worst prognosis [41]. Therefore, p16-positive OPSCC occurring in smokers represents a complex phenomenon where the role of HPV and tobacco in the carcinogenic process is difficult to evaluate, and where the tumor biology can mix together genetic alterations induced by HPV and by tobacco consumption [42]. This type of tumor does not represent a rare situation, particularly in Latin European countries, where tobacco consumption is still frequent and where HPV-positive OPSCC have experienced a drastic rise over the past 20 years [27]. At the time of personalized medicine, advances in molecular characterization of the tumor could make it possible, in the near future, to precisely assess the specific prognosis of each OPSCC patient. Table 1 summarizes the main clinical characteristics of HPV-positive and HPV-negative OPSCC.

Table 1. Main usual characteristics of HPV-positive vs. HPV-negative oropharyngeal squamous cell carcinomas (OPSCC).

Main Characteristics	HPV-Positive OPSCC	HPV-Negative OPSCC
Gender	Male >> female	Male >> female
Alcohol/tobacco	Low consumption	High consumption
General health status	Good	Poor, high comorbidity level
Educ./economic level	High	Low
Tumor location	Tongue base and tonsils	All parts of the oropharynx
Primary tumor	T1/T2, superficial/exophytic tumor	T3/T4, ulcerative and infiltrative tumor
Lymph-node involvement	Extremely frequent, multiple, cystic neck mass(es)	Moderately frequent, limited number of metastases
Second primary cancer	Very low risk	10 to 15% (head and neck, lung, esophagus +++)
Sensitivity to RT/CT	High	Variable, low to moderate
Prognosis	Good	Poor to intermediate

Educ.: educational; RT: radiation therapy; CT: chemotherapy.

3. Standard Therapeutic Options in OPSCC Patients

American and European guidelines on the management of OPSCC patients do not differ according to the HPV status of the tumor [8,43,44]. Indeed, two therapeutic options can be considered: one based on upfront surgery with or without adjuvant (C)RT, the other on definitive (C)RT. Early-stage (T1–T2, N0) OPSCCs can be managed by either primary surgery or definitive RT alone. Locally advanced (T3–T4, N0 and T1–T4, N1–N3) OPSCCs require multimodal therapy, including upfront surgery followed by RT or CRT according to pathological findings (surgical margins, extranodal extension), or definitive CRT.

3.1. Surgical Treatment

3.1.1. Evolution of Surgical Techniques

OPSCC oncologic surgery has undergone an intense transformation over the past 30 years. Although complete tumor removal with free surgical margins remains the cornerstone of surgical treatment, surgical techniques have evolved from radical non-conservative open surgery to functional organ preservation surgery [45–47]. Since the beginning of the 2000s, the classical transmandibular approach has been replaced, in most cases, by a double transoral and transcervical approach, preventing the complications related to mandibular osteotomy [45]. Considerable efforts have been made to avoid the functional sequelae of pharyngotomy by expanding the indications for exclusive transoral approach in oropharyngeal oncologic surgery [12,48]. These advances have been made possible by the development of appropriate retractors and specific instruments as well as by the use of CO_2 laser and especially robotic surgery (da Vinci® Surgical System) [49,50]. Transoral robotic surgery (TORS) for OPSCC has been used mainly for small T1–T2 primary tumor of the tonsils or the tongue base and has demonstrated satisfactory oncologic outcomes with a rate of free surgical margins comparable to conventional open surgery [49]. Some authors have shown that TORS could also achieve complete resection of locally advanced OPSCC in selected cases with the most experienced TORS surgeons [48].

Similar to primary tumor resection, neck surgical treatment has evolved into more conservative procedures, from radical neck dissection to modified and selective neck dissection [51]. With the development of minimally-invasive surgical techniques and similarly to oral cavity cancers, the sentinel node biopsy (SNB) has been developed in patients with early-stage OPSCC and N0 neck [47]. In this regard, a recent randomized trial comparing SNB and neck dissection in T1–T2, N0 oral, and oropharyngeal cancer demonstrated the oncologic equivalence of the two approaches, with lower morbidity in the SNB arm during the first 6 months after surgery [52].

Along with the development of more conservative surgical procedures, considerable advances have been made in head and neck reconstructive surgery. This progress is mainly linked to the development and refinements of microvascular surgical techniques [16,53,54]. The fibular free-flap is considered as the gold standard for mandibular reconstruction, and the development of three-dimensional preoperative virtual planning has considerably facilitated the flap-shaping process, which was recognized as a critical point of this particularly complex surgical procedure [55,56]. Radial forearm and anterolateral thigh free-flaps are the two main technical options for reconstruction of large oropharyngeal soft-tissues defects [16]. Anterolateral thigh flap thinning techniques have enabled its use, as the radial forearm flap, when a thin and pliable flap is needed, with less morbidity to the donor site [53].

3.1.2. Therapeutic Strategies Involving Upfront Surgery

Early-stage OPSCC (T1–T2, N0) can be managed by either surgery or RT alone [8,44]. When primary surgery has been performed, indication for adjuvant therapy is based on pathological findings. Surgery alone is sufficient after complete surgical resection of pT1–T2, N0 OPSCC, with free surgical margins (>5 mm) and without deleterious pathological features such as perineural invasion and vascular embolism. Postoperative RT has to be considered in cases of close surgical margins (1 to 5 mm), lymph node metastases, or perineural/vascular invasion. Postoperative concurrent CRT is indicated in patients less than 70 years of age with positive surgical margins or extranodal extension [57].

In patients with locally advanced (T3–T4, N0 and T1–T4, N1–N3) OPSCC treated by upfront surgery, postoperative RT is almost always indicated. A low proportion of patients with a pT3N0 tumor or with a small unique metastatic lymph node in the upper neck without any other adverse pathological feature may avoid postoperative RT [8,44]. Postoperative concurrent CRT is indicated in patients less than 70 years of age with positive surgical margins or extranodal extension [57]. Postoperative concurrent CRT should also be discussed in patients less than 70 years of age with close surgical margins, multiple lymph node metastases, and/or perineural/vascular invasion [57]. Although there is a large international consensus in favor of adapting cervical lymph node treatment to the primary therapy modality chosen for the primary tumor, primary upfront neck dissection before RT or CRT may be of interest in selected patients with small primary tumors but bulky nodal disease [10,58]. Indeed, although they have found no clear benefit in terms of overall survival (OS), some studies have shown improved disease-specific survival (DSS) and regional control rates with such a therapeutic strategy [59,60].

3.2. Non-Surgical Therapeutic Strategies

Non-surgical treatment of patients with OPSCC is mainly based on definitive RT. RT alone on the primary tumor and neck is sufficient for early-stage OPSCC, whereas it should be potentiated by a systemic therapy for locally advanced OPSCC [8,44].

Similar to head and neck surgery, RT techniques have largely evolved over the past 20 years. The use of intensity-modulated RT (IMRT) has become the gold standard in patients with OPSCC and has demonstrated an improved preservation of salivary function compared with conventional RT, without compromising locoregional control or survival [61]. IMRT also appears to have a favorable impact on swallowing and quality of life (QoL) outcomes [62]. With the rapid advances in medical physics, RT techniques are constantly evolving. Further technical refinements in RT of head and neck tumor and particularly of OPSCC have been recently evaluated and are currently being tested in clinical trials (Helical Tomotherapy, Volumetric Vodulated Arc Therapy, stereotactic RT, and proton RT) [63].

Three-weekly (100 mg/m^2) cisplatin-based concurrent CRT is the gold standard non-surgical treatment of locally advanced OPSCC [8,63]. In patients who are not fit enough to receive this standard therapeutic regimen, weekly cisplatin-based CRT has been shown to be a reasonable alternative [64]. Since the results of Bonner's study, cetuximab-based RT has been recognized as a valid therapeutic option in patients with locally advanced HNSCC [65]. A direct comparison with the standard of care, i.e., cisplatin-based CRT, was not available since the results of de-escalation prospective trials on HPV-positive OPSCC. These studies have shown that, when tested head-to-head, cisplatin was far more effective in terms of OS and locoregional control, with a different profile of toxicity but surprisingly comparable rates of grade 3 or 4 toxicity (grade 3: severe but not immediately life-threatening adverse event; grade 4: life-threatening adverse event according to the Common Terminology Criteria for Adverse Events-CTCAE v4.0) [38,66]. Therefore, cetuximab-based RT should be reserved to patients that are unfit for cisplatin-based CRT.

In contrast to de-escalation studies conducted in HPV-positive OPSCC, other studies have examined the opportunity to enhance treatment intensity by combining additional therapy with the conventional cisplatin-based CRT [67,68]. These studies did not produce encouraging results, which explains that cisplatin-based concurrent CRT remains the standard of care even for patients with unresectable OPSCC [8]. Indeed, the RTOG 0522 randomized phase III trial compared concurrent accelerated cisplatin-based CRT with or without cetuximab in patients with locally advanced HNSCC (70% of OPSCC, 73% of which were p16-positive) [68]. The study showed that adding cetuximab to cisplatin-based RT did not improve oncologic outcomes (3-year progression-free survival: PFS and OS, locoregional failure, and distant metastasis) but resulted in more grade 3 to 4 acute toxicities [68]. Two phase III randomized trials compared definitive CRT to induction CT (TPF: docetaxel, cisplatin, 5-fluorouracil, or PF) followed by CRT but failed to show any advantage of induction CT plus CRT over CRT alone [67,69]. Other prospective randomized studies have compared induction CT (TPF) followed by cetuximab-based RT to definitive cisplatin-based CRT but did not show any survival differences between the two therapeutic approaches [70]. Several studies are currently investigating the role of immunotherapy (anti-PD1/PD-L1 antibodies) added before or concomitantly to conventional CRT [71]. Although final data have yet to be released, preliminary results of the phase III JAVELIN head and neck 100 study, which were presented in the 2020 ESMO virtual congress, did not demonstrate statistically significant improvement in PFS with avelumab plus CRT compared with placebo plus CRT [71].

4. Impact of the HPV Tumor Status on Therapeutic Strategy

4.1. Early-Stage OPSCC

Early-stage (T1–T2, N0) OPSCC can be treated by either surgery or definitive RT alone. There is no demonstrated survival advantage with primary surgery compared to definitive RT for early-stage HPV-positive OPSCC [72,73]. Indeed, in a recent retrospective multicentric study conducted by the GETTEC collaborative study group, Culie et al. showed no significant differences in oncologic outcomes (OS, DSS, and recurrence-free survival: RFS) between the surgical and non-surgical treatment groups in 44 early-stage p16-positive OPSCC patients [72]. In a prospective phase II study (ORATOR) on 68 patients randomly assigned to primary TORS or definitive RT, Nichols et al. demonstrated no significant difference in OS or RFS between the two therapeutic strategies, but the trial was not designed for this purpose [73]. Despite a lower rate of tinnitus, hearing loss and neutropenia in patients receiving upfront surgery, one-year swallowing-related QoL scores were higher in patients treated by primary RT, although this improvement did not represent a clinically meaningful change [73].

Whatever the therapeutic strategy, the overall prognosis of these patients is excellent and the main objective should be therefore to preserve functions and QoL. Consequently, primary surgery should not be the first therapeutic option if the surgeon is not confident that it will provide optimal functional results. This depends mainly on the anatomical subsite and extension of the tumor. If surgery is selected, a transoral approach should be preferred. Indeed, minimally invasive surgery (TORS and elective neck dissection or SNB) has demonstrated promising results in terms of swallowing function and could be an interesting option to avoid late side-effects of RT [74,75]. Several phase III clinical trials (Best Of and TORPHYNX; ClinicalTrials.gov Identifiers: NCT02984410 and NCT04224389, respectively) comparing TORS and RT in terms of swallowing function in patients with early-stage OPSCC are currently ongoing. Hence, for patients with early-stage HPV-positive OPSCC, given that similar oncologic and functional results are obtained regardless of the therapeutic strategy, discussions between patients and tumor board (surgeon, radiation oncologist) remain the gold standard of the therapeutic decision-making process.

At the opposite, several retrospective studies showed that, for HPV-negative OPSCC, upfront surgery was associated with improved oncologic outcomes, including for early-stage tumors [6,15]. Indeed, in a retrospective multicentric analysis of 103 p16-negative early-stage OPSCC patients, Culie et al. showed significantly higher OS and DSS rates in patients treated by upfront surgery compared to those treated by definitive RT [15]. Similarly, the multicentric Papillophar French study showed that upfront surgery was independently associated with an improved PFS compared to non-surgical treatment in HPV-negative OPSCC patients [6]. Indeed, even after multivariate analysis taking into account performance status, alcohol/tobacco consumption, tumor stage, HPV status, and type of treatment, definitive RT was associated with worse OS (HR = 1.88; 95% CI: 1.10–3.21) and PFS (HR = 1.86; 95% CI: 1.19–2.92) [6]. Moreover, the possibility offered by primary surgery to reserve RT in case of second primary tumor has to be considered, particularly in patients with high alcohol/tobacco consumption [19]. Altogether, these data support the use of primary surgery in patients with early-stage HPV-negative OPSCC [10]. Figure 1 summarizes the therapeutic strategy for patients with early-stage OPSCC.

4.2. Locally Advanced Resectable OPSCC

In locally advanced (T3–T4, N0 and T1–T4, N1–N3) resectable OPSCC, primary surgery is associated with significant functional impairments depending on the anatomical subsite and tumor extensions [16,76]. Although TORS can be used in carefully selected cases (T1–T2 primary tumors, selected T3 primary tumors with adequate tumor exposition, and experienced robotic surgeon), most patients will require open surgery using a combined transoral/transcervical, or more rarely a transmandibular approach [10,45]. In most cases, a microvascular free-flap reconstruction will also be necessary. Since postoperative adjuvant therapy is required, upfront surgery will not prevent the use of RT. Compared with definitive CRT, primary surgery followed by RT or CRT is associated with longer treatment duration, higher costs, and possibly greater functional impairment [77]. Therefore, primary surgery should only be used if this therapeutic strategy is likely to improve survival outcomes.

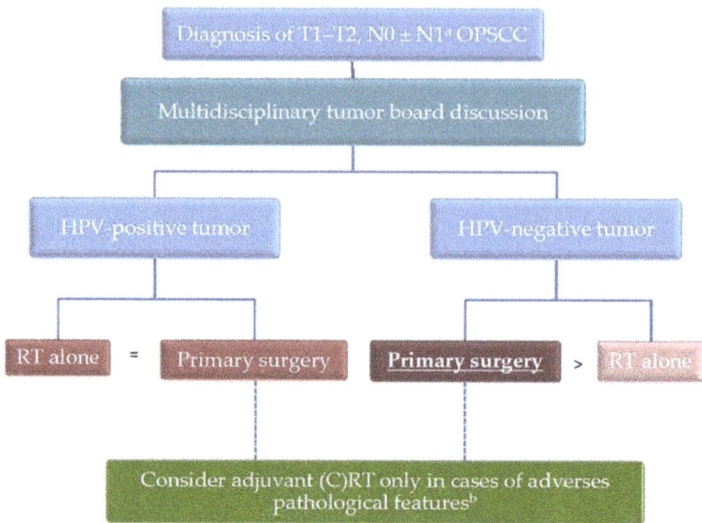

Figure 1. Therapeutic strategy for early-stage OPSCC. [a] some T1–T2, N1 OPSCC patients with a small unique ipsilateral metastatic lymph node can be classified in this category. [b] adverse pathological features include close/positive surgical margins, perineural or vascular invasion, metastatic lymph node(s), and extracapsular spread. The preferred therapeutic option, if any, is in bold and underlined.

In HPV-positive locally advanced OPSCC, there is no clear benefit in terms of survival of primary surgery followed by adjuvant (C)RT compared with definitive CRT [6,72,78]. Indeed, the French Papillophar study showed similar OS and PFS rates for HPV-positive OPSCC, whatever the primary treatment modality [6]. Similarly, Kelly et al., in a study investigating the outcomes of each treatment strategy using the American National Cancer Database, found that upfront surgery followed by adjuvant (C)RT and definitive CRT yielded comparable 3-year OS rates [79]. In the retrospective multicentric study of Culie et al. involving 338 p16-positive locally advanced OPSCC patients, there was no significant difference in OS between the surgical and non-surgical therapeutic strategies (5-year OS rates of 93.7% and 87.8%, respectively, $p = 0.10$) [72]. Of note, RFS was significantly higher in the surgical group than in the non-surgical group of patients (5-year RFS rates of 81.3% and 69.6%, respectively, $p = 0.002$). However, the high rate of successful surgical salvage for locoregional recurrence in the non-surgical group (17 successful surgical salvages for 26, local/regional recurrences) explained the absence of significant impact on OS [72]. Considering the lack of survival advantage, the additional costs, and the potential additional functional impairments, most patients with HPV-positive locally advanced OPSCC should be referred to definitive CRT, with surgery being reserved as a salvage procedure [10].

Conversely, although there is no randomized controlled study comparing surgery followed by adjuvant (C)RT and definitive CRT in patients with HPV-negative locally advanced OPSCC, most recent cohort studies suggested that primary surgery provided a clear benefit in terms of oncologic outcomes in this population [6,15,80]. Despite significant functional impairment, long-term clinical outcomes and QoL are acceptable given the survival advantage [16,81]. Indeed, in a recent study evaluating OS from the American National Cancer Database and involving 6,872 locally advanced OPSCC patients with a documented HPV status, Kamran et al. showed that patients treated with primary surgery followed by adjuvant (C)RT have improved survival compared with those treated with definitive CRT (HR = 0.79, 95% CI: 0.69–0.91, $p = 0.001$ for the whole cohort; HR = 0.74, 95% CI: 0.60–0.91, $p = 0.005$ in the HPV-negative group; and HR = 0.85, 95% CI: 0.70–1.03, $p = 0.098$ for the HPV-positive group) [80]. Similarly, in a prospective follow-up of 340 OPSCC patients with a previously determined HPV status, the French Papillophar study reported by Lacau St

Guily et al. found, after multivariate analysis, a benefit in terms of OS and PFS for upfront surgery [6]. In the HPV negative cohort, 2-year PFS rates were 64% and 42% in the surgical and non-surgical cohorts, respectively [6]. In a retrospective multicentric analysis of 371 patients with a p16-negative locally advanced OPSCC, Culie et al. showed that upfront surgery was significantly associated with improved OS (p = 0.01), DSS (p = 0.02), and RFS (p = 0.02), compared with non-surgical treatment (5-year OS: 71.9 vs. 46.5%; DSS: 76.8 vs. 57.7%; RFS: 60.2 vs. 42.2%) [15]. In another retrospective study involving 3674 patients with an HPV-negative stage III–IVa (T1–2, N1–2b, and M0) OPSCC from the American National Cancer Database and Surveillance, Epidemiology, and End Results (SEER) program between 2010 and 2016, Jacobs et al. showed that, on weighted multivariable Cox regression, patients recommended to receive frontline surgery had improved OS compared with those recommended to receive CRT alone (HR = 0.77; 95% CI: 0.68–0.86) [82]. Altogether, these data support the use of upfront surgery with risk-based addition of adjuvant therapy in patients with HPV-negative locally advanced OPSCC [10].

HPV-positive OPSCC occurring in smokers (>10 pack-years) exhibit an intermediate prognosis between HPV-positive tumors in non-smokers, which are associated with the best prognosis, and HPV-negative tumors, which are associated with the worst prognosis [6,83,84]. Interestingly, in a recent prospective nonrandomized longitudinal study on 279 patients with OPSCC, Seikaly et al. showed that primary surgery offered the best survival outcomes, in comparison with definitive RT with or without CT, in smokers with p16-positive OPSCC and in patients with p16-negative cancers, whereas there was no survival advantage in non-smokers with p16-positive tumors [84]. Although these results have to be reinforced by larger studies, they support the use of primary surgery followed by adjuvant therapy in smokers with HPV-positive OPSCC, in particular if surgery is feasible with minimal morbidity. Figure 2 summarizes the therapeutic strategy for patients with locally advanced resectable OPSCC.

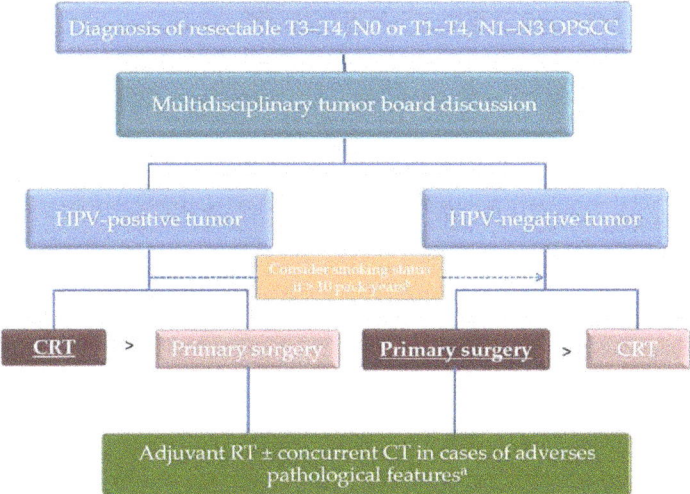

Figure 2. Therapeutic strategy for locally advanced resectable OPSCC. [a] adverse pathological features include positive surgical margins; extracapsular spread; or combination of several pejorative criteria such as close surgical margins, perineural or vascular invasion, multiple/bilateral metastatic lymph nodes. [b] when tobacco consumption is greater than 10 pack-years, HPV-positive OPSCC could be managed as HPV-negative OPSCC. The preferred therapeutic option is in bold and underlined. Primary surgery is only considered if an acceptable functional outcome can be reasonably expected.

4.3. Locally-Advanced Unresectable OPSCC

In addition to oropharyngeal tumors invading the pterygoid process, the skull base, the nasopharynx, or the carotid artery, those with a large tongue base involvement crossing the midline have to be classified in this category because primary surgery would lead to unacceptable functional impairment (definitive enteral nutrition, unintelligible speech) [10,85].

Definitive cisplatin-based concurrent CRT is the gold standard treatment for locally advanced unresectable OPSCC, whatever the HPV-status [8,86].

Patients with HPV-negative unresectable OPSCC bear a poor prognosis with reported 5-year OS rates inferior to 35% [69,86,87]. As mentioned previously, intensifying the therapeutic strategy by adding induction CT before CRT demonstrated no survival advantage, despite a possible benefit in terms of distant metastasis in patients with large or multiple node metastases [67].

At the opposite, even with a T4 unresectable tumor, HPV-positive OPSCC patients display satisfactory survival rates, particularly if they are non-smokers [88,89]. However, there is no alternative to the conventional cisplatin-based concurrent CRT in patients who are fit enough to receive this CT [88,89]. Indeed, in a recent retrospective review of 93 consecutive patients who underwent definitive CRT for HPV-positive OPSCC with clinical T4 disease, Bhattasali et al. found 3-year OS and DSS rates of 79% and 86%, respectively, and showed that, on multivariable analysis, the only prognostic factor was the CT regimen [88]. In a randomized, multicenter, non-inferiority trial of RT plus cetuximab or cisplatin in HPV-positive OPSCC (NRG Oncology RTOG 1016), Gillison et al. found that cisplatin-based CRT was associated with higher OS rate (estimated 5-year OS was 77.9%, 95% CI: 73.4–82.5, in the cetuximab group versus 84.6%, 95% CI: 80.6–88.6, in the cisplatin group). Of note, in the subgroup of patients with T4 and/or N3 disease treated by RT plus cisplatin, estimated 5-year OS was 66.1% [89].

4.4. Recurrent and/or Metastatic OPSCC

Treatment of recurrent and/or metastatic OPSCC is similar to that of other recurrent and/or metastatic HNSCC. There is no specific recommendation for oropharyngeal tumors and no particularities according to the HPV status [8,44,90]. However, even with a metastatic disease, HPV-positive OPSCC patients still harbor a better prognosis than HPV-negative OPSCC patients [90,91].

Briefly, salvage surgery, when feasible, is the gold standard therapy for loco-regional recurrence [33,92]. Whereas salvage neck dissection produced relatively favorable oncologic outcomes for nodal residual or recurrent disease, salvage surgery of local recurrences is associated with poor oncologic outcomes, particularly in HPV-negative OPSCC, and with substantial functional impairment [33,92]. (C)RT can be used in patients who did not receive RT before, if salvage surgery is not feasible or as adjuvant therapy after surgical salvage. Reirradiation of previously irradiated tumor sites can be delivered in highly selected cases [93].

Local therapy (surgery, stereotactic RT) is a valid therapeutic option for patients with a single metastatic or oligometastatic disease [94]. In other cases, systemic therapies will be delivered according to previous treatments received, general health status (PS) and comorbidities, tumor spread and patient symptoms, and PD-L1 tumor expression. The combination of cisplatin and cetuximab with 5-fluorouracil (EXTREME) or docetaxel (TPEx) are two standard systemic therapy regimens [91]. Alternatively, pembrolizumab (anti-PD1) can be used (alone or with CT: cisplatin + 5-FU) as first-line therapy since the phase III randomized study demonstrated improved OS with pembrolizumab alone in patients whose tumor expresses PD-L1 (combined positive score: CPS $\geq$ 1) or with pembrolizumab + CT independently of PD-L1 tumor expression [95]. In this regard, immunotherapy has been reported to be potentially more effective in HPV-positive patients, but its molecular mechanism is still unclear. However, to date, the HPV status has no impact on the indications for immunotherapy in patients with recurrent/metastatic OPSCC.

5. Current Research and Future Directions

The three main perspectives in the treatment of OPSCC can be summarized as follows: 1—to determine the optimal therapeutic strategy between primary surgery and RT alone in patients with early-stage OPSCC; 2—to improve oncologic outcomes in patients with HPV-negative locally advanced OPSCC with an intensified therapeutic regimen that does not raise acute and chronic treatment-related toxicities; 3—to reduce long-term functional impairment and improve QoL in HPV-positive locally advanced OPSCC patients through de-escalation therapeutic strategies without compromising survival.

As mentioned previously, primary surgery and definitive RT lead to satisfactory and comparable oncologic outcomes in patients with early-stage OPSCC [15,72,73,96]. The main goal for these patients is to reduce treatment-related morbidity in order to maintain QoL. Several prospective studies are currently ongoing with the objective to compare these two therapeutic approaches in terms of swallowing function. For example, the currently ongoing randomized phase III «best of» study (ClinicalTrials.gov Identifier: NCT02984410) compares IMRT vs. TORS in patients with T1–T2, N0–N1 OPSCC with patient-reported swallowing function at 1 year as the primary end point.

Approximately half of patients with HPV-negative locally advanced OPSCC will present tumor recurrence and will die from their cancer [15]. There is still, therefore, a crucial need to improve oncologic outcomes. Since maximum tolerable toxicity level is already reached with CRT, it is unlikely that adding conventional therapy to standard treatment will result in improved patient outcomes. Several attempts have been made in this direction but have failed to improve survival or have led to unacceptable toxicity [67,68]. In this context, there are two credible options to intensify the therapeutic approach. The first one would be to combine with conventional CRT a new therapeutic agent without cross-toxicity but that is able to potentiate the anti-tumor effects of concurrent CRT. Preliminary results of the phase III JAVELIN head and neck 100 trial have shown no benefit in terms of PFS of Avelumab (anti PD-L1) plus CRT followed by Avelumab maintenance vs. CRT despite similar tolerability [71]. The currently recruiting phase III NIVOPOSTOP study evaluates the addition of nivolumab (anti PD1) to CRT as adjuvant therapy after primary surgery (clinicalTrials.gov Identifier: NCT03576417). What is probably more promising is the phase III randomized study comparing Debio 1143 (Xevinapant), an antagonist of apoptosis proteins inhibitor, combined with cisplatin-based CRT vs. CRT alone, with event-free survival as the primary end-point (clinicalTrials.gov Identifier: NCT04459715) [97]. The second one would be to replace concurrent cisplatin by a new combination of innovative therapeutic agents. This is the case of the phase III randomized GORTEC-REACH study that compared the combination of avelumab, cetuximab, and RT with standard of care CRT [98]. However, preliminary results of this as yet unpublished study demonstrated that this new combination did not improve outcomes in patients fit to receive cisplatin-based CRT [98].

Given the favorable prognosis of HPV-positive OPSCC patients, several studies have investigated the possibility to reduce treatment intensity without compromising oncologic outcomes (treatment de-escalation) [38,99,100]. As already mentioned, replacement of cisplatin by cetuximab in association with definitive RT showed decreased survival outcomes without any benefit in terms of toxicity (de-escalate study) [66]. Since most treatment failures in HPV-positive patients correspond to distant metastasis while loco regional control is achieved in most patients, it is not logical to decrease the intensity of the systemic treatment. More promising would be to reduce the RT dose intensity. This approach would be interesting in the context of adjuvant (C)RT to take benefit from an upfront surgery that would be followed by a less toxic adjuvant treatment compared with definitive CRT. In this regard, the currently recruiting phase III PATHOS study assesses whether swallowing function can be improved following TORS for HPV-positive OPSCC, by reducing the intensity of adjuvant therapeutic protocols, with 50 Gy adjuvant RT alone as the experimental arm (clinicalTrials.gov Identifier: NCT02215265). The other strategy would be to reduce the RT dose intensity in definitive CRT protocols with or without adding a systemic treatment to conventional CRT to compensate this RT dose reduction. In this regard, a recent observational study using the National Cancer Database, by Gabani et al., showed that, in HPV-positive OPSCC patients, the use of RT doses inferior to 66 Gy did not result in reduced OS compared to standard RT doses (66 to 70 Gy) [101]. The currently recruiting phase II/III NRG HN005 trial (ClinicalTrials.gov Identifier: NCT03952585) compares a standard CRT arm (full dose IMRT, 70 Gy, with cisplatin) with two de-escalation experimental arms of either reduced-dose IMRT (60 Gy) with cisplatin or reduced-dose IMRT (60 Gy) with nivolumab in non-smoking patients with T1–2, N1, M0 or T3, N0–N1, M0 (AJCC, 8th edition) p16-positive OPSCC.

6. Conclusions

The role of tumor HPV-status on therapeutic decision-making in OPSCC patients is not yet well defined. However, the tumor HPV status will have, in the near future, a major impact on the therapeutic management of OPSCC patients (surgical vs. non-surgical strategy, RT doses, and RT-associated therapies). There is no published randomized phase III clinical trial comparing surgical vs. non-surgical therapeutic strategies in OPSCC patients. Nevertheless, there are convergent data supporting the use of primary surgery in patients with HPV-negative OPSCC since it is associated with improved oncologic outcomes, if an acceptable functional result can be reasonably expected. In patients with HPV-negative unresectable OPSCC, cisplatin-based CRT remains the gold standard treatment since recent studies aiming at intensifying therapeutic strategy have failed to improve both oncologic and functional outcomes. In patients with early-stage HPV-positive OPSCC, surgery and RT lead to comparable survival outcomes and treatment selection should be mainly based on treatment-related morbidity and preservation of swallowing function and QoL. In patients with HPV-positive locally advanced OPSCC, upfront surgery plus adjuvant (C)RT is associated with increased morbidity and functional impairment and no substantial gain in terms of survival compared with definitive CRT. In these patients, cisplatin-based concurrent CRT remains the cornerstone of the treatment but research is being undertaken to assess new therapeutic regimens (reduction in RT doses, and other combinations of systemic therapy) in order to minimize treatment-related toxicities.

Author Contributions: Conceptualization: A.B. and D.C.; writing—original draft preparation: A.B., G.P., F.D. and O.D.; writing—review and editing: A.B., G.P., F.D. and O.D. All authors have read and agreed to the published version of the manuscript.

Funding: This research received no external funding.

Acknowledgments: The authors acknowledge Christine Lovera for her administrative support.

Conflicts of Interest: The authors declare no conflict of interest.

References

1. Mahal, B.A.; Catalano, P.J.; Haddad, R.I.; Hanna, G.J.; Kass, J.I.; Schoenfeld, J.D.; Tishler, R.B.; Margalit, D.N. Incidence and Demographic Burden of HPV-Associated Oropharyngeal Head and Neck Cancers in the United States. *Cancer Epidemiol. Biomark. Prev.* **2019**, *28*, 1660–1667. [CrossRef] [PubMed]
2. Megwalu, U.C.; Sirjani, D.; Devine, E.E. Oropharyngeal squamous cell carcinoma incidence and mortality trends in the United States, 1973–2013. *Laryngoscope* **2017**, *128*, 1582–1588. [CrossRef]
3. Zevallos, J.P.; Kramer, J.R.; Sandulache, V.C.; Massa, S.T.; Hartman, C.M.; Mazul, A.L.; Wahle, B.M.; Gerndt, S.P.; Sturgis, E.M.; Chiao, E.Y. National trends in oropharyngeal cancer incidence and survival within the Veterans Affairs Health Care System. *Head Neck* **2020**, *43*, 108–115. [CrossRef] [PubMed]
4. Osazuwa-Peters, N.; Simpson, M.C.; Massa, S.T.; Boakye, E.A.; Antisdel, J.L.; Varvares, M.A. 40-year incidence trends for oropharyngeal squamous cell carcinoma in the United States. *Oral Oncol.* **2017**, *74*, 90–97. [CrossRef]
5. Timbang, M.R.; Sim, M.W.; Bewley, A.F.; Farwell, D.G.; Mantravadi, A.; Moore, M.G. HPV-related oropharyngeal cancer: A review on burden of the disease and opportunities for prevention and early detection. *Hum. Vaccines Immunother.* **2019**, *15*, 1920–1928. [CrossRef] [PubMed]
6. Guily, J.L.S.; Rousseau, A.; Baujat, B.; Périé, S.; Schultz, P.; Barry, B.; Dufour, X.; Malard, O.; Pretet, J.-L.; Clavel, C.; et al. Oropharyngeal cancer prognosis by tumour HPV status in France: The multicentric Papillophar study. *Oral Oncol.* **2017**, *67*, 29–36. [CrossRef]

7. Bhatia, A.; Burtness, B. Human Papillomavirus–Associated Oropharyngeal Cancer: Defining Risk Groups and Clinical Trials. *J. Clin. Oncol.* **2015**, *33*, 3243–3250. [CrossRef]
8. Mehanna, H.; Evans, M.; Beasley, M.; Chatterjee, S.; Dilkes, M.; Homer, J.; O'Hara, J.; Robinson, M.; Shaw, R.; Sloan, P. Oropharyngeal cancer: United Kingdom National Multidisciplinary Guidelines. *J. Laryngol. Otol.* **2016**, *130*, S90–S96. [CrossRef]
9. Maschio, F.; Lejuste, P.; Ilankovan, V. Evolution in the management of oropharyngeal squamous cell carcinoma: Systematic review of outcomes over the last 25 years. *Br. J. Oral Maxillofac. Surg.* **2019**, *57*, 101–115. [CrossRef]
10. Bozec, A.; Culié, D.; Poissonnet, G.; Dassonville, O. Current role of primary surgical treatment in patients with head and neck squamous cell carcinoma. *Curr. Opin. Oncol.* **2019**, *31*, 138–145. [CrossRef] [PubMed]
11. Culié, D.; Garrel, R.; Viotti, J.; Schiappa, R.; Chamorey, E.; Fakhry, N.; Lallemant, B.; Vergez, S.; Dupret-Bories, A.; Dassonville, O.; et al. Impact of HPV-associated p16-expression and other clinical factors on therapeutic decision-making in patients with oropharyngeal cancer: A GETTEC multicentric study. *Eur. J. Surg. Oncol. (EJSO)* **2018**, *44*, 1908–1913. [CrossRef] [PubMed]
12. Haigentz, M.; Silver, C.E.; Corry, J.; Genden, E.M.; Takes, R.P.; Rinaldo, A.; Ferlito, A. Current trends in initial management of oropharyngeal cancer: The declining use of open surgery. *Eur. Arch. Oto-Rhino-Laryngol.* **2009**, *266*, 1845–1855. [CrossRef]
13. Price, J.; West, C.; Mistry, H.; Betts, G.; Bishop, P.; Kennedy, J.; Dixon, L.; Homer, J.; Garcez, K.; Lee, L.; et al. Improved survival prediction for oropharyngeal cancer beyond TNMv8. *Oral Oncol.* **2021**, *115*, 105140. [CrossRef] [PubMed]
14. Boscolo-Rizzo, P.; Gava, A.; Baggio, V.; Marchiori, C.; Stellin, M.; Fuson, R.; Lamon, S.; DA Mosto, M.C. Matched Survival Analysis in Patients with Locoregionally Advanced Resectable Oropharyngeal Carcinoma: Platinum-Based Induction and Concurrent Chemoradiotherapy Versus Primary Surgical Resection. *Int. J. Radiat. Oncol.* **2011**, *80*, 154–160. [CrossRef] [PubMed]
15. Culié, D.; Viotti, J.; Modesto, A.; Schiappa, R.; Chamorey, E.; Dassonville, O.; Poissonnet, G.; Guelfucci, B.; Bizeau, A.; Vergez, S.; et al. Upfront surgery or definitive radiotherapy for patients with p16-negative oropharyngeal squamous cell carcinoma. A GETTEC multicentric study. *Eur. J. Surg. Oncol. (EJSO)* **2020**, *47*, 367–374. [CrossRef] [PubMed]
16. Bozec, A.; Demez, P.; Gal, J.; Chamorey, E.; Louis, M.-Y.; Blanchard, D.; De Raucourt, D.; Merol, J.-C.; Brenet, E.; Dassonville, O.; et al. Long-term quality of life and psycho-social outcomes after oropharyngeal cancer surgery and radial forearm free-flap reconstruction: A GETTEC prospective multicentric study. *Surg. Oncol.* **2018**, *27*, 23–30. [CrossRef] [PubMed]
17. Kumar, A.; Laskar, S.G.; Thiagarajan, S. Is Transoral Robotic Surgery (TORS) for oropharyngeal squamous cell carcinoma being done more often than actually indicated? *Head Neck* **2021**, *43*, 1376–1377. [CrossRef]
18. Dahlstrom, K.R.; Bell, D.; Hanby, D.; Li, G.; Wang, L.-E.; Wei, Q.; Williams, M.D.; Sturgis, E.M. Socioeconomic characteristics of patients with oropharyngeal carcinoma according to tumor HPV status, patient smoking status, and sexual behavior. *Oral Oncol.* **2015**, *51*, 832–838. [CrossRef]
19. Milliet, F.; Bozec, A.; Schiappa, R.; Viotti, J.; Modesto, A.; Dassonville, O.; Poissonnet, G.; Guelfucci, B.; Bizeau, A.; Vergez, S.; et al. Metachronous second primary neoplasia in oropharyngeal cancer patients: Impact of tumor HPV status. A GETTEC multicentric study. *Oral Oncol.* **2021**, *122*, 105503. [CrossRef]
20. Milliet, F.; Bozec, A.; Schiappa, R.; Viotti, J.; Modesto, A.; Dassonville, O.; Poissonnet, G.; Guelfucci, B.; Bizeau, A.; Vergez, S.; et al. Synchronous primary neoplasia in patients with oropharyngeal cancer: Impact of tumor HPV status. A GETTEC multicentric study. *Oral Oncol.* **2020**, *112*, 105041. [CrossRef]
21. Martel, M.; Alemany, L.; Taberna, M.; Mena, M.; Tous, S.; Bagué, S.; Castellsagué, X.; Quer, M.; León, X. The role of HPV on the risk of second primary neoplasia in patients with oropharyngeal cancer. *Oral Oncol.* **2016**, *64*, 37–43. [CrossRef] [PubMed]
22. Wang, J.; Xi, X.; Shang, W.; Acharya, A.; Li, S.; Savkovic, V.; Li, H.; Haak, R.; Schmidt, J.; Liu, X.; et al. The molecular differences between human papillomavirus-positive and -negative oropharyngeal squamous cell carcinoma: A bioinformatics study. *Am. J. Otolaryngol.* **2019**, *40*, 547–554. [CrossRef]
23. McLaughlin-Drubin, M.E.; Crum, C.P.; Munger, K. Human papillomavirus E7 oncoprotein induces KDM6A and KDM6B histone demethylase expression and causes epigenetic reprogramming. *Proc. Natl. Acad. Sci. USA* **2011**, *108*, 2130–2135. [CrossRef] [PubMed]
24. Shinn, J.R.; Davis, S.J.; Lang-Kuhs, K.A.; Rohde, S.; Wang, X.; Liu, P.; Dupont, W.D.; Plummer, D., Jr.; Thorstad, W.L.; Chernock, R.D.; et al. Oropharyngeal Squamous Cell Carcinoma with Discordant p16 and HPV mRNA Results: Incidence and Characterization in a Large, Contemporary United States Cohort. *Am. J. Surg. Pathol.* **2021**, *45*, 951–961.
25. Mirghani, H.; Amen, F.; Moreau, F.; Guigay, J.; Ferchiou, M.; Melkane, A.E.; Hartl, D.M.; Guily, J.L.S. Human papilloma virus testing in oropharyngeal squamous cell carcinoma: What the clinician should know. *Oral Oncol.* **2014**, *50*, 1–9. [CrossRef]
26. Cancer Genome Atlas, N. Comprehensive genomic characterization of head and neck squamous cell carcinomas. *Nature* **2015**, *517*, 576–582. [CrossRef] [PubMed]
27. Mirghani, H.; Bellera, C.; Delaye, J.; Dolivet, G.; Fakhry, N.; Bozec, A.; Garrel, R.; Malard, O.; Jegoux, F.; Maingon, P.; et al. Prevalence and characteristics of HPV-driven oropharyngeal cancer in France. *Cancer Epidemiol.* **2019**, *61*, 89–94. [CrossRef]
28. Huang, Y.-H.; Yeh, C.-H.; Cheng, N.-M.; Lin, C.-Y.; Wang, H.-M.; Ko, S.-F.; Toh, C.-H.; Yen, T.-C.; Liao, C.-T.; Ng, S.-H. Cystic nodal metastasis in patients with oropharyngeal squamous cell carcinoma receiving chemoradiotherapy: Relationship with human papillomavirus status and failure patterns. *PLoS ONE* **2017**, *12*, e0180779. [CrossRef]
29. Mirghani, H.; Amen, F.; Tao, Y.; Deutsch, E.; Levy, A. Increased radiosensitivity of HPV-positive head and neck cancers: Molecular basis and therapeutic perspectives. *Cancer Treat. Rev.* **2015**, *41*, 844–852. [CrossRef] [PubMed]

30. Liu, C.; Mann, D.; Sinha, U.K.; Kokot, N.C. The molecular mechanisms of increased radiosensitivity of HPV-positive oropharyngeal squamous cell carcinoma (OPSCC): An extensive review. *J. Otolaryngol. Head Neck Surg.* **2018**, *47*, 59. [CrossRef] [PubMed]
31. Culié, D.; Lisan, Q.; Leroy, C.; Modesto, A.; Schiappa, R.; Chamorey, E.; Dassonville, O.; Poissonnet, G.; Guelfucci, B.; Bizeau, A.; et al. Oropharyngeal cancer: First relapse description and prognostic factor of salvage treatment according to p16 status, a GETTEC multicentric study. *Eur. J. Cancer* **2020**, *143*, 168–177. [CrossRef]
32. Wendt, M.; Hammarstedt-Nordenvall, L.; Zupancic, M.; Friesland, S.; Landin, D.; Munck-Wikland, E.; Dalianis, T.; Näsman, A.; Marklund, L. Long-Term Survival and Recurrence in Oropharyngeal Squamous Cell Carcinoma in Relation to Subsites, HPV, and p16-Status. *Cancers* **2021**, *13*, 2553. [CrossRef]
33. Culié, D.; Benezery, K.; Chamorey, E.; Ettaiche, M.; Fernandez, J.; Poissonnet, G.; Riss, J.-C.; Hannoun-Lévi, J.-M.; Chand, M.-E.; Leysalle, A.; et al. Salvage surgery for recurrent oropharyngeal cancer: Post-operative oncologic and functional outcomes. *Acta Oto-Laryngol.* **2015**, *135*, 1323–1329. [CrossRef] [PubMed]
34. Willenbrink, T.J.; Ruiz, E.S.; Cornejo, C.M.; Schmults, C.D.; Arron, S.T.; Jambusaria-Pahlajani, A. Field cancerization: Definition, epidemiology, risk factors, and outcomes. *J. Am. Acad. Dermatol.* **2020**, *83*, 709–717. [CrossRef] [PubMed]
35. Dickey, B.L.; Fan, W.; Bettampadi, D.; Reich, R.R.; Sirak, B.; Abrahamsen, M.; Baggio, M.L.; Galan, L.; Silva, R.C.; Salmerón, J.; et al. Sequential acquisition of human papillomavirus infection between genital and oral anatomic sites in males. *Int. J. Cancer* **2021**, *149*, 1483–1494. [CrossRef]
36. Larish, A.; Yin, L.; Glaser, G.; Moore, E.; Bakkum-Gamez, J.; Routman, D.; Ma, D.; Price, D.; Janus, J.; Price, K.; et al. Human Papillomavirus–Associated Anogenital Pathology in Females with HPV-Positive Oropharyngeal Squamous Cell Carcinoma. *Otolaryngol. Neck Surg.* **2020**, *164*, 369–374. [CrossRef]
37. Nauta, I.; Rietbergen, M.; van Bokhoven, A.; Bloemena, E.; Lissenberg-Witte, B.; Heideman, D.; de Jong, R.B.; Brakenhoff, R.; Leemans, C. Evaluation of the eighth TNM classification on p16-positive oropharyngeal squamous cell carcinomas in the Netherlands and the importance of additional HPV DNA testing. *Ann. Oncol.* **2018**, *29*, 1273–1279. [CrossRef]
38. Rühle, A.; Grosu, A.-L.; Nicolay, N. De-Escalation Strategies of (Chemo)Radiation for Head-and-Neck Squamous Cell Cancers—HPV and Beyond. *Cancers* **2021**, *13*, 2204. [CrossRef]
39. Chen, S.Y.; Last, A.; Ettyreddy, A.; Kallogjeri, D.; Wahle, B.; Chidambaram, S.; Mazul, A.; Thorstad, W.; Jackson, R.S.; Zevallos, J.P.; et al. 20 pack-year smoking history as strongest smoking metric predictive of HPV-positive oropharyngeal cancer outcomes. *Am. J. Otolaryngol.* **2021**, *42*, 102915. [CrossRef] [PubMed]
40. Bouland, C.; Dequanter, D.; Lechien, J.R.; Hanssens, C.; Aubain, N.D.S.; Digonnet, A.; Javadian, R.; Yanni, A.; Rodriguez, A.; Loeb, I.; et al. Prognostic Significance of a Scoring System Combining p16, Smoking, and Drinking Status in a Series of 131 Patients with Oropharyngeal Cancers. *Int. J. Otolaryngol.* **2021**, *2021*, 1–6. [CrossRef]
41. Xiao, R.; Pham, Y.; Ward, M.C.; Houston, N.; Reddy, C.A.; Joshi, N.P.; Greskovich, J.F., Jr.; Woody, N.M.; Chute, D.J.; Lamarre, E.D.; et al. Impact of active smoking on outcomes in HPV+ oropharyngeal cancer. *Head Neck* **2019**, *42*, 269–280. [CrossRef]
42. House, R.; Majumder, M.; Janakiraman, H.; Ogretmen, B.; Kato, M.; Erkul, E.; Hill, E.; Atkinson, C.; Barth, J.; Day, T.A.; et al. Smoking-induced control of miR-133a-3p alters the expression of EGFR and HuR in HPV-infected oropharyngeal cancer. *PLoS ONE* **2018**, *13*, e0205077. [CrossRef] [PubMed]
43. Mesia, R.; Iglesias, L.; Lambea, J.; Martínez-Trufero, J.; Soria, A.; Taberna, M.; Trigo, J.; Chaves, M.; García-Castaño, A.; Cruz, J. SEOM clinical guidelines for the treatment of head and neck cancer (2020). *Clin. Transl. Oncol.* **2021**, *23*, 913–921. [CrossRef]
44. Colevas, A.D.; Yom, S.; Pfister, D.G.; Spencer, S.; Adelstein, D.; Adkins, D.; Brizel, D.; Burtness, B.; Busse, P.M.; Caudell, J.J.; et al. NCCN Guidelines Insights: Head and Neck Cancers, Version 1.2018. *J. Natl. Compr. Cancer Netw.* **2018**, *16*, 479–490. [CrossRef]
45. Bozec, A.; Poissonnet, G.; Chamorey, E.; Sudaka, A.; Laout, C.; Vallicioni, J.; Demard, F.; Dassonville, O. Transoral and cervical approach without mandibulotomy for oropharynx cancer with fasciocutaneous radial forearm free flap reconstruction. *Ann. Otolaryngol. Chir. Cervicofac.* **2009**, *126*, 182–189. [CrossRef] [PubMed]
46. De Virgilio, A.; Costantino, A.; Mercante, G.; Pellini, R.; Ferreli, F.; Malvezzi, L.; Colombo, G.; Cugini, G.; Petruzzi, G.; Spriano, G. Transoral robotic surgery and intensity-modulated radiotherapy in the treatment of the oropharyngeal carcinoma: A systematic review and meta-analysis. *Eur. Arch. Oto-Rhino-Laryngol.* **2020**, *278*, 1321–1335. [CrossRef]
47. Garrel, R.; Poissonnet, G.; Temam, S.; Dolivet, G.; Fakhry, N.; de Raucourt, D. Review of sentinel node procedure in cN0 head and neck squamous cell carcinomas. Guidelines from the French evaluation cooperative subgroup of GETTEC. *Eur. Ann. Otorhinolaryngol. Head Neck Dis.* **2017**, *134*, 89–93. [CrossRef] [PubMed]
48. Qureshi, H.A.; Abouyared, M.; Barber, B.; Houlton, J.J. Surgical Options for Locally Advanced Oropharyngeal Cancer. *Curr. Treat. Options Oncol.* **2019**, *20*, 36. [CrossRef]
49. Moore, E.J.; Van Abel, K.M.; Price, D.L.; Lohse, C.M.; Olsen, K.D.; Jackson, R.; Martin, E.J. Transoral robotic surgery for oropharyngeal carcinoma: Surgical margins and oncologic outcomes. *Head Neck* **2018**, *40*, 747–755. [CrossRef] [PubMed]
50. Gorphe, P.; Von Tan, J.; El Bedoui, S.; Hartl, D.M.; Auperin, A.; Qassemyar, Q.; Moya-Plana, A.; Janot, F.; Julieron, M.; Temam, S. Early assessment of feasibility and technical specificities of transoral robotic surgery using the da Vinci Xi. *J. Robot. Surg.* **2017**, *11*, 455–461. [CrossRef]
51. López, F.; Fernández-Vañes, L.; García-Cabo, P.; Grilli, G.; Álvarez-Marcos, C.; Llorente, J.L.; Rodrigo, J.P. Selective neck dissection in the treatment of head and neck squamous cell carcinoma patients with a clinically positive neck. *Oral Oncol.* **2020**, *102*, 104565. [CrossRef]

52. Garrel, R.; Poissonnet, G.; Plana, A.M.; Fakhry, N.; Dolivet, G.; Lallemant, B.; Sarini, J.; Vergez, S.; Guelfucci, B.; Choussy, O.; et al. Equivalence Randomized Trial to Compare Treatment on the Basis of Sentinel Node Biopsy Versus Neck Node Dissection in Operable T1-T2N0 Oral and Oropharyngeal Cancer. *J. Clin. Oncol.* **2020**, *38*, 4010–4018. [CrossRef]
53. Gorphe, P.; Temam, S.; Kolb, F.; Qassemyar, Q. Cervical-transoral robotic oropharyngectomy and thin anterolateral thigh free flap. *Eur. Ann. Otorhinolaryngol. Head Neck Dis.* **2018**, *135*, 71–74. [CrossRef]
54. Melan, J.-B.; Philouze, P.; Pradat, P.; Benzerdjeb, N.; Blanc, J.; Ceruse, P.; Fuchsmann, C. Functional outcomes of soft palate free flap reconstruction following oropharyngeal cancer surgery. *Eur. J. Surg. Oncol. (EJSO)* **2021**, *47*, 2265–2271. [CrossRef]
55. Camuzard, O.; Dassonville, O.; Ettaiche, M.; Chamorey, E.; Poissonnet, G.; Berguiga, R.; Leysalle, A.; Benezery, K.; Peyrade, F.; Saada, E.; et al. Primary radical ablative surgery and fibula free-flap reconstruction for T4 oral cavity squamous cell carcinoma with mandibular invasion: Oncologic and functional results and their predictive factors. *Eur. Arch. Oto-Rhino-Laryngol.* **2016**, *274*, 441–449. [CrossRef] [PubMed]
56. Culié, D.; Dassonville, O.; Poissonnet, G.; Riss, J.-C.; Fernandez, J.; Bozec, A. Virtual planning and guided surgery in fibular free-flap mandibular reconstruction: A 29-case series. *Eur. Ann. Otorhinolaryngol. Head Neck Dis.* **2016**, *133*, 175–178. [CrossRef]
57. Bernier, J.; Vermorken, J.B.; Koch, W.M. Adjuvant Therapy in Patients with Resected Poor-Risk Head and Neck Cancer. *J. Clin. Oncol.* **2006**, *24*, 2629–2635. [CrossRef] [PubMed]
58. Boros, A.; Blanchard, P.; Dade, A.; Gorphe, P.; Breuskin, I.; Even, C.; Nguyen, F.; Deutsch, E.; Bidault, F.; Janot, F.; et al. Outcomes in N3 Head and Neck Squamous Cell Carcinoma and Role of Upfront Neck Dissection. *Laryngoscope* **2020**, *131*, E846–E850. [CrossRef] [PubMed]
59. Paximadis, P.A.; Christensen, M.E.; Dyson, G.; Kamdar, D.P.; Sukari, A.; Lin, H.-S.; Yoo, G.H.; Kim, H.E. Up-front neck dissection followed by concurrent chemoradiation in patients with regionally advanced head and neck cancer. *Head Neck* **2012**, *34*, 1798–1803. [CrossRef]
60. Klausner, G.; Troussier, I.; Fabiano, E.; Kreps, S.; Laccourreye, O.; Giraud, P. 881P Impact of neck dissection in N2-3 oropharyngeal squamous-cell carcinomas treated with definitive chemo-radiotherapy: An observational real-life study. *Ann. Oncol.* **2021**, *32*, S794–S795. [CrossRef]
61. Gupta, T.; Sinha, S.; Ghosh-Laskar, S.; Budrukkar, A.; Mummudi, N.; Swain, M.; Phurailatpam, R.; Prabhash, K.; Agarwal, J.P. Intensity-modulated radiation therapy versus three-dimensional conformal radiotherapy in head and neck squamous cell carcinoma: Long-term and mature outcomes of a prospective randomized trial. *Radiat. Oncol.* **2020**, *15*, 1–9. [CrossRef]
62. Tribius, S.; Bergelt, C. Intensity-modulated radiotherapy versus conventional and 3D conformal radiotherapy in patients with head and neck cancer: Is there a worthwhile quality of life gain? *Cancer Treat. Rev.* **2011**, *37*, 511–519. [CrossRef]
63. Mazzola, R.; Fiorentino, A.; Ricchetti, F.; Gregucci, F.; Corradini, S.; Alongi, F. An update on radiation therapy in head and neck cancers. *Expert Rev. Anticancer. Ther.* **2018**, *18*, 359–364. [CrossRef]
64. De Felice, F.; Belgioia, L.; Alterio, D.; Bonomo, P.; Maddalo, M.; Paiar, F.; Denaro, N.; Corvò, R.; Merlotti, A.; Bossi, P.; et al. Survival and toxicity of weekly cisplatin chemoradiotherapy versus three-weekly cisplatin chemoradiotherapy for head and neck cancer: A systematic review and meta-analysis endorsed by the Italian Association of Radiotherapy and Clinical Oncology (AIRO). *Crit. Rev. Oncol.* **2021**, *162*, 103345. [CrossRef]
65. Bonner, J.A.; Harari, P.M.; Giralt, J.; Cohen, R.B.; Jones, C.U.; Sur, R.K.; Raben, D.; Baselga, J.; Spencer, S.A.; Zhu, J.; et al. Radiotherapy plus cetuximab for locoregionally advanced head and neck cancer: 5-year survival data from a phase 3 randomised trial, and relation between cetuximab-induced rash and survival. *Lancet Oncol.* **2010**, *11*, 21–28. [CrossRef]
66. Mehanna, H.; Robinson, M.; Hartley, A.; Kong, A.; Foran, B.; Fulton-Lieuw, T.; Dalby, M.; Mistry, P.; Sen, M.; O'Toole, L.; et al. Radiotherapy plus cisplatin or cetuximab in low-risk human papillomavirus-positive oropharyngeal cancer (De-ESCALaTE HPV): An open-label randomised controlled phase 3 trial. *Lancet* **2019**, *393*, 51–60. [CrossRef]
67. Haddad, R.; O'Neill, A.; Rabinowits, G.; Tishler, R.; Khuri, F.R.; Adkins, D.; Clark, J.; Sarlis, N.; Lorch, J.; Beitler, J.J.; et al. Induction chemotherapy followed by concurrent chemoradiotherapy (sequential chemoradiotherapy) versus concurrent chemoradiotherapy alone in locally advanced head and neck cancer (PARADIGM): A randomised phase 3 trial. *Lancet Oncol.* **2013**, *14*, 257–264. [CrossRef]
68. Ang, K.K.; Zhang, Q.; Rosenthal, D.; Nguyen-Tan, P.F.; Sherman, E.J.; Weber, R.S.; Galvin, J.M.; Bonner, J.A.; Harris, J.; El-Naggar, A.K.; et al. Randomized Phase III Trial of Concurrent Accelerated Radiation Plus Cisplatin with or Without Cetuximab for Stage III to IV Head and Neck Carcinoma: RTOG 0522. *J. Clin. Oncol.* **2014**, *32*, 2940–2950. [CrossRef] [PubMed]
69. Hitt, R.; Grau, J.J.; López-Pousa, A.; Berrocal, A.; García-Girón, C.; Irigoyen, A.; Sastre, J.; Martínez-Trufero, J.; Castelo, J.A.B.; Verger, E.; et al. A randomized phase III trial comparing induction chemotherapy followed by chemoradiotherapy versus chemoradiotherapy alone as treatment of unresectable head and neck cancer. *Ann. Oncol.* **2013**, *25*, 216–225. [CrossRef] [PubMed]
70. Merlano, M.C.; Denaro, N.; Vecchio, S.; Licitra, L.; Curcio, P.; Benasso, M.; Bagicalupo, A.; Numico, G.; Russi, E.; Corvo', R.; et al. Phase III Randomized Study of Induction Chemotherapy Followed by Definitive Radiotherapy + Cetuximab Versus Chemoradiotherapy in Squamous Cell Carcinoma of Head and Neck: The INTERCEPTOR-GONO Study (NCT00999700). *Oncology* **2020**, *98*, 763–770. [CrossRef]
71. Yu, Y.; Lee, N.Y. JAVELIN Head and Neck 100: A Phase III trial of avelumab and chemoradiation for locally advanced head and neck cancer. *Future Oncol.* **2019**, *15*, 687–694. [CrossRef]

72. Culié, D.; Schiappa, R.; Modesto, A.; Viotti, J.; Chamorey, E.; Dassonville, O.; Poissonnet, G.; Bizeau, A.; Vergez, S.; Dupret-Bories, A.; et al. Upfront surgery or definitive radiotherapy for p16+ oropharyngeal cancer. A GETTEC multicentric study. *Eur. J. Surg. Oncol. (EJSO)* **2020**, *47*, 1389–1397. [CrossRef]
73. Nichols, A.C.; Theurer, J.; Prisman, E.; Read, N.; Berthelet, E.; Tran, E.; Fung, K.; de Almeida, J.R.; Bayley, A.; Goldstein, D.P.; et al. Radiotherapy versus transoral robotic surgery and neck dissection for oropharyngeal squamous cell carcinoma (ORATOR): An open-label, phase 2, randomised trial. *Lancet Oncol.* **2019**, *20*, 1349–1359. [CrossRef]
74. Charters, E.; Wu, R.; Milross, C.; Bogaardt, H.; Freeman-Sanderson, A.; Ballard, K.; Davies, S.; Oates, J.; Clark, J. Swallowing and communication outcomes following primary transoral robotic surgery. *Head Neck* **2021**, *43*, 2013–2023. [CrossRef]
75. Feng, A.L.; Holcomb, A.J.; Abt, N.B.; Mokhtari, T.E.; Suresh, K.; McHugh, C.I.; Parikh, A.S.; Holman, A.; Kammer, R.E.; Goldsmith, T.A.; et al. Feeding Tube Placement Following Transoral Robotic Surgery for Oropharyngeal Squamous Cell Carcinoma. *Otolaryngol. Neck Surg.* **2021**, 01945998211020302. [CrossRef]
76. Pierre, C.S.; Dassonville, O.; Chamorey, E.; Poissonnet, G.; Ettaiche, M.; Santini, J.; Peyrade, F.; Benezery, K.; Sudaka, A.; Bozec, A. Long-term quality of life and its predictive factors after oncologic surgery and microvascular reconstruction in patients with oral or oropharyngeal cancer. *Eur. Arch. Oto-Rhino-Laryngol.* **2013**, *271*, 801–807. [CrossRef]
77. Rizzo, P.B.; Stellin, M.; Fuson, R.; Marchiori, C.; Gava, A.; Da Mosto, M.C. Long-term quality of life after treatment for locally advanced oropharyngeal carcinoma: Surgery and postoperative radiotherapy versus concurrent chemoradiation. *Oral Oncol.* **2009**, *45*, 953–957. [CrossRef]
78. Kelly, J.R.; Park, H.S.; An, Y.; Yarbrough, W.G.; Contessa, J.N.; Decker, R.; Mehra, S.; Judson, B.L.; Burtness, B.; Husain, Z. Upfront surgery versus definitive chemoradiotherapy in patients with human Papillomavirus-associated oropharyngeal squamous cell cancer. *Oral Oncol.* **2018**, *79*, 64–70. [CrossRef] [PubMed]
79. Kelly, J.; Husain, Z.A.; Burtness, B. Treatment de-intensification strategies for head and neck cancer. *Eur. J. Cancer* **2016**, *68*, 125–133. [CrossRef] [PubMed]
80. Kamran, S.C.; Qureshi, M.M.; Jalisi, S.; Salama, A.; Grillone, G.; Truong, M.T. Primary surgery versus primary radiation-based treatment for locally advanced oropharyngeal cancer. *Laryngoscope* **2017**, *128*, 1353–1364. [CrossRef]
81. Ranta, P.; Kinnunen, I.; Jouhi, L.; Vahlberg, T.; Back, L.J.J.; Halme, E.; Koivunen, P.; Autio, T.; Pukkila, M.; Irjala, H. Long-term Quality of Life After Treatment of Oropharyngeal Squamous Cell Carcinoma. *Laryngoscope* **2020**, *131*. [CrossRef] [PubMed]
82. Jacobs, D.; Torabi, S.J.; Park, H.S.; Rahmati, R.; Young, M.R.; Mehra, S.; Judson, B.L. Revisiting the Radiation Therapy Oncology Group 1221 Hypothesis: Treatment for Stage III/IV HPV-Negative Oropharyngeal Cancer. *Otolaryngol. Neck Surg.* **2020**, *164*, 1240–1248. [CrossRef] [PubMed]
83. Trinh, J.-M.; Thomas, J.; Salleron, J.; Henrot, P. Differences in clinical and imaging characteristics between p16-positive non-smokers and p16-positive smokers or p16-negative patients in oropharyngeal carcinoma. *Sci. Rep.* **2021**, *11*, 1–11. [CrossRef]
84. Seikaly, H.; Biron, V.L.; Zhang, H.; O'Connell, D.A.; Côté, D.W.J.; Ansari, K.; Williams, D.C.; Puttagunta, L.; Harris, J.R. Role of primary surgery in the treatment of advanced oropharyngeal cancer. *Head Neck* **2015**, *38*, E571–E579. [CrossRef]
85. Mazarro, A.; de Pablo, A.; Puiggròs, C.; Velasco, M.M.; Saez, M.; Pamias, J.; Bescós, C. Indications, reconstructive techniques, and results for total glossectomy. *Head Neck* **2016**, *38*, E2004–E2010. [CrossRef]
86. Fulcher, C.D.; Haigentz, M.; Ow, T.J. The Education Committee of the American Head and Neck Society (AHNS) AHNS Series: Do you know your guidelines? Principles of treatment for locally advanced or unresectable head and neck squamous cell carcinoma. *Head Neck* **2017**, *40*, 676–686. [CrossRef]
87. Soba, E.; Budihna, M.; Smid, L.; Gale, N.; Lesnicar, H.; Zakotnik, B.; Strojan, P. Prognostic value of some tumor markers in unresectable stage IV oropharyngeal carcinoma patients treated with concomitant radiochemotherapy. *Radiol. Oncol.* **2015**, *49*, 365–370. [CrossRef]
88. Bhattasali, O.; Ryoo, J.J.; Thompson, L.; Abdalla, I.A.; Chen, J.; Iganej, S. Impact of chemotherapy regimen on treatment outcomes in patients with HPV-associated oropharyngeal cancer with T4 disease treated with definitive concurrent chemoradiation. *Oral Oncol.* **2019**, *95*, 74–78. [CrossRef]
89. Gillison, M.L.; Trotti, A.M.; Harris, J.; Eisbruch, A.; Harari, P.M.; Adelstein, D.J.; Jordan, R.C.K.; Zhao, W.; Sturgis, E.M.; Burtness, B.; et al. Radiotherapy plus cetuximab or cisplatin in human papillomavirus-positive oropharyngeal cancer (NRG Oncology RTOG 1016): A randomised, multicentre, non-inferiority trial. *Lancet* **2018**, *393*, 40–50. [CrossRef]
90. Wang, H.; Zhao, Q.; Zhang, Y.; Zhang, Q.; Zheng, Z.; Liu, S.; Liu, Z.; Meng, L.; Xin, Y.; Jiang, X. Immunotherapy Advances in Locally Advanced and Recurrent/Metastatic Head and Neck Squamous Cell Carcinoma and Its Relationship with Human Papillomavirus. *Front. Immunol.* **2021**, *12*, 2333. [CrossRef]
91. Guigay, J.; Aupérin, A.; Fayette, J.; Saada-Bouzid, E.; Lafond, C.; Taberna, M.; Geoffrois, L.; Martin, L.; Capitain, O.; Cupissol, D.; et al. Cetuximab, docetaxel, and cisplatin versus platinum, fluorouracil, and cetuximab as first-line treatment in patients with recurrent or metastatic head and neck squamous-cell carcinoma (GORTEC 2014-01 TPExtreme): A multicentre, open-label, randomised, phase 2 trial. *Lancet Oncol.* **2021**, *22*, 463–475. [CrossRef] [PubMed]
92. Zafereo, M. Surgical Salvage of Recurrent Cancer of the Head and Neck. *Curr. Oncol. Rep.* **2014**, *16*, 1–6. [CrossRef] [PubMed]
93. Bagley, A.F.; Garden, A.S.; Reddy, J.P.; Moreno, A.C.; Frank, S.J.; Rosenthal, D.I.; Morrison, W.H.; Gunn, G.B.; Fuller, C.D.; Shah, S.J.; et al. Highly conformal reirradiation in patients with prior oropharyngeal radiation: Clinical efficacy and toxicity outcomes. *Head Neck* **2020**, *42*, 3326–3335. [CrossRef] [PubMed]

94. Szturz, P.; Nevens, D.; Vermorken, J.B. Oligometastatic Disease Management: Finding the Sweet Spot. *Front. Oncol.* **2020**, *10*, 617793. [CrossRef]
95. Burtness, B.; Harrington, K.; Greil, R.; Soulières, D.; Tahara, M.; de Castro, G.; Psyrri, A.; Basté, N.; Neupane, P.; Bratland, Å.; et al. Pembrolizumab alone or with chemotherapy versus cetuximab with chemotherapy for recurrent or metastatic squamous cell carcinoma of the head and neck (KEYNOTE-048): A randomised, open-label, phase 3 study. *Lancet* **2019**, *394*, 1915–1928. [CrossRef]
96. Nichols, A.C.; Lang, P.; Prisman, E.; Berthelet, E.; Tran, E.; Hamilton, S.; Wu, J.; Fung, K.; De Almeida, J.R.; Bayley, A.; et al. Treatment de-escalation for HPV-associated oropharyngeal squamous cell carcinoma with radiotherapy vs. trans-oral surgery (ORATOR2): Study protocol for a randomized phase II trial. *BMC Cancer* **2020**, *20*, 1–13. [CrossRef]
97. Sun, X.-S.; Tao, Y.; Le Tourneau, C.; Pointreau, Y.; Sire, C.; Kaminsky, M.-C.; Coutte, A.; Alfonsi, M.; Boisselier, P.; Martin, L.; et al. Debio 1143 and high-dose cisplatin chemoradiotherapy in high-risk locoregionally advanced squamous cell carcinoma of the head and neck: A double-blind, multicentre, randomised, phase 2 study. *Lancet Oncol.* **2020**, *21*, 1173–1187. [CrossRef]
98. Tao, Y.; Aupérin, A.; Sun, X.; Sire, C.; Martin, L.; Coutte, A.; Lafond, C.; Miroir, J.; Liem, X.; Rolland, F.; et al. Avelumab–cetuximab–radiotherapy versus standards of care in locally advanced squamous-cell carcinoma of the head and neck: The safety phase of a randomised phase III trial GORTEC 2017-01 (REACH). *Eur. J. Cancer* **2020**, *141*, 21–29. [CrossRef]
99. Mirghani, H.; Amen, F.; Blanchard, P.; Moreau, F.; Guigay, J.; Hartl, D.; Guily, J.L.S. Treatment de-escalation in HPV-positive oropharyngeal carcinoma: Ongoing trials, critical issues and perspectives. *Int. J. Cancer* **2014**, *136*, 1494–1503. [CrossRef]
100. Wotman, M.T.; Miles, B.A.; Bakst, R.L.; Posner, M.R. A proposal for risk-based and strategy-adapted de-escalation in human papillomavirus-positive oropharyngeal squamous cell carcinoma. *Cancer* **2021**, in press. [CrossRef]
101. Gabani, P.; Lin, A.J.; Barnes, J.; Oppelt, P.; Adkins, D.R.; Rich, J.T.; Zevallos, J.P.; Daly, M.D.; Gay, H.A.; Thorstad, W.L. Radiation therapy dose de-escalation compared to standard dose radiation therapy in definitive treatment of HPV-positive oropharyngeal squamous cell carcinoma. *Radiother. Oncol.* **2019**, *134*, 81–88. [CrossRef] [PubMed]

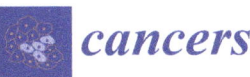

Hypothesis

Potential of Farnesyl Transferase Inhibitors in Combination Regimens in Squamous Cell Carcinomas

Linda Kessler, Shivani Malik, Mollie Leoni and Francis Burrows *

Kura Oncology, Inc., San Diego, CA 92130, USA; linda@kuraoncology.com (L.K.); smalik@kuraoncology.com (S.M.); mleoni@kuraoncology.com (M.L.)
* Correspondence: francis@kuraoncology.com; Tel.: +1-858-500-8854

Simple Summary: Current therapies for recurrent and metastatic squamous cell carcinomas (SCCs) are associated with poor patient outcomes, and options for later lines of treatment are very limited. In cases where single-agent therapy may be insufficient to eradicate the tumor, thus allowing outgrowth of resistant cells, a well-chosen combination of therapeutic agents may enable improved outcomes. Tipifarnib, a farnesyl transferase inhibitor, is a small molecule drug candidate that has demonstrated promising clinical activity in HRAS-mutant head and neck squamous cell carcinoma (HNSCC). New molecular analyses suggest that HRAS may also be important in some HNSCC cases where it is not mutated, which might allow tipifarnib to be active in a broader population of HNSCC patients when used in combination with other agents such as cisplatin, cetuximab, or alpelisib. Other non-HRAS oncoproteins that can also be blocked by tipifarnib may offer alternative approaches to combination regimens for SCCs.

Abstract: Current therapies for recurrent and metastatic SCC are associated with poor outcomes, and options for later lines of treatment are limited. Insights into potential therapeutic targets, as well as mechanisms of resistance to available therapies, have begun to be elucidated, creating the basis for exploration of combination approaches to drive better patient outcomes. Tipifarnib, a farnesyl transferase inhibitor (FTI), is a small molecule drug that has demonstrated encouraging clinical activity in a genetically-defined subset of head and neck squamous cell carcinoma (HNSCC)–specifically, tumors that express a mutation in the *HRAS* protooncogene. More recently, bioinformatic analyses and results from patient-derived xenograft modeling indicate that HRAS pathway dependency may extend to a broader subpopulation of SCCs beyond HRAS mutants in the context of combination with agents such as cisplatin, cetuximab, or alpelisib. In addition, tipifarnib can also inactivate additional farnesylated proteins implicated in resistance to approved therapies, including immunotherapies, through a variety of distinct mechanisms, suggesting that tipifarnib could serve as an anchor for combination regimens in SCCs and other tumor types.

Keywords: HNSCC; farnesyl transferase; tipifarnib; combination regimen

1. Tipifarnib in HRAS-Mutant HNSCC—History, Preclinical Validation, and Clinical Development

The RAS family is a group of low molecular weight guanosine triphosphate (GTP)-binding proteins localized to the cell membrane that play a pivotal role in the transduction of cell growth-stimulating signals. Well-established effectors of RAS are the protein kinase RAF and the lipid kinase PI3-kinase (PI3K). Following recruitment by RAS to the plasma membrane and activation by phosphorylation, RAF induces a phosphorylation cascade that drives the transcription of genes associated with cell proliferation [1]. PI3K activation leads to increased cell motility, invasiveness, and suppression of apoptosis [2,3]. RAS-driven downstream effector pathways also regulate the cell cycle and integrin signaling [4,5].

Approximately 30% of human tumors express a mutation in one of three *RAS* protooncogenes (*KRAS*, *NRAS*, and *HRAS*) encoding four RAS proteins (KRAS4A, KRAS4B,

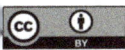

NRAS, and HRAS) [6]. The frequency of *RAS* mutation and the dominant isoform vary depending on the tissue and tumor type [7]. The majority of these mutations are localized to codons 12, 13, or 61 and defined as "activating mutations" because they encode RAS proteins with suppressed GTPase activity that allows RAS to remain in the GTP-bound active state [8,9]. The critical role of RAS in oncogenic transformation was characterized by expression of dominant-negative forms of RAS and homologous recombination to disrupt mutated, active *RAS* genes in various human cancer cell lines [10,11].

RAS isoforms must associate with the inner surface of the plasma membrane to transduce extracellular signals. To become active, RAS undergoes several post-translational modifications. The first step is the farnesylation of the cysteine in the CAAX box at the C-terminal end (where C represents cysteine, A represents an aliphatic amino acid, and X represents any amino acid) [6]. The enzyme farnesyltransferase (FTase) recognizes the CAAX motif and transfers a 15-carbon farnesyl isoprenoid from farnesyl diphosphate to the cysteine residue. The AAX amino acids subsequently are cleaved by RAS-converting enzyme I, and the farnesylated cysteine is carboxymethylated by isoprenylcysteine carboxyl methyltransferase [12]. Further palmitoylation (KRAS4A, NRAS, and HRAS or the presence of a polybasic domain (KRAS4B) leads to anchoring of the protein in the plasma membrane [13].

With the elucidation of this RAS post-translational modification pathway in the late 1980s, FTase became a viable pharmacological target to affect RAS function in cancer. Preliminary strategies were directed towards CAAX tetrapeptide inhibitors, which were competitive with the protein substrate [14]. However, such tetrapeptides were not efficiently taken up into cells, and the drug discovery efforts shifted toward more stable, peptidomimetic inhibitors [15–18]. Small molecule inhibitors were identified through high-throughput screening efforts and aided by crystallographic structures [19]. One such drug candidate, which later advanced into clinical evaluation, was R115777, also known as tipifarnib, a heterocyclic non-peptidomimetic that inhibits the FTase prenylation of KRAS in vitro with an IC_{50} of 7.9 nM [20].

Tipifarnib was the first FTI to enter clinical development in 1997, and its safety and efficacy have been assessed in more than 70 clinical studies [21–25]. Observations that mutations within *KRAS* are most common in lung, colorectal, and pancreatic tumors; *NRAS* mutations typically observed in human myeloid cancers; and *HRAS* mutations found in bladder, thyroid, and head and neck tumors [8] helped guide the clinical development program. However, Phase 3 trials in non-enriched patient populations resulted in no significant antitumor effect in patients with advanced colorectal cancer [26]. In addition, no significant increase in response rate was observed in patients with pancreatic carcinoma when tipifarnib was combined with gemcitabine [27]. Overall, tipifarnib failed to achieve clinically meaningful improvements in two solid tumors known to highly express mutations in *KRAS*. Subsequently, it was discovered that certain farnesylated proteins—including KRAS and NRAS—can be rescued from membrane displacement in the presence of FTIs by an alternative prenylation by the enzyme geranylgeranyltransferase (GGTase) [28,29]. Conversely, the third family member, HRAS, is not a GGTase substrate, and therefore its membrane localization and cellular function are diminished by FTIs [29]. Thus, it was hypothesized that using tipifarnib to target enriched patient populations of tumors harboring *HRAS* mutations via a classical precision medicine approach might yield more favorable clinical outcomes.

Despite being comparatively less frequent than those of *KRAS* and *NRAS*, mutations in *HRAS* are highly expressed in follicular thyroid cell-derived and in medullary thyroid carcinomas, as well as in head and neck and bladder cancers [30–34]. In a dedifferentiated thyroid cancer model, Untch et al. demonstrated that mice harboring flox-and-replace $HRAS^{G12V}$ and floxed p53 alleles developed aggressive tumors and 50% mortality after 40 weeks [35]. Treatment of these mice with tipifarnib significantly improved survival and reduced tumor volume relative to vehicle-treated controls at 14 days. However, a subset of mice presented persistent, albeit diminished, tumor growth, occurring despite appropriate HRAS defarnesylation, suggesting an adaptive response to FTI treatment. To confirm this hypothesis, the investigators treated human and murine *HRAS* mutant cell lines with tipifarnib and observed increased GTP loading of wild-type KRAS and NRAS, a mechanism by which the efficacy of blunting oncogenic HRAS signaling could be circumvented. The authors further demonstrated that prolonged treatment of *HRAS* mutant tumors with tipifarnib elicited the emergence of nonsense mutations in *Nf1*, which encodes a GTPase-activating protein that is a negative regulator of RAS. Notably, loss of function mutations in *Nf1* have also been shown to confer resistance to other therapies for melanoma and lung cancer [36–38]. In addition to the *Nf1* loss, an activating mutation was found in *Gnas*, a complex locus whose most well-characterized transcript is the stimulatory G-protein alpha subunit ($G_{\alpha s}$). Similar findings have been described in the resistance to RAF inhibitors in melanoma cells, indicating that this mechanism may be common in cells that are dependent on cAMP for differentiated function [39]. Collectively, these adaptations to HRAS inhibition may limit the effectiveness of therapies for certain patients with *HRAS* mutant malignancies, although other concurrent oncogenomic abnormalities may also impact the response.

More recently, the efficacy of tipifarnib was examined in a series of cell- and patient-derived xenograft models of head and neck squamous cell carcinoma (HNSCC) [40]. Genomic analyses have revealed that *HRAS* mutations occur in 6% of HNSCC at initial diagnosis [41] and in 15% of patients during acquisition of resistance to cetuximab [42], and *HRAS* mutations have been demonstrated to correlate with reduced response of HNSCC patients to cetuximab treatment [43]. Gilardi et al. reported that both tipifarnib and *HRAS* knockdown significantly reduced the growth of *HRAS* mutated cell lines with no effects observed in *HRAS* wild-type cells. The investigators also demonstrated that tipifarnib induced selective anti-tumor activity, with *HRAS* wild-type tumors growing progressively on tipifarnib treatment but *HRAS* mutant tumors being highly sensitive to tipifarnib when compared to control groups. In addition, tipifarnib significantly reduced angiogenesis, as shown previously [44–46], and inhibited cell cycle progression while inducing squamous cell differentiation. Indeed, the anti-tumor activity of tipifarnib shown by Gilardi and colleagues in these HNSCC *HRAS* mutant models was equivalent to or exceeded that reported with a combination of MAPK and PI3K inhibitors in a *HRAS* mutant lung cancer model [47]. Collectively, these findings highlight mutant *HRAS* as a targetable oncogene that can be inhibited by tipifarnib, resulting in either consistent stasis or tumor regression in vivo in multiple preclinical models.

Despite these promising results, the clinical efficacy of tipifarnib during its initial evaluation in the late 1990s and early 2000s was limited and response rates were insufficient to support registrational trials. However, since its reintroduction to the clinic in 2015, findings from several trials have supported mutant *HRAS* as a target for the treatment of a subset of patients with HNSCC. Most recently, Ho et al. reported data from a Phase 2 clinical trial (KO-TIP-001, NCT02383927) investigating the efficacy of tipifarnib in second line and beyond recurrent and/or metastatic (R/M) head and neck squamous cell carcinomas, among others [48]. Patients received a starting dose of tipifarnib of either 600 or 900 mg administered orally twice daily on days 1–7 and 15–21 of 28-day treatment cycles until progression of disease or unacceptable toxicity. At the time of data analysis, 21 HNSCC patients with HRAS mutations with a variant allele frequency (VAF) of at least 20% had been treated with tipifarnib, of whom 18 were efficacy evaluable. The objective response rate among these evaluable patients was 50%; those patients that did not have an objective response did obtain a best overall response of stable disease. Progression-free survival on tipifarnib was 5.9 months versus 3.6 months on the patients' most recent prior therapy. Safety was evaluated in all 30 treated HNSCC patients, regardless of VAF. The most frequently observed treatment-emergent adverse events (TEAEs) of any grade observed in >10% of patients were hematological-related events (anemia, neutropenia, leukopenia, lymphopenia) and gastrointestinal disturbances (nausea). Three patients experienced TEAEs leading to tipifarnib discontinuation. All three events were not related to tipifarnib and possibly related to disease. Based on this encouraging clinical activity, an international, multi-center, open-label, single-arm, pivotal study of tipifarnib after failure of platinum-based therapy in recurrent or metastatic HNSCC with *HRAS* mutations, AIM-HN, is under way (NCT03719690). Furthermore, encouraging results in urothelial carcinoma and salivary gland tumors were also reported. Twenty-four percent of HRAS mutant metastatic urothelial carcinoma patients treated with tipifarnib experienced an objective response. In addition, of 13 patients with recurrent/metastatic salivary gland tumors (SGT) treated with tipifarnib, one experienced an objective response and an additional seven patients had stable disease as best response.

The recent completion of The Cancer Genome Atlas (TCGA) [41] has enabled the identification of patient populations harboring *HRAS* mutations that may benefit from tipifarnib therapy. Gilardi et al. performed a detailed analysis of genomic information in the TCGA database focused on revealing *HRAS* expression levels and mutational status in an array of cancer types [40]. The study showed that relatively few cancers harbor *HRAS* mutations, particularly thyroid cancer, pheochromocytoma and paraganglioma, and HNSCC, with HNSCC expressing the highest levels of *HRAS* transcripts. In agreement with previous findings, *HRAS* mutations are characterized, in most cases, by coincident loss-of-function mutations in caspase-8 and by the absence of *TP53* mutations. Moreover, *HRAS* mutant HNSCC cases are of low overall mutational burden and respond poorly to standard-of-care immuno-oncology therapies [41]. In summary, preclinical murine studies, in-depth oncogenic analyses, and ongoing clinical investigation in patients with mutant *HRAS* tumors may support tipifarnib as a novel precision therapeutic approach for HNSCC and other cancers.

2. HRAS Dependency: Role of Unmutated HRAS in Progression and Chemoresistance in HNSCC

Driver oncoproteins are commonly hyperactive forms of signaling molecules that regulate cellular proliferation and survival. This hyperactivity may be achieved by mutation leading to constitutive activation and/or by overexpression of the wild-type protein due to fusion with a highly expressed gene, genetic amplification or transcriptional dysregulation. Given that activating point mutations render the protein activity independent of upstream signaling, it is not surprising that mutations of a given tumor driver pack a greater oncogenic punch than either amplification or overexpression of the wild-type form. However, the protein need not be mutated to represent a valuable therapeutic target. Indeed, increasing preclinical and clinical data suggest that targeting wild-type oncoproteins has potential therapeutic value in the era of personalized medicine, particularly in the context of the combination regimens that are increasingly becoming the standard of care in cancer therapy [49].

Oncogene amplification and overexpression are common phenomena in solid tumors, particularly in SCCs. For example, *KRAS* is mutated in approximately 30% of cases of lung adenocarcinoma (ADC) in TCGA's PanCancer Atlas but amplified at a rate of only around 5%; in lung SCC, the relative frequencies are reversed (1% vs. 4%). Similarly, *EGFR* is mutated in twice as many lung ADCs as it is amplified, compared to a threefold excess of amplification vs. mutation in LSCC, where frequencies of high polysomy and amplification may be up to 40% [50]. *EGFR* is very rarely mutated in HNSCC but is amplified 10–30% of cases [51] and overexpressed at high frequency [52]. Perhaps the most compelling evidence for the importance of unmutated oncogenic driver proteins in SCCs is the approval and widespread use of the chimeric anti-EGFR antibody cetuximab as a standard of care treatment for HNSCC [53,54]. EGFR and MET are examples of receptor tyrosine kinases (RTK) that can become hyperactive through receptor clustering when overexpressed in HNSCC, but non-RTK oncogenes can also drive HNSCC, including *PIK3CA*, which is mutated and amplified at a higher prevalence, around 35%, in HNSCC [55], and the oncogenic chloride channel ANO1/TMEM16, a core element of the 11q13 amplicon, is found in a quarter of HNSCCs and more than half of ESCCs [56,57].

Despite—or perhaps because of—the high prevalence of *EGFR* amplification and overexpression in HNSCC, several clinical studies failed to demonstrate enhanced sensitivity to cetuximab in amplified or overexpressing populations [49,58]. Therefore, although cetuximab is the first and the only FDA-approved targeted therapy in HNSCC to date, the prescribing information makes no reference to EGFR. The picture is less clear in other SCCs: preclinical studies showed superior activity of cetuximab in *EGFR*-amplified and overexpressing esophageal SCC (ESCC) xenografts [59], and *EGFR*-amplified and overexpressing lung SCC patients responded better to gefitinib [49] and cetuximab and chemotherapy [54,60,61] than their EGFR^{low} counterparts. The FLEX trial compared chemotherapy (cisplatin and vinorelbine) with and without cetuximab in a cohort of first-line NSCLC patients, 35% of whom were SCC [61]. Addition of cetuximab to the regimen resulted in a 38% reduction in risk of death and a 2.3-month net increase in median survival among those with *EGFR* overexpression with no difference in overall survival (OS) among those with low *EGFR* expression [61]; but in a similar trial with a different cocktail of chemotherapeutics (paclitaxel and carboplatin), outcomes were not associated with EGFR mutation, increase in *EGFR* gene copy number, or EGFR protein [62].

To begin exploring the therapeutic potential of HRAS inhibition via farnesyltransferase inhibition beyond the HRAS mutant fraction of HNSCC, we reasoned that the biology of tumors driven by hyperactivity of wild-type oncoproteins is likely to resemble that of their corresponding mutant counterparts more than that of tumors with unrelated driver pathways. Intriguingly, several groups have reported that HRAS-mutant SCCs co-cluster in unbiased genomic and epigenomic profiling analyses. Indeed, genomic clustering suggests that HRAS mutations define a unique subset of HNSCC, characterized in most cases by coincident loss of function mutations in caspase 8 and enrichment for absence (near-mutual exclusivity) of TP53 mutations [40,55,63]. Furthermore, a recent systematic analysis of TCGA SCC cohorts by Campbell and colleagues reported that *HRAS*-mutant HNSCCs also cluster on the basis of copy number variations (CNVs, i.e. chromosomal alterations) and methylation pattern [64]. Closer inspection of TCGA PanCancer Atlas cohorts revealed that, although amplification at the *HRAS* locus is surprisingly rare, SCCs express significantly higher levels of HRAS than adenocarcinomas, and HRAS mRNA is overexpressed in around 30%, 25%, and 10% of cases of HNSCC, UC, and LSCC, respectively (Figure 1). The large majority of HRAS mutants are also found in the overexpressing population. Interestingly, the methylation cluster described in Campbell et al. is also significantly enriched for HRAS-overexpressing HNSCC cases, suggesting that HRAS expression levels could be used as a biomarker to explore the potential role of the wild-type form of the oncoprotein in HNSCC progression and drug resistance.

We tested tipifarnib (80 mg/kg, BID) as a single agent in a panel of around 20 *HRAS* mutant and wild-type HNSCC patient-derived xenograft (PDX) models with mixed results. As reported previously [40], tipifarnib was highly active in the *HRAS* mutant setting and displayed weak activity in the majority of *HRAS* wild-type models, but we observed unexpectedly robust inhibition of tumor growth in a minority of *HRAS* wild-type cases, all of which expressed high levels of the *HRAS* gene (Figure 2). These hints of activity, while encouraging, were sporadic and variable in nature and did not extend to tumor regression, indicating that these tumors could tolerate HRAS depletion in isolation, but might also be rendered hypersensitive to other stressors.

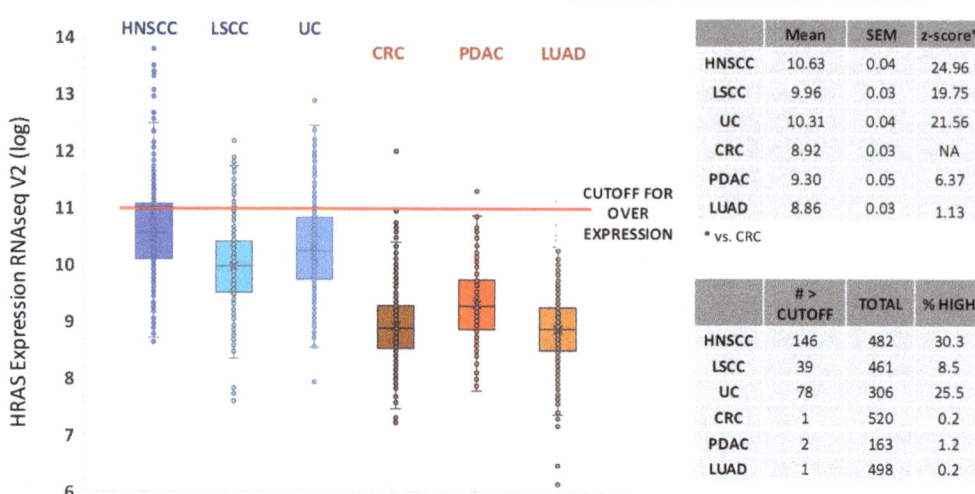

Figure 1. HRAS is overexpressed in squamous cell carcinomas. Data from TCGA PanCancer Atlas accessed at http://www.cbioportal.org/ (accessed on: 9 November 2020. Comparison of HRAS mRNA expression between the major adenocarcinomas, colorectal (CRC), pancreatic (PDAC), and lung (LUAD), and squamous cell carcinomas of the head and neck (HNSCC), lung (LSCC), and urothelium (UC). * vs. CRC.

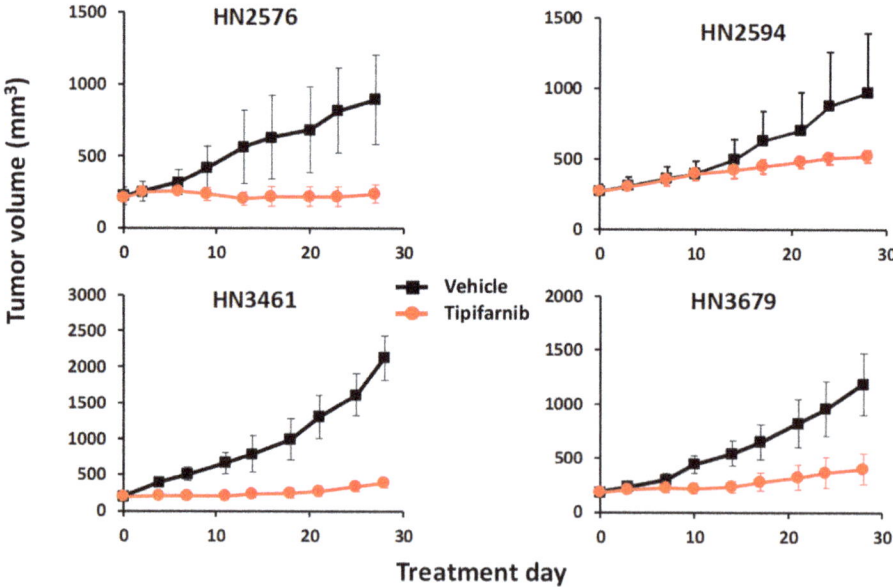

Figure 2. Some HRAS-overexpressing HNSCC PDX models are sensitive to tipifarnib. BALB/c nu/nu or SCID mice were inoculated subcutaneously with 2–3 mm tumor fragments, the PDX were allowed to establish to 250–350 mm^3, the animals were randomized into groups of three and treated orally BID with vehicle or tipifarnib (60 mg/kg for SCID, 80 mg/kg for nu/nu) for 25–30 days. Tumor volumes were measured twice weekly in two dimensions using a caliper, and the volume was expressed in mm3 using the formula: $V = (L \times W \times W)/2$, where V is tumor volume, L is tumor length (the longest tumor dimension), and W is tumor width (the longest tumor dimension perpendicular to L).

With the notable exception of Herceptin and other HER2 antagonists, few drugs directed against non-mutated oncoprotein targets have proven effective as single agents [43], but it is more likely that clinically-actionable dependencies on overexpressed wild-type drivers will emerge in the context of synthetic lethal interactions with other therapies. Indeed, cetuximab demonstrated enhanced activity in EGFR-amplified HNSCC PDX models in combination with fractionated irradiation [65]. Our preliminary data in HNSCC models spurred interest in a possible role of wild-type HRAS in innate resistance to standard-of-care drugs such as cisplatin and cetuximab as well as targeted agents in clinical development in HNSCC, including CDK4/6 inhibitors and PI3K pathway drugs. As shown in Figure 3, tipifarnib co-treatment sensitized the HRAS-overexpressing HN2594 PDX model to all four classes of drugs, inducing consistent regressions in all combination regimens, despite only the CDK4/6 inhibitor palbociclib being significantly active as a single agent in this experiment. In expanded tests, tipifarnib enhanced cisplatin activity in 3/12 HRAS wild-type models examined, all of which overexpressed the HRAS gene, as described previously [66]. Tipifarnib also increased tumor growth inhibition with palbociclib in the majority of HRAS^{high} models tested, but cetuximab was highly active in all four PDX studied, precluding assessment of this combination in these models; previous work suggests that HRAS signaling is a key driver of cetuximab resistance in experimental models and in the clinic [61]. In a third study focused on PI3K pathway combinations, synergy was noted with both the mTOR kinase inhibitor TAK-228 (sapanisertib) and the PI3Kα inhibitor BYL-719 (alpelisib), including in *HRAS* or *PIK3CA* mutant (20% of HNSCC) [67], *PIK3CA*-amplified (15%) [68] or HRAS-overexpressing (30%) (Figure 3) models, and this combination has previously been shown to be synergistic in CDX systems [69], suggesting that simultaneous blockade of these two prominent oncogenic pathways could offer potential benefit in a broad population of HNSCC patients.

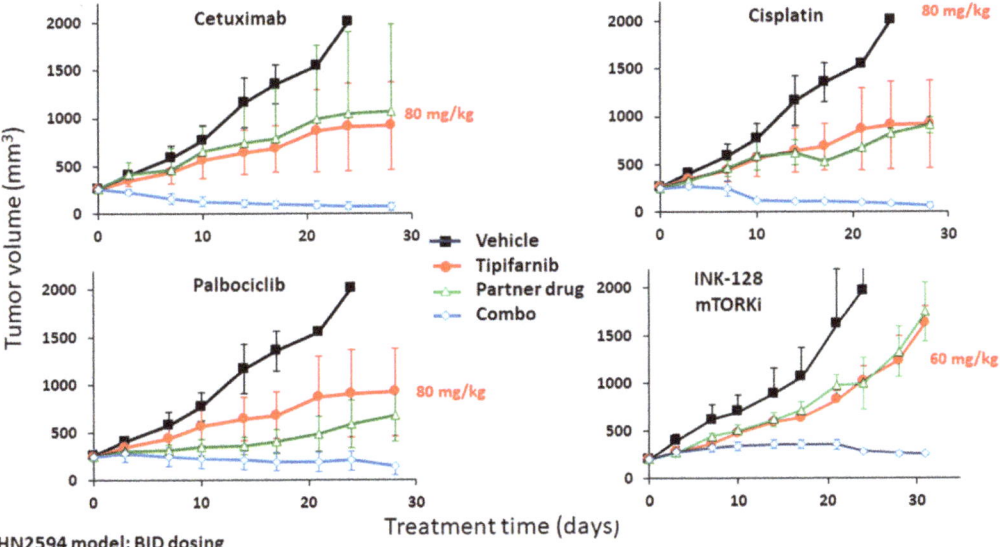

Figure 3. Tipifarnib displays additive or synergistic anti-tumor activity with a variety of partner drugs in HRAS-overexpressing patient-derived xenograft (PDX) models. BALB/c nu/nu or SCID mice were inoculated subcutaneously with 2–3 mm tumor fragments, the PDX were allowed to establish to 250–350 mm^3 and the animals were randomized into groups of three before being dosed with vehicle or tipifarnib (60–80 mg/kg BID as labeled above) alone or in combination with cetuximab (1 mg/mouse IP QW), cisplatin (5 mg/kg Q3D PO), palbociclib (40 mg/kg QD PO), or INK-128 (2 mg/kg QD PO).

In summary, extensive studies in panels of PDX models indicate that both mutant and overexpressed HRAS contribute significantly to the proliferation, survival, and innate drug resistance of HNSCC cells in vivo. HRAS is the predominant RAS isoform in squamous epithelial cells and the SCCs derived from them [55] and so may play a wider role. Although HRAS activity has previously been reported to contribute to most hallmarks of cancer [40] and to drive clinical resistance to cetuximab [42,43], it is also likely that HRAS-independent mechanisms contribute, at least in part, to the antitumor activity of tipifarnib in HNSCC models. Dozens of proteins are dependent upon farnesylation for membrane insertion and function [70]. In the next section, we explore the potential of farnesyltransferase inhibition to anchor combination regimens through mechanisms independent of HRAS.

3. Combination Approaches with FTIs in SCCs and Other Solid Tumors

Although RAS is known to play a key role in innate resistance to a variety of therapeutics used in SCCs, including platinum-based chemotherapy and anti-EGFR antibodies [43,66], and HRAS inactivation sensitizes HNSCC PDX tumors to a range of drugs in mice (Figure 3), it has been established that much of the documented antineoplastic activity of FTIs is mediated by effects on proteins other than RAS [71,72]. For example, several lines of evidence suggest that RHOB farnesylation may have contextual roles in tumor progression and survival. RHOB expression in Rat1 cells induces proliferation, which can be inhibited by FTIs [73]. RHOB has also been shown to be a direct regulator of phosphatase 2A (PP2A) activity via recruitment of the B55 subunit [74]. During lung cancer progression, downregulation of RHOB may inhibit PP2A activity, leading to activation of the Akt1-Trio-Rac1 axis, triggering cell migration and invasion. Furthermore, an AKT-dependent mechanism has been suggested to underlie RHOB-driven resistance to EGFR inhibitors in EGFR-mutant NSCLC models [75]. Another potential target of FTIs is RHEB (RAS homolog enriched in brain), a GTPase with two isoforms (RHEB1 and RHEB2) that are commonly upregulated in transformed cells and human cancer cell lines. RHEB binds and activates the mechanistic target of rapamycin (mTOR), a regulator of tumor cell growth, survival, and metabolism [76,77]. It is thought that mTOR is activated via farnesylation-dependent transient interactions of RHEB with the mTORC1 complex in lysosomal membranes [78]. Human RHEB1 and RHEB2 have been shown in vitro to be substrates for FTase, and treatment of cells with FTIs inhibits RHEB prenylation. Basso et al. demonstrated that treatment of MCF-7 cells with lonafarnib inhibited RHEB farnesylation, resulting in inhibition of DNA synthesis and S6 kinase activation. Furthermore, it was found that lonafarnib enhanced tamoxifen- and taxane-driven apoptosis, supporting the combination of FTIs with standard-of-care agents. RHEB-mTOR signaling has also been implicated in resistance to antineoplastic therapies [79]; thus, combination approaches may bypass these resistance mechanisms [80]. Recent findings by Mahkov et al. demonstrated that 786-O renal carcinoma cells expressing prenylation-incompetent RHEB display robust apoptosis in response to sunitinib treatment [81]. Moreover, the investigators examined the anti-tumor effect of sunitinib in combination with lonafarnib using mice bearing clear cell renal cell carcinoma (ccRCC) xenograft tumors. Monotherapy with either sunitinib or lonafarnib showed a moderate decrease in tumor growth; however, co-administration resulted in impressive reductions in tumor volume. Thus, FTIs may offer a means to circumvent sunitinib resistance, perhaps through prevention of RHEB localization to lysosomal membranes and subsequent downstream activation of mTOR signaling.

Several additional families of proteins with functional roles in proliferation, invasion and other hallmarks of cancer are dependent upon farnesylation for appropriate intracellular localization and activity. Centromere protein-E (CENP-)E and CENP-F have also been shown to be FTI targets. CENP-E is a centromere-associated kinesin motor protein that functions in microtubule attachment to kinetochores, which is required for the separation of sister chromatids during mitosis [82,83]. CENP-F is a cell cycle-regulated passenger protein which also has mitotic function [84]. Both CENP-E and CENP-F are farnesylated proteins whose prenylation is inhibited by FTI treatment [85], subsequently preventing CENP-E association with microtubules and reducing levels of CENP-F at the kinetochores [85,86]. Similarly, the PRL family of protein tyrosine phosphatases (PTPS), also known as PTP-CAAX proteins, are a unique subfamily of PTPs that regulate cell growth and mitosis and have been shown to be upregulated in numerous human tumor cell lines and implicated in progression of several tumor types [87–89]. The PRL family includes three members, all of which are farnesylated. Al three forms traffic to the plasma membrane in transfected CHO cells, localization of which is inhibited by FTIs [90].

Some farnesylated substrates carry unknown significance for cancer but may still provide clinical utility, such as the DnaJ homologs which serve as co-chaperones and stimulate the ATPase activity of Hsp70, a cancer-associated protein [91]. One homolog, HDJ2, is a farnesylated protein whose prenylation status is used as a pharmacodynamic (PD) biomarker for FTase inhibition in clinical trials [92]. The functional significance of HDJ2 farnesylation remains unclear. Nuclear lamins (e.g., lamin A, lamin B), proteins that are required for nuclear envelope assembly, were some of the first proteins shown to be prenylated [93]. Similar to HDJ2, the functional consequence of lamin prenylation is unknown but may assist in the targeting of prelamins to the nuclear membrane. A mutation in *prelamin A* occurs in children with Hutchinson-Gilford progeria syndrome (HGPS), a debilitating and fatal disease characterized by premature aging. FTIs have been shown to reverse the abnormal nuclear phenotype in cells derived from HGPS patients [94], and the FTI lonafarnib was recently approved for therapy of this devastating rare disease [95].

In some instances, farnesyltransferase inhibition has been found to mediate antitumor activity, but the farnesylated substrate underlying the effect remains to be confirmed. For instance, tipifarnib and other FTIs have been suggested to act as antiangiogenic agents in several tumor types including HNSCC [40,46], but the mechanisms are yet to be elucidated [44] and may be hard to delineate from indirect downstream consequences of inhibiting another target, such as HRAS [40]. Similarly, FTIs have been shown to rapidly trigger the production of reactive oxygen species (ROS) [96]. Though the mechanism of ROS generation remains unclear, the consequences include DNA damage responses, such as activation of DNA repair proteins and induction of RHOB [96]. In turn, RHOB may sensitize cancer cells to DNA damage-induced apoptosis following genotoxic stress [97]. FTIs may also offer the potential to modulate antitumor immunity. RAS-MAPK signaling drives expression of the *CD274* gene leading to PDL-1 overexpression [98] but also downregulates MHC Class I expression, reducing immunogenicity and undermining the effectiveness of immune checkpoint inhibitors [99]. Therefore, FTI treatment might enhance responsiveness of HRAS-dependent SCCs to immunotherapy.

CXCL12 (or SDF1) is a potent immunoregulatory chemokine and CXCL12-CXCR4 signaling is associated with resistance to immunotherapy in HNSCC [100]. Intriguingly, we have recently reported that CXCL12 production by stromal fibroblasts, the predominant CXCL12-producing cell in solid tumors, can be inhibited by tipifarnib in vitro [101]. Further studies are ongoing in our laboratory to characterize this novel FTI activity and the potential of FTIs to enhance immunotherapy in SCC models. CXCL12 also shows promise as a biomarker guiding FTI therapy in T-cell lymphoma patients. Recently, the effect of tipifarnib on the CXCL12 axis was investigated in an open-label, Phase 2 study in relapsed or refractory peripheral T-cell lymphoma [102]. Tumor gene expression data were available for 12 of the 18 evaluable patients. Five of those patients had elevated CXCL12 expression and experienced tumor size reductions and >6-month median time to progress following tipifarnib treatment. Thus, tipifarnib may be a promising therapeutic approach in this patient population.

It is likely that protein farnesylation plays an actionable role in many oncogenic signaling pathways. Indeed, there are hundreds of proteins with CAAX motifs that are potentially farnesylated [72], although the true number of farnesylation-dependent proteins is probably several dozen in most cell types [70]. Given this pleiotropy, it is perhaps counterintuitive that tipifarnib has been evaluated in more than 5000 patients and has been generally well-tolerated with a clearly delineated toxicity profile when used at doses that sharply reduce farnesylation of several PD biomarkers in vivo [92]. Several mitigating factors, including redundancy with farnesylation-independent orthologs or collateral signaling pathways, varying sensitivity to FTase activity between substrates [70], and pharmacokinetic compartmentalization, may render FTIs more selective in vivo, but mounting evidence supports the notion that farnesylated target oncoproteins including HRAS, RHEB, and RHOB could be exploited as part of FTI-anchored combination regimens in SCCs and a range of other tumor types.

4. Conclusions

In summary, preclinical murine studies, in-depth oncogenic analyses, and ongoing clinical investigation in patients with mutant HRAS tumors may support tipifarnib as a novel precision therapeutic approach for HNSCC and other cancers. Recent advances in genomic and cellular studies have led to the identification of HRAS mutations as drivers of tumor growth in a subset of HNSCC. These mutations in an oncogene that is uniquely sensitive to inhibition of farnesylation appear to sensitize the tumors to farnesyl transferase inhibitors such as tipifarnib, as supported by animal models and ongoing clinical trials. In addition, preclinical studies in PDX models overexpressing HRAS have demonstrated that tipifarnib sensitizes these tumors to several drugs in clinical use in SCCs, suggesting that the benefit of tipifarnib may be extended to include those patients with HRAS overexpressing tumors when used in combination with drugs such as cetuximab, alpelisib, and cisplatin. Furthermore, inhibition of other farnesylated proteins, such as RHEB and RHOB, may help overcome resistance to standard therapies in SCCs and additional tumor types.

Author Contributions: M.L. provided clinical data content and overview of tipifarnib as in Section 1; F.B. provided content and overview of Section 2; S.M. and L.K. provided content and overview of Section 3 and the conclusions, as well as final editing. All authors have read and agreed to the published version of the manuscript.

Funding: This was supported by research funding from Kura Oncology.

Acknowledgments: JetPub Scientific Communications LLC, supported by Kura Oncology, Inc., assisted in the preparation of this manuscript, in accordance with Good Publication Practice (GPP3) guidelines.

Conflicts of Interest: All authors are full-time employees of Kura Oncology.

References

1. Stokoe, D.; Macdonald, S.G.; Cadwallader, K.; Symons, M.; Hancock, J.F. Activation of Raf as a result of recruitment to the plasma membrane. *Science* **1994**, *264*, 1463–1467. [CrossRef] [PubMed]
2. Keely, P.J.; Westwick, J.K.; Whitehead, I.P.; Der, C.J.; Parise, L.V. Cdc42 and Rac1 induce integrin-mediated cell motility and invasiveness through PI(3)K. *Nature* **1997**, *390*, 632–636. [CrossRef] [PubMed]
3. Kennedy, S.G.; Wagner, A.J.; Conzen, S.D.; Jordán, J.; Bellacosa, A.; Tsichlis, P.N.; Hay, N. The PI 3-kinase/Akt signaling pathway delivers an anti-apoptotic signal. *Genes Dev.* **1997**, *11*, 701–713. [CrossRef] [PubMed]
4. Gille, H.; Downward, J. Multiple Ras effector pathways contribute to G1 cell cycle progression. *J. Biol. Chem.* **1999**, *274*, 22033–22040. [CrossRef]
5. Keely, P.J.; Rusyn, E.V.; Cox, A.D.; Parise, L.V. R-Ras signals through specific integrin α cytoplasmic domains to promote migration and invasion of breast epithelial cells. *J. Cell Biol.* **1999**, *145*, 1077–1088. [CrossRef]
6. Rowinsky, E.K.; Windle, J.J.; Von Hoff, D.D. Ras protein farnesyltransferase: A strategic target for anticancer therapeutic development. *J. Clin. Oncol.* **1999**, *17*, 3631–3652. [CrossRef]
7. Adjei, A.A. Blocking oncogenic ras signaling in cancer. *Rev. J. Natl. Cancer Inst.* **2001**, *93*, 1062–1074. [CrossRef]
8. Bos, J.L. Ras oncogenes in human cancer: A review. *Cancer Res.* **1989**, *49*, 4682–4689.
9. Moore, A.R.; Rosenberg, S.C.; McCormick, F.; Malek, S. RAS-targeted therapies: Is the undruggable drugged? *Nat. Rev. Drug Discov.* **2020**, *19*, 533–552. [CrossRef]
10. Mulcahy, L.S.; Smith, M.R.; Stacey, D.W. Requirement for ras proto-oncogene function during serum-stimulated growth of NIH 3T3 cells. *Nature* **1985**, *313*, 241–243. [CrossRef]
11. Shirasawa, S.; Furuse, M.; Yokoyama, N.; Sasazuki, T. Altered growth of human colon cancer cell lines disrupted at activated Ki-ras. *Science* **1993**, *260*, 85–88. [CrossRef]
12. Prior, I.A.; Hancock, J.F. Compartmentalization of Ras proteins. *J. Cell Sci.* **2001**, *114*, 1603–1608. [CrossRef]

13. Hancock, J.F.; Paterson, H.; Marshall, C.J. A polybasic domain or palmitoylation is required in addition to the CAAX motif to localize p21ras to the plasma membrane. *Cell* **1990**, *63*, 133–139. [CrossRef]
14. Reiss, Y.; Goldstein, J.L.; Seabra, M.C.; Casey, P.J.; Brown, M.S. Inhibition of purified p21ras farnesyl:protein transferase by Cys-AAX tetrapeptides. *Cell* **1990**, *62*, 81–88. [CrossRef]
15. James, G.L.; Goldstein, J.L.; Brown, M.S.; Rawson, T.E.; Somers, T.C.; McDowell, R.S.; Crowley, C.W.; Lucas, B.K.; Levinson, A.D.; Marsters, J.C. Benzodiazepine peptidomimetics: Potent inhibitors of Ras farnesylation in animal cells. *Science* **1993**, *260*, 1937–1942. [CrossRef] [PubMed]
16. Qian, Y.; Blaskovich, M.A.; Saleem, M.; Seong, C.M.; Wathen, S.P.; Hamilton, A.D.; Sebti, S.M. Design and structural requirements of potent peptidomimetic inhibitors of p21(ras) farnesyltransferase. *J. Biol. Chem.* **1994**, *269*, 12410–12413. [CrossRef]
17. Vogt, A.; Qian, Y.; Blaskovich, M.A.; Fossum, R.D.; Hamilton, A.D.; Sebti, S.M. A non-peptide mimetic of Ras-CAAX: Selective inhibition of farnesyltransferase and Ras processing. *J. Biol. Chem.* **1995**, *270*, 660–664. [CrossRef]
18. Nigam, M.; Seong, C.M.; Qian, Y.; Hamilton, A.D.; Sebti, S.M. Potent inhibition of human tumor p21(ras) farnesyltransferase by A1A2- lacking p21(ras) CA1A2X peptidomimetics. *J. Biol. Chem.* **1993**, *268*, 20695–20698. [CrossRef]
19. Long, S.B.; Hancock, P.J.; Kral, A.M.; Hellinga, H.W.; Beese, L.S. The crystal structure of human protein farnesyltransferase reveals the basis for inhibition by CaaX tetrapeptides and their mimetics. *Proc. Natl. Acad. Sci. USA* **2001**, *98*, 12948–12953. [CrossRef]
20. End, D.W.; Smets, G.; Todd, A.V.; Applegate, T.L.; Fuery, C.J.; Angibaud, P.; Venet, M.; Sanz, G.; Poignet, H.; Skrzat, S.; et al. Characterization of the antitumor effects of the selective farnesyl protein transferase inhibitor R115777 in vivo and in vitro. *Cancer Res.* **2001**, *61*, 131–137.
21. Crul, M.; de Klerk, G.J.; Swart, M.; van't Veer, L.J.; de Jong, D.; Boerrigter, L.; Palmer, P.A.; Bol, C.J.; Tan, H.; de Gast, G.C.; et al. Phase I clinical and pharmacologic study of chronic oral administration of the farnesyl protein transferase inhibitor R115777 in advanced cancer. *J. Clin. Oncol.* **2002**, *20*, 2726–2735. [CrossRef]
22. Zujewski, J.; Horak, I.D.; Bol, C.J.; Woestenborghs, R.; Bowden, C.; End, D.W.; Piotrovsky, V.K.; Chiao, J.; Belly, R.T.; Todd, A.; et al. Phase I and pharmacokinetic study of farnesyl protein transferase inhibitor R115777 in advanced cancer. *J. Clin. Oncol.* **2000**, *18*, 927–941. [CrossRef]
23. Cohen, S.J.; Ho, L.; Ranganathan, S.; Abbruzzese, J.L.; Alpaugh, R.K.; Beard, M.; Lewis, N.L.; McLaughlin, S.; Rogatko, A.; Perez-Ruixo, J.J.; et al. Phase II and pharmacodynamic study of the farnesyltransferase inhibitor R115777 as initial therapy in patients with metastatic pancreatic adenocarcinoma. *J. Clin. Oncol.* **2003**, *21*, 1301–1306. [CrossRef]
24. Alsina, M.; Fonseca, R.; Wilson, E.F.; Belle, A.N.; Gerbino, E.; Price-Troska, T.; Overton, R.M.; Ahmann, G.; Bruzek, L.M.; Adjei, A.A.; et al. Farnesyltransferase inhibitor tipifarnib is well tolerated, induces stabilization of disease, and inhibits farnesylation and oncogenic/tumor survival pathways in patients with advanced multiple myeloma. *Blood* **2004**, *103*, 3271–3277. [CrossRef]
25. Adjei, A.A.; Mauer, A.; Bruzek, L.; Marks, R.S.; Hillman, S.; Geyer, S.; Hanson, L.J.; Wright, J.J.; Erlichman, C.; Kaufmann, S.H.; et al. Phase II study of the farnesyl transferase inhibitor R115777 in patients with advanced non-small-cell lung cancer. *J. Clin. Oncol.* **2003**, *21*, 1760–1766. [CrossRef]
26. Rao, S.; Cunningham, D.; de Gramont, A.; Scheithauer, W.; Smakal, M.; Humblet, Y.; Kourteva, G.; Iveson, T.; Andre, T.; Dostalova, J.; et al. Phase III double-blind placebo-controlled study of farnesyl transferase inhibitor R115777 in patients with refractory advanced colorectal cancer. *J. Clin. Oncol.* **2004**, *22*, 3950–3957. [CrossRef]
27. Van Cutsem, E.; van de Velde, H.; Karasek, P.; Oettle, H.; Vervenne, W.L.; Szawlowski, A.; Schoffski, P.; Post, S.; Verslype, C.; Neumann, H.; et al. Phase III trial of gemcitabine plus tipifarnib compared with gemcitabine plus placebo in advanced pancreatic cancer. *J. Clin. Oncol.* **2004**, *22*, 1430–1438. [CrossRef] [PubMed]
28. Zhang, F.L.; Kirschmeier, P.; Carr, D.; James, L.; Bond, R.W.; Wang, L.; Patton, R.; Windsor, W.T.; Syto, R.; Zhang, R.; et al. Characterization of Ha-Ras, N-Ras, Ki-Ras4A, and Ki-Ras4B as in vitro substrates for farnesyl protein transferase and geranylgeranyl protein transferase type I. *J. Biol. Chem.* **1997**, *272*, 10232–10239. [CrossRef] [PubMed]
29. Whyte, D.B.; Kirschmeier, P.; Hockenberry, T.N.; Nunez-Oliva, I.; James, L.; Catino, J.J.; Bishop, W.R.; Pai, J.K. K- and N-Ras are geranylgeranylated in cells treated with farnesyl protein transferase inhibitors. *J. Biol. Chem.* **1997**, *272*, 14459–14464. [CrossRef] [PubMed]
30. Fukahori, M.; Yoshida, A.; Hayashi, H.; Yoshihara, M.; Matsukuma, S.; Sakuma, Y.; Koizume, S.; Okamoto, N.; Kondo, T.; Masuda, M.; et al. The associations between ras mutations and clinical characteristics in follicular thyroid tumors: New insights from a single center and a large patient cohort. *Thyroid* **2012**, *22*, 683–689. [CrossRef]
31. Volante, M.; Rapa, I.; Gandhi, M.; Bussolati, G.; Giachino, D.; Papotti, M.; Nikiforov, Y.E. RAS mutations are the predominant molecular alteration in poorly differentiated thyroid carcinomas and bear prognostic impact. *J. Clin. Endocrinol. Metab.* **2009**, *94*, 4735–4741. [CrossRef]
32. Ricarte-Filho, J.C.; Ryder, M.; Chitale, D.A.; Rivera, M.; Heguy, A.; Ladanyi, M.; Janakiraman, M.; Solit, D.; Knauf, J.A.; Tuttle, R.M.; et al. Mutational profile of advanced primary and metastatic radioactive iodine-refractory thyroid cancers reveals distinct pathogenetic roles for BRAF, PIK3CA, and AKT1. *Cancer Res.* **2009**, *69*, 4885–4893. [CrossRef]
33. Moura, M.M.; Cavaco, B.M.; Pinto, A.E.; Leite, V. High prevalence of RAS mutations in RET-negative sporadic medullary thyroid carcinomas. *J. Clin. Endocrinol. Metab.* **2011**, *96*, 863–868. [CrossRef]
34. Agrawal, N.; Frederick, M.J.; Pickering, C.R.; Bettegowda, C.; Chang, K.; Li, R.J.; Fakhry, C.; Xie, T.X.; Zhang, J.; Wang, J.; et al. Exome sequencing of head and neck squamous cell carcinoma reveals inactivating mutations in NOTCH1. *Science* **2011**, *333*, 1154–1157. [CrossRef] [PubMed]

35. Untch, B.R.; Dos Anjos, V.; Garcia-Rendueles, M.E.R.; Knauf, J.A.; Krishnamoorthy, G.P.; Saqcena, M.; Bhanot, U.K.; Socci, N.D.; Ho, A.L.; Ghossein, R.; et al. Tipifarnib inhibits HRAS-driven dedifferentiated thyroid cancers. *Cancer Res.* **2018**, *78*, 4642–4657. [CrossRef]
36. de Bruin, E.C.; Cowell, C.; Warne, P.H.; Jiang, M.; Saunders, R.E.; Melnick, M.A.; Gettinger, S.; Walther, Z.; Wurtz, A.; Heynen, G.J.; et al. Reduced NF1 expression confers resistance to EGFR inhibition in lung cancer. *Cancer Discov.* **2014**, *4*, 606–619. [CrossRef] [PubMed]
37. Whittaker, S.R.; Theurillat, J.P.; Van Allen, E.; Wagle, N.; Hsiao, J.; Cowley, G.S.; Schadendorf, D.; Root, D.E.; Garraway, L.A. A genome-Scale RNA interference screen implicates NF1 loss in resistance to RAF inhibition. *Cancer Discov.* **2013**, *3*, 351–362. [CrossRef]
38. Beauchamp, E.M.; Woods, B.A.; Dulak, A.M.; Tan, L.; Xu, C.; Gray, N.S.; Bass, A.J.; Wong, K.K.; Meyerson, M.; Hammerman, P.S. Acquired resistance to dasatinib in lung cancer cell lines conferred by DDR2 gatekeeper mutation and NF1 loss. *Mol. Cancer Ther.* **2014**, *13*, 475–482. [CrossRef] [PubMed]
39. Johannessen, C.M.; Johnson, L.A.; Piccioni, F.; Townes, A.; Frederick, D.T.; Donahue, M.K.; Narayan, R.; Flaherty, K.T.; Wargo, J.A.; Root, D.E.; et al. A melanocyte lineage program confers resistance to MAP kinase pathway inhibition. *Nature* **2013**, *504*, 138–142. [CrossRef]
40. Gilardi, M.; Wang, Z.; Proietto, M.; Chilla, A.; Calleja-Valera, J.L.; Goto, Y.; Vanoni, M.; Janes, M.R.; Mikulski, Z.; Gualberto, A.; et al. Tipifarnib as a precision therapy for HRAS-mutant head and neck squamous cell carcinomas. *Mol. Cancer Ther.* **2020**, *19*, 1784–1796. [CrossRef]
41. Hoadley, K.A.; Yau, C.; Hinoue, T.; Wolf, D.M.; Lazar, A.J.; Drill, E.; Shen, R.; Taylor, A.M.; Cherniack, A.D.; Thorsson, V.; et al. Cell-of-origin patterns dominate the molecular classification of 10,000 tumors from 33 types of cancer. *Cell* **2018**, *173*, 291–304.e6. [CrossRef]
42. Braig, F.; Voigtlaender, M.; Schieferdecker, A.; Busch, C.J.; Laban, S.; Grob, T.; Kriegs, M.; Knecht, R.; Bokemeyer, C.; Binder, M. Liquid biopsy monitoring uncovers acquired RAS-mediated resistance to cetuximab in a substantial proportion of patients with head and neck squamous cell carcinoma. *Oncotarget* **2016**, *7*, 42988–42995. [CrossRef] [PubMed]
43. Rampias, T.; Giagini, A.; Siolos, S.; Matsuzaki, H.; Sasaki, C.; Scorilas, A.; Psyrri, A. RAS/PI3K crosstalk and cetuximab resistance in head and neck squamous cell carcinoma. *Clin. Cancer Res.* **2014**, *20*, 2933–2946. [CrossRef] [PubMed]
44. Scott, A.N.; Hetheridge, C.; Reynolds, A.R.; Nayak, V.; Hodivala-Dilke, K.; Mellor, H. Farnesyltransferase inhibitors target multiple endothelial cell functions in angiogenesis. *Angiogenesis* **2008**, *11*, 337–346. [CrossRef]
45. Han, J.Y.; Oh, S.H.; Morgillo, F.; Myers, J.N.; Kim, E.; Hong, W.K.; Lee, H.Y. Hypoxia-inducible factor 1α and antiangiogenic activity of farnesyltransferase inhibitor SCH66336 in human aerodigestive tract cancer. *J. Natl. Cancer Inst.* **2005**, *97*, 1272–1286. [CrossRef]
46. Oh, S.H.; Kim, W.Y.; Kim, J.H.; Younes, M.N.; El-Naggar, A.K.; Myers, J.N.; Kies, M.; Cohen, P.; Khuri, F.; Hong, W.K.; et al. Identification of insulin-like growth factor binding protein-3 as a farnesyl transferase inhibitor SCH66336-induced negative regulator of angiogenesis in head and neck squamous cell carcinoma. *Clin. Cancer Res.* **2006**, *12*, 653–661. [CrossRef]
47. Kiessling, M.; Curioni Fontecedro, A.; Samaras, P.; Scharl, M.; Rogler, G. Mutant HRAS as novel target for MEK and mTOR inhibitors. *J. Clin. Oncol.* **2015**, *33*, 11082. [CrossRef]
48. Ho, A.L.; Hanna, G.J.; Scholz, C.R.; Gualberto, A.; Park, S.H. Preliminary activity of tipifarnib in tumors of the head and neck, salivary gland and urothelial tract with HRAS mutations. *J. Clin. Oncol.* **2020**, *38*, 6504. [CrossRef]
49. Takano, T.; Ohe, Y.; Sakamoto, H.; Tsuta, K.; Matsuno, Y.; Tateishi, U.; Yamamoto, S.; Nokihara, H.; Yamamoto, N.; Sekine, I.; et al. Epidermal growth factor receptor gene mutations and increased copy numbers predict gefitinib sensitivity in patients with recurrent non-small-cell lung cancer. *J. Clin. Oncol.* **2005**, *23*, 6829–6837. [CrossRef] [PubMed]
50. Smrdel, U.; Kovač, V. Erlotinib in previously treated non-small-cell lung cancer. *Radiol. Oncol.* **2006**, *40*. [CrossRef]
51. Temam, S.; Kawaguchi, H.; El-Naggar, A.K.; Jelinek, J.; Tang, H.; Liu, D.D.; Lang, W.; Issa, J.P.; Lee, J.J.; Mao, L. Epidermal growth factor receptor copy number alterations correlate with poor clinical outcome in patients with head and neck squamous cancer. *J. Clin. Oncol.* **2007**, *25*, 2164–2170. [CrossRef] [PubMed]
52. Hansen, A.R.; Siu, L.L. Epidermal growth factor receptor targeting in head and neck cancer: Have we been just skimming the surface? *J. Clin. Oncol.* **2013**, *31*, 1381–1383. [CrossRef] [PubMed]
53. Byeon, H.K.; Ku, M.; Yang, J. Beyond EGFR inhibition: Multilateral combat strategies to stop the progression of head and neck cancer. *Exp. Mol. Med.* **2019**, *51*, 1–14. [CrossRef] [PubMed]
54. Juergens, R.A.; Bratman, S.V.; Tsao, M.S.; Laurie, S.A.; Sara Kuruvilla, M.; Razak, A.R.A.; Hansen, A.R. Biology and patterns of response to EGFR-inhibition in squamous cell cancers of the lung and head & neck. *Cancer Treat. Rev.* **2017**, *54*, 43–57. [PubMed]
55. Cancer genome atlas network comprehensive genomic characterization of head and neck squamous cell carcinomas. *Nature* **2015**, *517*, 576–582. [CrossRef] [PubMed]
56. Kulkarni, S.; Bill, A.; Godse, N.R.; Khan, N.I.; Kass, J.I.; Kemp, C.; Davis, K.; Bertrand, C.A.; Vyas, A.R.; Douglas, E.; et al. TMEM16A/ANO1 suppression improves response to antibody-mediated targeted therapy of EGFR and HER2/ERBB2. *Genes Chromosomes Cancer* **2017**, *56*, 460–471. [CrossRef]
57. Hermida-Prado, F.; Menéndez, S.; Albornoz-Afanasiev, P.; Granda-Diaz, R.; Álvarez-Teijeiro, S.; Villaronga, M.; Allonca, E.; Alonso-Durán, L.; León, X.; Alemany, L.; et al. Distinctive expression and amplification of genes at 11q13 in relation to HPV status with impact on survival in head and neck cancer patients. *J. Clin. Med.* **2018**, *7*, 501. [CrossRef]

58. Rabinowits, G.; Haddad, R.I. Overcoming resistance to EGFR inhibitor in head and neck cancer: A review of the literature. *Oral Oncol.* **2012**, *48*, 1085–1089. [CrossRef]
59. Zhu, H.; Wang, C.; Wang, J.; Chen, D.; Deng, J.; Deng, J.; Fan, J.; Badakhshi, H.; Huang, X.; Zhang, L.; et al. A subset of esophageal squamous cell carcinoma patient-derived xenografts respond to cetuximab, which is predicted by high EGFR expression and amplification. *J. Thorac. Dis.* **2018**, *10*, 5328–5338. [CrossRef]
60. Bonomi, P.D.; Gandara, D.; Hirsch, F.R.; Kerr, K.M.; Obasaju, C.; Paz-Ares, L.; Bellomo, C.; Bradley, J.D.; Bunn, P.A.; Culligan, M.; et al. Predictive biomarkers for response to EGFR-directed monoclonal antibodies for advanced squamous cell lung cancer. *Ann. Oncol.* **2018**, *29*, 1701–1709. [CrossRef]
61. Pirker, R.; Pereira, J.R.; Von Pawel, J.; Krzakowski, M.; Ramlau, R.; Park, K.; De Marinis, F.; Eberhardt, W.E.E.; Paz-Ares, L.; Störkel, S.; et al. EGFR expression as a predictor of survival for first-line chemotherapy plus cetuximab in patients with advanced non-small-cell lung cancer: Analysis of data from the phase 3 FLEX study. *Lancet Oncol.* **2012**, *13*, 33–42. [CrossRef]
62. Khambata-Ford, S.; Harbison, C.T.; Hart, L.L.; Awad, M.; Xu, L.A.; Horak, C.E.; Dakhil, S.; Hermann, R.C.; Lynch, T.J.; Weber, M.R. Analysis of potential predictive markers of cetuximab benefit in BMS099, a phase III study of cetuximab and first-line taxane/carboplatin in advanced non-small-cell lung cancer. *J. Clin. Oncol.* **2010**, *28*, 918–927. [CrossRef]
63. Su, S.C.; Lin, C.W.; Liu, Y.F.; Fan, W.L.; Chen, M.K.; Yu, C.P.; Yang, W.E.; Su, C.W.; Chuang, C.Y.; Li, W.H.; et al. Exome sequencing of oral squamous cell carcinoma reveals molecular subgroups and novel therapeutic opportunities. *Theranostics* **2017**, *7*, 1088–1099. [CrossRef]
64. Campbell, J.D.; Yau, C.; Bowlby, R.; Liu, Y.; Brennan, K.; Fan, H.; Taylor, A.M.; Wang, C.; Walter, V.; Akbani, R.; et al. Genomic, Pathway Network, and Immunologic Features Distinguishing Squamous Carcinomas. *Cell Rep.* **2018**, *23*, 194–212.e6. [CrossRef]
65. Koi, L.; Löck, S.; Linge, A.; Thurow, C.; Hering, S.; Baumann, M.; Krause, M.; Gurtner, K. EGFR-amplification plus gene expression profiling predicts response to combined radiotherapy with EGFR-inhibition: A preclinical trial in 10 HNSCC-tumour-xenograft models. *Radiother. Oncol.* **2017**, *124*, 496–503. [CrossRef] [PubMed]
66. Rampias, T.; Hoxhallari, L.; Avgeris, M.; Kanaki, Z.; Telios, D.; Giotakis, E.; Giotakis, I.; Scorilas, A.; Psyrri, A.; Klinakis, A. Sensitizing HRAS overexpressing head and neck squamous cell carcinoma (HNSCC) to chemotherapy. *Ann. Oncol.* **2019**, *30*, v462–v463. [CrossRef]
67. Mountzios, G.; Rampias, T.; Psyrri, A. The mutational spectrum of squamous-cell carcinoma of the head and neck: Targetable genetic events and clinical impact. *Ann. Oncol. Off. J. Eur. Soc. Med. Oncol.* **2014**, *25*, 1889–1900. [CrossRef] [PubMed]
68. Lui, V.W.Y.; Hedberg, M.L.; Li, H.; Vangara, B.S.; Pendleton, K.; Zeng, Y.; Lu, Y.; Zhang, Q.; Du, Y.; Gilbert, B.R.; et al. Frequent mutation of the PI3K pathway in head and neck cancer defines predictive biomarkers. *Cancer Discov.* **2013**, *3*, 761–769. [CrossRef]
69. Ruicci, K.M.; Pinto, N.; Khan, M.I.; Yoo, J.; Fung, K.; MacNeil, D.; Mymryk, J.S.; Barrett, J.W.; Nichols, A.C. ERK-TSC2 signalling in constitutively-active HRAS mutant HNSCC cells promotes resistance to PI3K inhibition. *Oral Oncol.* **2018**, *84*, 95–103. [CrossRef] [PubMed]
70. Storck, E.M.; Morales-Sanfrutos, J.; Serwa, R.A.; Panyain, N.; Lanyon-Hogg, T.; Tolmachova, T.; Ventimiglia, L.N.; Martin-Serrano, J.; Seabra, M.C.; Wojciak-Stothard, B.; et al. Dual chemical probes enable quantitative system-wide analysis of protein prenylation and prenylation dynamics. *Nat. Chem.* **2019**, *11*, 552–561. [CrossRef]
71. Basso, A.D.; Kirschmeier, P.; Bishop, W.R. Farnesyl transferase inhibitors. *J. Lipid Res.* **2006**, *47*, 15–31. [CrossRef] [PubMed]
72. Pan, J.; Yeung, S.J. Recent advances in understanding the antineoplastic mechanisms of farnesyltransferase inhibitors. *Cancer Res.* **2005**, 9109–9113. [CrossRef] [PubMed]
73. Lebowitz, P.F.; Davide, J.P.; Prendergast, G.C. Evidence that farnesyltransferase inhibitors suppress Ras transformation by interfering with Rho activity. *Mol. Cell. Biol.* **1995**, *15*, 6613–6622. [CrossRef] [PubMed]
74. Bousquet, E.; Calvayrac, O.; Mazières, J.; Lajoie-Mazenc, I.; Boubekeur, N.; Favre, G.; Pradines, A. RhoB loss induces Rac1-dependent mesenchymal cell invasion in lung cells through PP2A inhibition. *Oncogene* **2016**, *35*, 1760–1769. [CrossRef]
75. Calvayrac, O.; Mazières, J.; Figarol, S.; Marty-Detraves, C.; Raymond-Letron, I.; Bousquet, E.; Farella, M.; Clermont-Taranchon, E.; Milia, J.; Rouquette, I.; et al. The RAS -related GTP ase RHOB confers resistance to EGFR -tyrosine kinase inhibitors in non-small-cell lung cancer via an AKT -dependent mechanism. *EMBO Mol. Med.* **2017**, *9*, 238–250. [CrossRef]
76. Smith, E.M.; Finn, S.G.; Tee, A.R.; Brownei, G.J.; Proud, C.G. The tuberous sclerosis protein TSC2 is not required for the regulation of the mammalian target of rapamycin by amino acids and certain cellular stresses. *J. Biol. Chem.* **2005**, *280*, 18717–18727. [CrossRef]
77. Long, X.; Lin, Y.; Ortiz-Vega, S.; Yonezawa, K.; Avruch, J. Rheb binds and regulates the mTOR kinase. *Curr. Biol.* **2005**, *15*, 702–713. [CrossRef]
78. Angarola, B.; Ferguson, S.M.; Gruenberg, J.E. Weak membrane interactions allow Rheb to activate mTORC1 signaling without major lysosome enrichment. *Mol. Biol. Cell* **2019**, *30*, 2750–2760. [CrossRef]
79. Guri, Y.; Hall, M.N. mTOR signaling confers resistance to targeted cancer drugs. *Trends Cancer* **2016**, *2*, 688–697. [CrossRef]
80. Basso, A.D.; Mirza, A.; Liu, G.; Long, B.J.; Bishop, W.R.; Kirschmeier, P. The farnesyl transferase inhibitor (FTI) SCH66336 (lonafarnib) inhibits Rheb farnesylation and mTOR signaling: Role in FTI enhancement of taxane and tamoxifen anti-tumor activity. *J. Biol. Chem.* **2005**, *280*, 31101–31108. [CrossRef]
81. Makhov, P.; Sohn, J.A.; Serebriiskii, I.G.; Fazlieva, R.; Khazak, V.; Boumber, Y.; Uzzo, R.G.; Kolenko, V.M. CRISPR/Cas9 genome-wide loss-of-function screening identifies druggable cellular factors involved in sunitinib resistance in renal cell carcinoma. *Br. J. Cancer* **2020**, *123*, 1749–1756. [CrossRef]

82. Yao, X.; Anderson, K.L.; Cleveland, D.W. The microtubule-dependent motor centromere-associated protein E (CENP-E) is an integral component of kinetochore corona fibers that link centromeres to spindle microtubules. *J. Cell Biol.* **1997**, *139*, 435–447. [CrossRef]
83. Wood, K.W.; Sakowicz, R.; Goldstein, L.S.B.; Cleveland, D.W. CENP-E is a plus end–directed kinetochore motor required for metaphase chromosome alignment. *Cell* **1997**, *91*, 357–366. [CrossRef]
84. Liao, H.; Winkfein, R.J.; Mack, G.; Rattner, J.B.; Yen, T.J. CENP-F is a protein of the nuclear matrix that assembles onto kinetochores at late G2 and is rapidly degraded after mitosis. *J. Cell Biol.* **1995**, *130*, 507–518. [CrossRef]
85. Ashar, H.R.; James, L.; Gray, K.; Carr, D.; Black, S.; Armstrong, L.; Bishop, W.R.; Kirschmeier, P. Farnesyl transferase inhibitors block the farnesylation of CENP-E and CENP-F and alter the association of CENP-E with the microtubules. *J. Biol. Chem.* **2000**, *275*, 30451–30457. [CrossRef]
86. Hussein, D.; Taylor, S.S. Farnesylation of Cenp-F is required for G2/M progression and degradation after mitosis. *J. Cell Sci.* **2002**, *115*, 3403–3414. [CrossRef] [PubMed]
87. Cates, C.A.; Michael, R.L.; Stayrook, K.R.; Harvey, K.A.; Burke, Y.D.; Randall, S.K.; Crowell, P.L.; Crowell, D.N. Prenylation of oncogenic human PTPcaax protein tyrosine phosphatases. *Cancer Lett.* **1996**, *110*, 49–55. [CrossRef]
88. Hassan, N.M.M.; Hamada, J.I.; Kameyama, T.; Tada, M.; Nakagawa, K.; Yoshida, S.; Kashiwazaki, H.; Yamazaki, Y.; Suzuki, Y.; Sasaki, A.; et al. Increased expression of the PRL-3 gene in human oral squamous cell carcinoma and dysplasia tissues. *Asian Pacific J. Cancer Prev.* **2011**, *12*, 947–951.
89. Wei, M.; Korotkov, K.V.; Blackburn, J.S. Targeting phosphatases of regenerating liver (PRLs) in cancer. *Pharmacol. Ther.* **2018**, *190*, 128–138. [CrossRef] [PubMed]
90. Zeng, Q.; Dong, J.-M.; Guo, K.; Li, J.; Tan, H.-X.; Koh, V.; Pallen, C.J.; Manser, E.; Hong, W. PRL-3 and PRL-1 promote cell migration, invasion, and metastasis. *Cancer Res.* **2003**, *63*, 2716–2722.
91. Murphy, M.E. The HSP70 family and cancer. *Carcinogenesis* **2013**, *34*, 1181–1188. [CrossRef]
92. Karp, J.E.; Lancet, J.E.; Kaufmann, S.H.; End, D.W.; Wright, J.J.; Bol, K.; Horak, I.; Tidwell, M.L.; Liesveld, J.; Kottke, T.J.; et al. Clinical and biologic activity of the farnesyltransferase inhibitor R115777 in adults with refractory and relapsed acute leukemias: A phase 1 clinical-laboratory correlative trial. *Blood* **2001**, *97*, 3361–3369. [CrossRef] [PubMed]
93. Wolda, S.L.; Glomsets, J.A. Evidence for modification of lamin B by a product of mevalonic acid. *J. Biol. Chem.* **1988**, *263*, 5997–6000. [CrossRef]
94. Meta, M.; Yang, S.H.; Bergo, M.O.; Fong, L.G.; Young, S.G. Protein farnesyltransferase inhibitors and progeria. *Trends Mol. Med.* **2006**, *12*, 480–487. [CrossRef] [PubMed]
95. Dhillon, S. Lonafarnib: First approval. *Drugs* **2021**, *81*, 283–289. [CrossRef] [PubMed]
96. Pan, J.; She, M.; Xu, Z.X.; Sun, L.; Yeung, S.C.J. Farnesyltransferase inhibitors induce DNA damage via reactive oxygen species in human cancer cells. *Cancer Res.* **2005**, *65*, 3671–3681. [CrossRef]
97. Liu, A.X.; Cerniglia, G.J.; Bernhard, E.J.; Prendergast, G.C. RhoB is required to mediate apoptosis in neoplastically transformed cells after DNA damage. *Proc. Natl. Acad. Sci. USA* **2001**, *98*, 6192–6197. [CrossRef]
98. Chen, J.; Jiang, C.C.; Jin, L.; Zhang, X.D. Regulation of PD-L1: A novel role of pro-survival signalling in cancer. *Ann. Oncol.* **2016**, *27*, 409–416. [CrossRef]
99. Ebert, P.J.R.; Cheung, J.; Yang, Y.; McNamara, E.; Hong, R.; Moskalenko, M.; Gould, S.E.; Maecker, H.; Irving, B.A.; Kim, J.M.; et al. MAP kinase inhibition promotes T cell and anti-tumor activity in combination with PD-L1 checkpoint blockade. *Immunity* **2016**, *44*, 609–621. [CrossRef]
100. Albert, S.; Riveiro, M.E.; Halimi, C.; Hourseau, M.; Couvelard, A.; Serova, M.; Barry, B.; Raymond, E.; Faivre, S. Focus on the role of the CXCL12/CXCR4 chemokine axis in head and neck squamous cell carcinoma. *Head Neck* **2013**, *35*, 1819–1828. [CrossRef]
101. Gualberto, A.; Scholz, C.; Mishra, V.; Janes, M.R.; Kessler, L.; Cutsem, E.; Van Ho, A.L.; Witzig, T. Abstract CT191: Mechanism of action of the farnesyltransferase inhibitor, tipifarnib, and its clinical applications. In *Proceedings of the Cancer Research*; American Association for Cancer Research (AACR): Philadelphia, PA, USA, 2019; Volume 79, p. CT191.
102. Witzig, T.; Sokol, L.; Jacobsen, E.; Advani, R.; Foss, F.; Mondejar, R.; Piris, M.A.; Bolognese, J.; Burrows, F.; Kessler, L.; et al. The CXCL12/CXCR4 pathway as a potential target of tipifarnib: Preliminary results from an open-label, phase II Study in relapsed or refractory peripheral T-Cell lymphoma. *Blood* **2017**, *130*, 2788. [CrossRef]

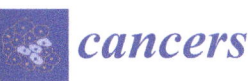

Review

The Balance between Differentiation and Terminal Differentiation Maintains Oral Epithelial Homeostasis

Yuchen Bai [1], Jarryd Boath [1], Gabrielle R. White [1], Uluvitike G. I. U. Kariyawasam [1], Camile S. Farah [1,2] and Charbel Darido [1,3,*]

1. Peter MacCallum Cancer Centre, 305 Grattan St., Melbourne, VIC 3000, Australia; yuchen.bai@petermac.org (Y.B.); jarryd.boath@petermac.org (J.B.); gabrielle.white@petermac.org (G.R.W.); imalki.kariyawasam@petermac.org (U.G.I.U.K.); camile@oralmedpath.com.au (C.S.F.)
2. Australian Centre for Oral Oncology Research & Education, Perth, WA 6009, Australia
3. Sir Peter MacCallum Department of Oncology, The University of Melbourne, Parkville, VIC 3010, Australia
* Correspondence: charbel.darido@petermac.org; Tel.: +61-3-8559-7111

Simple Summary: Oral cancer affecting the oral cavity represents the most common cancer of the head and neck region. Oral cancer develops in a multistep process in which normal cells gradually accumulate genetic and epigenetic modifications to evolve into a malignant disease. Mortality for oral cancer patients is high and morbidity has a significant long-term impact on the health and wellbeing of affected individuals, typically resulting in facial disfigurement and a loss of the ability to speak, chew, taste, and swallow. The limited scope to which current treatments are able to control oral cancer underlines the need for novel therapeutic strategies. This review highlights the molecular differences between oral cell proliferation, differentiation and terminal differentiation, defines terminal differentiation as an important tumour suppressive mechanism and establishes a rationale for clinical investigation of differentiation-paired therapies that may improve outcomes in oral cancer.

Abstract: The oral epithelium is one of the fastest repairing and continuously renewing tissues. Stem cell activation within the basal layer of the oral epithelium fuels the rapid proliferation of multipotent progenitors. Stem cells first undergo asymmetric cell division that requires tightly controlled and orchestrated differentiation networks to maintain the pool of stem cells while producing progenitors fated for differentiation. Rapidly expanding progenitors subsequently commit to advanced differentiation programs towards terminal differentiation, a process that regulates the structural integrity and homeostasis of the oral epithelium. Therefore, the balance between differentiation and terminal differentiation of stem cells and their progeny ensures progenitors commitment to terminal differentiation and prevents epithelial transformation and oral squamous cell carcinoma (OSCC). A recent comprehensive molecular characterization of OSCC revealed that a disruption of terminal differentiation factors is indeed a common OSCC event and is superior to oncogenic activation. Here, we discuss the role of differentiation and terminal differentiation in maintaining oral epithelial homeostasis and define terminal differentiation as a critical tumour suppressive mechanism. We further highlight factors with crucial terminal differentiation functions and detail the underlying consequences of their loss. Switching on terminal differentiation in differentiated progenitors is likely to represent an extremely promising novel avenue that may improve therapeutic interventions against OSCC.

Keywords: differentiation; terminal differentiation; oral epithelium; epithelial integrity; epithelial transformation; genetic alterations; oral cancer; therapy response biomarkers

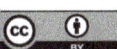

1. Introduction

Oral squamous cell carcinoma (OSCC) is the most commonly diagnosed head and neck cancer [1]. OSCC frequently affects the tongue and floor of the mouth within the oral cavity [2] and accounts for approximately 5% of cancer diagnoses in men and 2% in women, worldwide [3]. Among developing countries within Southeast Asia, OSCC represents a quarter of all cancers diagnosed [4], where in India and Sri Lanka, it is the leading cause of cancer death in men [3]. OSCC is the endpoint of a disease spectrum affecting oral epithelial cells and ranging from hyperplasia, dysplasia and carcinoma in-situ, to locally invasive and then metastatic disease. Within the oral cavity, the normal tongue mucosa comprises a connective tissue known as the lamina propria (LP) covered by squamous cell layers forming the oral epithelium (OE). The OE is constantly exposed to acute and chronic environmental insults including damage from mastication, exposure to dietary and airborne antigens, chemical carcinogens, and diverse commensal and pathogenic microorganisms [5]. Tongue OE basal cells attach to the basement membrane and continuously divide to replace damaged cells and to maintain tissue homeostasis. Similar to skin keratinocytes, OE differentiation begins in the basal layer where stem cells differentiate into progenitors, which migrate upward to form the spinous, granular, clear and superficial layers of the tongue, and undergo terminal differentiation to establish a functional protective outer barrier [6,7]. Mitotic figure orientation analyses showed that most daughter progenitor cells divide parallel to the basement membrane and initially remain within the basal layer [8]. Clonal analyses have revealed that up to half of the cells in the basal layer are post-mitotic. Lineage-committed, post-mitotic progenitor cells downregulate the expression of basal layer markers and start to express differentiation-associated genes to exit the basal layer [9]. While they migrate and mature, differentiated cells upregulate differentiation genes to further differentiate, terminally differentiate and eventually delaminate. Signalling circuitries regulating stem cell fate such as Notch, Hippo and TP63-dependent pathways and DNA and histone methylases are among the main mechanisms that allow stem cells to balance their regenerative potential, while initiating early differentiation programs [10]. The resultant progenitors are cells with potent expansion potential. Factors that end progenitor cell division and induce commitment to terminal differentiation in post-mitotic cells have attracted particular attention as their loss could facilitate the return to a progenitor state through a mechanism activated in response to acute damage or insult [11,12].

The balance between proliferation, differentiation and terminal differentiation is therefore key to maintaining OE homeostasis and securing the physical and physiological functions of the oral barrier [6,13]. Exposure to known risk factors of OSCC such as smoking tobacco and marijuana, betel quid chewing, frequent alcohol use, radiation exposure, immunosuppression, genetic predisposition, poor hygiene and Human Papilloma Virus (HPV) infections may impair the integrity of the OE and facilitate cellular transformation into hyperplastic lesions, dysplasia and even OSCC [1]. Considering its multifactorial origin, it is not surprising that OSCC is a highly heterogeneous disease at the molecular level [14].

2. Oral Homeostasis

The OE undergoes a rapid turnover (estimated 4.5 days) to eliminate cells damaged by constant exposure to environmental risk factors. Stem cells initiate this process through their proliferation and differentiation to repopulate the OE and to maintain its homeostasis [15]. Over the last few decades, several techniques have been developed to identify and characterise oral stem cells under different physiological and pathological conditions.

2.1. Oral Epithelial Stem Cells

Stem cells are referred to as a quiescent, infrequently dividing cell population with self-renewal properties. The identification and characterization of oral epithelial stem cells have been challenged for decades [16]. The *Bmi1*-expressing OE stem cells were first reported using multi-colour lineage tracing and label retention experiments in the dorsal tongue epithelium [17]. The results suggested that *Bmi1*-positive stem cells were slow-cycling and distributed at a low density within the basal layer. Their proliferation was shown to follow the invariant asymmetry model, supporting an asymmetrical division of long-lived cells that maintain stemness while producing highly proliferative, transit-amplifying daughter cells that differentiate incrementally to produce the clearly defined OE layers. However, using RNAscope on the dorsal tongue and buccal epithelium, Klein's group found that all basal cells, including progenitors, express *Bmi1*, albeit at low levels, contradicting the data suggesting that *Bmi1* marked rare, solitary stem cells in the suprabasal layers of the OE [9]. Furthermore, through label retention and single-cell sequencing experiments, the authors proposed a population asymmetry model of self-renewal in which half of all basal cells are highly proliferative and half are post-mitotic cells acquiring differentiation programs. In parallel, stochastic proliferation was identified in stem cells within the oral mucosa using the hard palate as a model [18]. Here, the OE is maintained by both symmetrical and asymmetrical divisions of stem cells. Cells expressing *Lrig1* infrequently divide in a symmetrical fashion then become quiescent while *Igfbp5+* cells undergo rapid asymmetrical division in the lead-up to differentiation. These studies underscore that our understanding of stem cell niche function within the OE is still confounded by various anatomical locations and technical limitations. Spatial single-cell sequencing will be crucial to identify and characterise specific stem cell populations within various head and neck regions and shed light on the mechanisms governing their maintenance and differentiation.

2.2. Damage-Induced Stem Cell Activation

The OE is equipped with an effective "catastrophe" response to damage induced by a variety of insults, such as wounding, masticatory stresses, chemical exposure and microbial pathogens. A transcriptional analysis of the OE during wound healing identified reduced differentiation and increased proliferation signatures in OE cells recruited to facilitate tissue repair [19]. This response mechanism is highly effective, and as a result, oral wounds heal rapidly without producing scars. Furthermore, different oral stem cell models show consistent wound healing phases: migration, stem cell expansion and re-epithelization. Upon puncture, irradiation or cytotoxic injuries, OE stem cells were able to migrate to wound-proximal areas, exit quiescence and divide symmetrically to close the wound, simultaneously reducing asymmetrical divisions and restricting differentiation within the OE [18,20]. As soon as proliferating stem cells repopulate the damaged site, a differentiation programme initiates to instate oral homeostasis in injured OE and to re-establish a functional oral epithelial barrier. Cooperative mechanisms linked to the breakdown of the OE basal layer such as the activation of $p16^{INK4A}$ may guide replicative senescence, limiting cellular migration and proliferation while retaining normal growth and differentiation characteristics [21–24]. In the event of chronic insult, stem cell activation persists in a state that is prone to acquire genetic/epigenetic alterations, which can eventually lead to senescence bypass and oncogenic transformation [25–28]. Hence, following the damage repair of oral tissue, the differentiation of committed progenitor cells is crucial for tissue remodelling and the prevention of oral diseases and carcinogenesis.

2.3. Oral Cancer Stem Cell

Cancer stem cells (CSCs) are believed to act as the drivers of OSCC [29]. These cells are highly tumourigenic with increased self-renewal and clonal capacities. They may originate from the accumulation of multiple oncogenic hits in normal stem cells, in differentiated or senescent cells, which result in their reprogramming into CSC [12,30]. In the context of OSCC, putative CSCs were first described as CD44-expressing cells which formed well-differentiated tumours in a patient-derived xenograft model [31]. CD44 protein expression and spatial regulation has been observed in a dermis-based organotypic 3D culture model of oral epithelium, with an increase in expression from normal OE through to dysplasia and then carcinoma, and with CD44 expression closely associated with the basal layer [32]. In addition to CD44, other characteristics including aldehyde dehydrogenase activation, spheroid-forming ability and the overexpression of CD133 have been proposed as CSC markers in OSCC [33]. Moreover, genetic lineage tracing experiments and carcinogen induced OSCC in mice confirmed the existence of OSCC

CSCs with deregulated *Bmi1* expression [34]. Bmi1+ cancer cells can form tumour clones with comparable architectural and molecular features seen in primary tumours. More importantly, slow-cycling Bmi1+ CSCs show increasing invasive and metastatic phenotypes as well as chemoresistance. Additionally, there has been an observed increased trend for the expression of Bmi1 and ABCG2 in dysplastic and malignant tissues compared to normal, highlighting the potential use of these stem cell markers in the malignant transformation of the oral epithelium [35]. Consequently, these CSCs are now recognised as the main drivers of OSCC development and progression, where future therapeutic strategies should aim at targeting their proliferative as well as quiescent states to achieve a complete therapeutic response.

3. Molecular Landscape of Oral Epithelial Differentiation

3.1. Signalling Pathways

As OE progenitor cells commit to differentiation programs and migrate upward, these cells are exposed to a dynamic gradient of Notch/Wnt ligands and growth factors. These gradients contribute profoundly to the strict regulation of basal-suprabasal compartmentalisation (Figure 1).

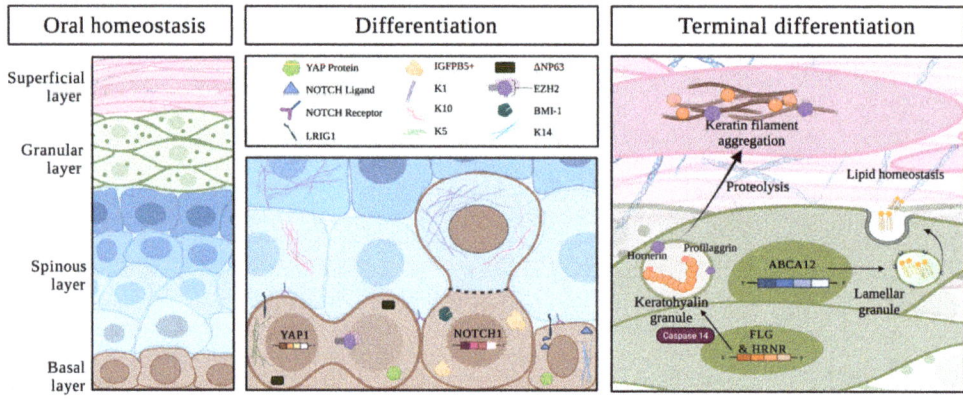

Figure 1. Schematic representation (original figure) of the oral layers in homeostasis (**left**) with a highlight of the basal layer depicting major players in epithelial differentiation (**middle**) and those regulating terminal differentiation in the superficial layer (**right**).

3.2. Notch Signalling

Notch signalling is regulated predominantly through cell–cell interactions. Notch ligands are expressed in basal cells while Notch receptors are present on suprabasal spinous cells. The activation of Notch signalling in differentiation-committed cells coincides with their detachment from the basement membrane and the expression of terminal differentiation program genes. Notch regulates cell fate commitment and governs the balance between basal progenitor proliferation and supra-basal differentiated cells within a process known as the basal-to-suprabasal switch [36]. In agreement with this, the deregulation of NOTCH signalling in basal cells results in increased tumour susceptibility and a shift towards tumours with poor differentiation [37,38]. This correlates with the proliferation–differentiation imbalance and the *Notch1*-driven terminal differentiation in supra-basal layers [39]. Loss of Notch signalling also synergised with both a *TP53* gain-of-function mutation or the expression of HPV oncogenes to induce high-grade carcinomas within the head and neck region [37]. Moreover, an in vivo CRISPR screen in OSCC identified oncogenic drivers that cooperate with rare mutations in 15 driver genes, all with activities that converge on *Notch* signalling [40]. These results highlight the important role played by Notch signalling in the suppression of OSCC through the promotion of progenitor differentiation. Moreover, aberrant NOTCH signalling was shown to contribute to deregulating the cell cycle, escaping cell death, and establishing a tumour-promoting microenvironment in SCC [41,42]. Recent data from exome sequencing and the Cancer Genome Atlas (TCGA) analyses identified a high frequency for *NOTCH1/2/3* mutations and truncations (~27%) which presumably lead to protein inactivation, disruption of differentiation and OSCC development [42–44]. More importantly, mutations of *NOTCH1* are commonly detected in precancerous lesions, highlighting its protective role against the early onset of OSCC in patients [21,40,45]. Contradictory, while *NOTCH1* mutations are mainly considered drivers of the disease, growing evidence points out to the hyperactivation of NOTCH signalling in a subset of OSCC, proposing an oncogenic potential to wild-type *NOTCH1* [40,46]. NOTCH1-targeting γ-secretase inhibitors, which prevent the cleavage of the Notch intracellular domain and consequently block its translocation to the nucleus, are being evaluated in pre-clinical and clinical trials [47,48]. However, no studies to date have evaluated these inhibitors specifically in OSCC, and due to the context and tissue-specific dependent role of NOTCH signalling, clinical application of NOTCH inhibitors may require further caution.

3.3. Hippo Pathway

The Hippo pathway controls organ size in *Drosophila* through cell fate determination, tissue regeneration and stem cell self-renewal and is mainly regulated through contact inhibition [49]. In the presence of cell–cell interactions, structural protein complexes activate Hippo kinases on the cell membrane, leading to cytosolic sequestration and proteasomal degradation of the downstream transcriptional factor YAP1 and its co-activator TAZ [50]. This mechanism maintains apical–basolateral polarity for the regulation of stemness and differentiation, and the inactivation of the Hippo pathway perturbs differentiation, promoting proliferation and tissue hyperplasia [49]. In the skin, YAP1 is mainly expressed in basal progenitors and its overexpression expands the proliferative basal cell pool and deregulates terminal differentiation, facilitating tumourigenesis [51]. Indeed, hyperactivation of YAP1 in the mouse oral cavity induces an early onset of OSCC, indicating that this pathway is a potent driver of the disease [52]. Furthermore, 8.6% of OSCC primary tumours show an amplification of the *YAP1* locus and 21.6% with truncated *FAT1* [53], an upstream membrane receptor protein in the Hippo kinase cascade, which results in increased YAP1 activity, malignant progression and poor patient prognosis [54,55]. YAP1 has also been shown to act as a potential biomarker for cetuximab resistance in head and neck cancer [56].

3.4. TP63-Regulated Transcription

TP63 belongs to the TP53 family of transcription factors and has two distinct isoforms: TAp63 and ΔNp63. TAp63 possesses a transactivation domain at N-terminal, while ΔNp63 contains a shorter activation domain. Despite the conservation in their structures and transcriptional activities, these isoforms are expressed in different tissues and have distinct roles in embryonic development and epithelial maintenance [57]. In stratified squamous epithelium, ΔNp63 is strongly expressed in basal cells where TAp63 is weak, indicating that ΔNp63 may play a major role in these epithelia. Interestingly, ΔNp63 null mice manifest with limb truncation, orofacial malformation and the defective maturation of stratified epithelia, while no obvious epidermal defects were noted in mice with targeted ablation of TAp63 [58]. Additionally, the loss of ΔNp63 induces the dysregulation of NOTCH and TGF-β signalling, linking ΔNp63 to epithelial cell fate specification and stem cell maintenance, and highlighting the notion that TP63 is the "guardian of the epithelial lineage" [59]. On the other hand, TP63 facilitates squamous cell carcinoma (SCC) formation and an in vivo deletion of the *TP63* gene in established SCC tumours leads to rapid tumour shrinkage, revealing a crucial function for TP63 in SCC maintenance [60]. Moreover, up to 80% of OSCC patients show overexpression and/or genomic amplification of *TP63*, and these events are associated with poor tumour differentiation and patient prognosis [61].

3.5. Epigenetic Regulators of the Commitment Switch to Epithelial Differentiation

During lineage specification, dynamic epigenetic modifications profoundly influence gene expression. The open chromatin conformation in stem cells enables active transcription of genes related to keratinocyte commitment and differentiation. This process is progressively accompanied by increased DNA methylation, the accumulation of various histone markers and chromatin remodelling, resulting in diminished chromatin accessibility and full inactivation of transcription in terminally differentiated cells [62]. These observations confirm an active role for the epigenome in fine tuning epithelial differentiation. An example of this process relates to EZH2, a component of the polycomb repressor complex 2 (PRC2), a key regulator of differentiation responsible for the trimethylation of lysine 27 on histone H3 (H3K27me3) in gene repression. EZH2 is highly expressed in basal progenitor cells and its expression correlates with cell proliferation and is thus gradually suppressed with the occurrence of epithelial differentiation. EZH2-induced H3K27me3 marker inhibits the binding of AP1 transcription activator to its target genes, leading to the repression of AP1-transcribed differentiation genes in basal cells. In addition, the loss of EZH2 in vitro and in vivo correlates with reduced proliferation of basal cells and accelerated differentiation suprabasally [63]. It was also shown that EZH2 is overexpressed in OSCC cell lines and primary tumours, and that a genetic or pharmacological inhibition of EZH2 attenuates tumour growth and restores differentiation gene expression in differentiation refractory OSCC xenografts [64]. Arguably, driver mutations in epigenetic modulators are often retained for the entire course of carcinogenesis, implying that their dysregulation is key to the loss of differentiation in OSCC tumourigenesis and an exciting area for therapeutic targeting.

Another level of regulation that follows the transcriptional control of differentiation genes depends on the post-transcriptional modifications that also influence the dynamics of protein abundance during differentiation [65]. One of the crucial post-transcriptional mechanisms is miRNA-mediated gene silencing. Small non-coding single stranded RNAs pair to target mRNAs, inhibiting translation and inducing mRNA decay. In mammalian epidermis, it was shown that the Grainy-head like 3 (GRHL3), an evolutionarily conserved transcription factor and a master regulator of terminal keratinocyte differentiation [66,67], is repressed by oncogenic miR-21 [68,69]. Importantly, an epidermal-specific loss of key miRNA processing machinery components, such as Dicer and Dgcr8, causes epidermal dehydration, hair follicle apoptosis and neonatal lethality [70]. These results underscore the importance of regulating protein expression associated with differentiation and invite further investigations of the multi-level controls of this process.

4. Terminal Differentiation in OSCC

Terminal differentiation programs are fully engaged in granular and cornified layers of the oral epithelium, leading to the establishment of a functional barrier that prevents against environmental insults. This outermost layer of the dorsal tongue epithelium is formed of corneocytes embedded in a lipid matrix that contains small vesicles of cholesterol, phospholipids and ceramides. In addition to protein cross-linking, the correct presence of lipid complexes is essential to maintain barrier function, preventing dehydration and infection [6]. Nevertheless, how the loss of terminal differentiation factors affects the integrity of the epithelium and the epithelial architecture are still poorly understood.

4.1. ABCA12

ABCA12 regulates vesicular trafficking in terminally differentiated cells and is one of the core components that preserve lipid homeostasis [6]. The loss of *Abca12* induces a failure of extracellular lipid deposition and premature differentiation, consequently leading to hyperkeratosis and impaired barrier function [71]. In humans, germline mutations in ABCA12 are linked to Harlequin Ichthyosis, a severe inherited disease causing high neonatal death, dehydrated skin and infections [72]. Interestingly, these mutations are present in 3.7% of OSCC patients with up to 27% of tumours losing ABCA12 expression [43], further proposing the loss of ABCA12 as an initiator of OSCC development.

4.2. FLG

Keratins and filaggrin contribute to 80–90% of the mass of the granular layer in stratified epithelia, where they are tightly cross-linked to establish a physiological epithelial barrier. Notably, filaggrin (filament aggregation protein) serves as an indispensable molecule for the aggregation process of keratin filaments. Filaggrin derives from the proteolytic maturation of profilaggrin (FLG), an S100 fused-type protein of approximately 500 kDa, histidine-rich with tandem repeats of filaggrin stored in the membrane-less protein deposits, known as keratohyalin granules (KGs) [73]. The disassembly of KGs leads to squame formation. The maturation of FLG depends on caspase-14 (CASP14), with Casp14 knockout mice showing increased *FLG* in KGs in conjunction with a striking glossy and scurfy epidermal phenotype, water loss and increased susceptibility of ultraviolet B damage [74]. Intriguingly, a decreased expression of *FLG* has been recorded in the autosomal semi-dominant disease ichthyosis vulgaris (IV) and in atopic dermatitis (AD), where the presence of loss-of-function mutations in *FLG* also predisposes to IV and AD as well as additional allergic diseases such as asthma [75]. Collectively, these observations demonstrate an essential role for filaggrin in the formation of epithelial barrier to protect against the outer environment. It is also noteworthy that *FLG* is one of the most frequently mutated genes (13%) in OSCC [43,44], and its loss disrupts OSCC differentiation and decreases therapy response [76].

4.3. HRNR

HRNR is also an S100 fused-type protein encoded in the epidermal differentiation complex same as FLG. The precursor of HRNR is approximately 280 kDa with a central tandem peptide repeats domain with calcium-binding sites, located in the periphery of KGs within the upper granular and cornified layers [77]. Similar to FLG, HRNR maturation proteolysis leads to releasing amino acids as natural moisturising factors for epithelial hydration and photo-protection, and to cross-linking keratins as part of the establishment of a functional barrier. *HRNR* expression is downregulated in the skin of AD patients, and a single-nucleotide polymorphism of HRNR was identified in people vulnerable to AD [78]. Importantly, 4.1% of OSCC patients show mutations in HRNR [44]. These observations suggest that defective HRNR-induced terminal differentiation may contribute to the pathophysiology of AD and OSCC (Figure 1).

5. Treatments for Patients with OSCC

Most OSCC patients present with advanced-stage disease, and treatment is met with high levels of recurrence and metastasis [79,80]. Moreover, OSCC patients are at high risk of developing a second primary malignancy [81]. Conventional OSCC treatment regimens include surgery, radiotherapy, chemotherapy, immunotherapy and targeted therapy [82]. The recent success of immune checkpoint blockade in cancer underlines the clinical importance of novel immunotherapy drug regimens [83], and antibodies against CTLA-4, PD-1 and PD-L1 have revolutionised OSCC care [84]. However, immunotherapy using the immune checkpoint inhibitor Pembrolizumab resulted in a relatively low (~20%) response rate, albeit in the absence of patient stratification [85,86]. The study recruited patients with advanced solid tumours over 18 years old. The archival tumour sample was obtained before the treatment and after 9 weeks of the treatment process, irrespective of PD-L1 or HPV status. Patients received 200 mg of the drug once every 3 weeks, for 24 months, and treatment response was assessed every 8 weeks by using computed tomography or magnetic resonance imaging. A significant proportion of these patients developed adaptive resistance due to the upregulation of additional immune checkpoints, whilst others experienced increased tumour growth kinetics (hyper-progressive disease) [87]. Nevertheless, OSCC with high PD-L1 expression were the most responsive, prompting the search for additional biomarkers, beyond PD-L1, that are still needed to inform the choice of therapy [88]. The interference with cancer cell-intrinsic signalling pathways was shown to modulate cancer sensitivity to immunotherapy [89]. While EGFR overexpression directly regulates immune checkpoint molecule expression and response to immunotherapy [90], the loss of *TP53* may render cancer cells resistant to T cell-mediated killing [91]. This suggests that combining immunotherapy with inhibitors of oncogenic signalling may provide greater therapeutic benefit and a rationale for a tailored OSCC-personalised targeted therapy. This approach is being investigated in a phase II clinical trial (NCT03544723) of the combination of an adenoviral p53 (Ad-p53) gene therapy administered intra-tumourally with approved immune checkpoint inhibitors in patients with recurrent or metastatic solid tumours [92], and has potential application in head and neck cancers.

6. Targeted Therapy against OSCC

The central concept of targeted therapy typically involves clinical testing to determine features of a patient's malignant disease that may inform treatment decisions. Why some patients respond well to targeted therapies, and other patients who appear to have the same type of cancer respond poorly or not at all, remains poorly understood. Genomic biomarkers paired with targeted therapies have proven highly efficacious in some cases, such as HER2 amplification and trastuzumab in breast cancer [93], BRAF mutation and combined BRAF/MEK inhibition in melanoma [94] and EML4-ALK fusions and Crizotinib in lung adenocarcinoma [95]. While many studies have focused on targeting oncogenic mechanisms, none have proven totally effective for predicting responsiveness. The resistance to targeted therapy can operate at the genomic level in many cancers. Key examples include EGFR-T790M mutations and resistance to EGFR inhibitors in EGFR-mutant lung cancer [96], ESR1 mutations in estrogen receptor positive breast cancer treated with endocrine therapy [97], and reversions of pathogenic mutations in BRCA1 and BRCA2 deficient cancers treated with PARP inhibitors [98]. However, no genetic tests are routinely incorporated into the management of OSCC, and patient stratification is largely done based on clinical features, even in the absence of HPV status, with a huge knowledge gap in response biomarkers [99,100]. One of the best attempts at treating recurrent or metastatic OSCC patients with targeted therapy was made using Cetuximab, a U.S. Food and Drug Administration (FDA)-approved monoclonal antibody that specifically binds and inhibits the activity of EGFR. Despite EGFR overexpression in ~90% of OSCC patients [101], only 10% of patients derived a beneficial response to combined Cetuximab and radiotherapy while the remainder were at higher risk of relapse [102]. In recent years, it has become clear that the prognostic value of EGFR overexpression or increased gene copy number does not correlate with Cetuximab response due to common alterations downstream of EGFR [103]. Somatic mutations, genetic and epigenetic alterations have been shown to drive senescence bypass, proliferation, continuous cancer cell survival and OSCC treatment resistance [25,104]. Such mechanisms render most OSCC patients difficult to cure and emphasise the urgent need to identify additional strategies to enhance therapy response [105].

7. Differentiation-Paired Targeted Therapy for OSCC

Large-scale genomic and transcriptomic sequencing of OSCC tumours showed very high (~90%) inactivating mutations in tumour suppressor genes, most of which encoded terminal differentiation factors [106]. TP53 was the most dominant (>74%) mutated gene while mutations in squamous differentiation factors (e.g., TP63, Notch1, IRF6 and RIPK4) were commonly observed and co-existed in the same cancers [106–108]. These mutations are likely to drive more proliferative basal-like OSCC phenotypes and correlate with poor patient survival [107,108]. Surprisingly, the incidence of oncogene-activating mutations was low (~20%) and suggests that the dysregulation of differentiation may act as the main driver of TP53 mutant OSCC.

The lack of effective targeted therapies for heterogeneous OSCC, particularly those with TP53 mutations, has hampered improvements in patient survival, which has remained virtually unchanged for the last 30 years [109]. Nonetheless, recombinant human p53 adenovirus vectors (such as Ad5RSV-p53 and AdCMV-p53) have been used to replace mutated *TP53* with wild-type gene in order to restore p53 functionality, with potential utility as a new treatment approach for head and neck cancers [110–112]. While much has been learned about the mutational landscape of OSCC (Table 1) through next-generation sequencing [113], a tremendous challenge remains in translating this genomic information into functional outcomes [106]. Integrated approaches leveraging both genetic and epigenetic data may determine whether functional differentiation factors affect the responses to targeted therapy. Since key terminal differentiation effectors have not been explored with regards to squamous differentiation and therapy response in OSCC, particularly in those exposed to differing aetiologies, novel strategies that combine targeted therapy with terminal differentiation could lead to optimizing patients' therapy response in a manner that is superior to traditional oncogene-targeting approaches. Innovative screening methods to stratify OSCC patients into specific subsets should enhance clinical outcomes for targeted therapies [114]. Of these, a potent switch that remains active and controls progenitor commitment to terminal differentiation and therefore induces growth arrest should be on the horizon. Such findings could open-up novel avenues for more accurate differentiation-guided treatment stratification of OSCC and could contribute to a strong evidence-based foundation for novel clinical applications.

Table 1. Frequency of genetic alterations targeting differentiation and terminal differentiation genes in HNSCC (original table).

Name of Genes	Frequency of Genetic Alterations in HNSCC	Functions in Epithelia	Evidence	Ref
ASXL1	Mutation, 2.90% CNA, 2.70%	Differentiation	IMP	[115]
DLG5	Mutation, 2.30%	Differentiation, cell polarity	IMP	[116]
DMBT1	Mutation, 2.70%	Differentiation, innate immunity	IDA	[117]
ERBB4	Mutation, 4.50%	Differentiation	IMP	[118]
FAT1	Mutation, 21.60%; CNA, 6.80%	Differentiation, hippo/Wnt signalling, EMT		[10,54,55]
GATA4	CNA, 3.10%; *HOMDEL*	Differentiation, transcription factor	IMP	[119]
MEF2C	Mutation, 2.70%	Differentiation, transcription factor, histone deacetylase	IMP	[120]
MYO9A	Mutation, 2.90%	Differentiation, cell junction	ISO	[121]
NOTCH1	Mutation, 17.10%; Fusion, 0.60%	Differentiation, notch pathway		[10,36,106–108,122]
NOTCH2	Mutation, 3.90% CNA, 2.50%	Differentiation, notch pathway		[10,36,43,44]
NOTCH4	Mutation, 1.90%	Differentiation, notch pathway		[10,36,106,108]
NUMA1	Mutation, 3.70% CNA, 8.10%	Differentiation, asymmetric cell division	IMP	[122]
ONECUT2	CNA, 2.90% *HOMDEL*	Early differentiation, specification	IMP	[123]
PTCH1	Mutation, 2.70%	Differentiation, SHH signalling	IGI	[124]

Table 1. Cont.

Name of Genes	Frequency of Genetic Alterations in HNSCC	Functions in Epithelia	Evidence	Ref
RARG	Mutation, 2.50%	Differentiation, specification, non-cornified	IGI	[125]
RHOA	Mutation, 1.90%	Differentiation, specification, cell junction	ISO	[126]
ROCK1	Mutation, 2.90% Fusion, 0.60% CNA, 1.90%	Differentiation, polarization	IGI	[127]
ROCK2	Mutation, 2.10%	Differentiation, polarization	ISO	[128]
ROS1	Mutation, 5.00%	Differentiation	IMP	[129]
SCRIB	Mutation, 2.30% CNA, 2.90%	Differentiation, polarization	TAS	[130]
SEC24B	Mutation, 1.90%	Differentiation, polarization	IMP, IGI	[131]
SMAD4	Mutation, 2.90% CNA, 3.50%	Differentiation, transcription factor	IMP	[132]
TJP1	Mutation, 1.90%	Differentiation, tight junction protein	IBA	[133]
TP63	Mutation, 2.30% CNA, 16.10%	Differentiation, transcription factor		[10,57–61,106,108]
TRIOBP	Mutation, 1.90%	Differentiation, junction, AJ formation	IMP	[134]
AGR2	CNA, 1.90% AMP	Differentiation	IDA	[135]
DLX5	CNA, 4.10% AMP	Differentiation, transcription factor	IGI	[136]
DLX6	CNA, 4.10% AMP	Differentiation, transcription factor	IGI	[136]
EHF	CNA, 2.70% AMP	Differentiation, transcription factor	IEA	[137]
ELF5	CNA, 2.50% AMP	Differentiation, anti-EMT	IGI	[138]
ESRP1	CNA, 2.70% AMP	Differentiation, splicing	IMP	[139]
EXT1	CNA, 5.80% AMP	Differentiation, mesenchymal development, regeneration	IMP	[140]
FAM20C	CNA, 1.90% AMP	Differentiation, secreted phosphoproteome, wound healing	IDA	[141]
FOXL2	CNA, 5.00% AMP	Differentiation, transcription factor	IMP	[142]
GSK3B	CNA, 2.90% AMP	Differentiation, notch pathway		[69]
IFNG	CNA, 4.10% AMP	Differentiation, polarization	ISO	[143]
KLF5	CNA, 2.90% AMP	Proliferation, early differentiation	IMP	[144]
NFIB	CNA, 3.30% AMP	Mesenchymal to epithelial differentiation	IMP	[145]
NKX2-1	CNA, 1.90% AMP	Differentiation, transcription factor	IGI	[146]
OVOL1	CNA, 4.10% AMP	Differentiation, transcription factor	IBA	[133]

Table 1. Cont.

Name of Genes	Frequency of Genetic Alterations in HNSCC	Functions in Epithelia	Evidence	Ref
PGR	CNA, 3.90% AMP	Differentiation	IMP	[147]
RFX3	CNA, 3.70% AMP	Differentiation, specification, transcription factor	IMP	[148]
SOX17	CNA, 2.90% AMP	Differentiation, specification	IGI	[149]
TBX1	CNA, 2.10% AMP	Differentiation, adhesion	IMP	[150]
ABCA12	Mutation, 3.70%	Terminal differentiation, lipid homeostasis		[6,43,71,72]
FLG	Mutation, 13.00%	Terminal differentiation, cornified envelop		[43,44,73,74,76,107]
HRNR	Mutation, 4.10%	Terminal differentiation, cornified envelop		[43,44,77,78,107]
MYO7A	Mutation, 1.90% CNA, 3.10%	Terminal differentiation	IMP	[151]

The genetic alteration data were extracted from HNSCC patients (n = 515) available through The Cancer Genome Atlas (TCGA, PanCancer Atlas). Three housekeeping genes were used to establish the percentage of base-level mutation—ACTB: 0.8%; GAPDH: 0.4%; HPRT: 0.4%. All genes with a frequency of genetic alterations that is equal or below 0.8% were omitted. References are evidence for the gene function in epithelia, suggesting a differentiation/terminal differentiation role for the selected genes with significant genetic alterations in HNSCC. Abbreviations: AMP, amplification; CNA, copy number alteration; IDA, inferred from direct assay; IMP, inferred from mutant phenotype; ISO, inferred from sequence orthology; IGI, inferred from genetic interaction; TAS, traceable author statement; IEA, inferred from electronic annotation; IBA, inferred from biological aspect of ancestor.

8. Conclusions

OSCC genomic alterations are dominated by the loss of terminal differentiation tumour suppressor genes, with 80% of patients harbouring at least one genomic alteration in a targetable gene [104]. This suggests that novel approaches to treatment may be possible for OSCC, particularly by identifying upstream signalling leading to the induction of functional terminal differentiation factors and subsequently, OE terminal differentiation to promote therapy response.

Author Contributions: Conceptualization, Y.B. and C.D.; literature and investigation, Y.B., J.B., C.S.F. and C.D.; data curation, Y.B., J.B. and C.D.; methodology, Y.B., J.B. and C.D.; software, Y.B. and J.B.; formal analysis, Y.B., J.B. and C.D.; figure and table preparation, Y.B., G.R.W., U.G.I.U.K.; writing—original draft preparation, Y.B. and C.D.; writing—review and editing, Y.B., J.B., G.R.W., U.G.I.U.K., C.S.F. and C.D.; supervision, C.D.; project administration, C.D. All authors have read and agreed to the published version of the manuscript.

Funding: This research received no external funding. Authors were funded by a Victorian Cancer Agency mid-career Fellowship (MCRF16017) to C.D., a research scholarship from the Garnett Passe and Rodney William Memorial Foundation to J.B., and a grant from the 2021 Medical Research Future Fund (MRFF 2008888) to C.S.F. and C.D.

Institutional Review Board Statement: Not applicable.

Informed Consent Statement: Not applicable.

Conflicts of Interest: The authors declare no conflict of interest.

References

1. Chi, A.C.; Day, T.A.; Neville, B.W. Oral cavity and oropharyngeal squamous cell carcinoma—An update. *CA Cancer J. Clin.* **2015**, *65*, 401–421. [CrossRef]
2. Tan, F.H.; Bai, Y.; Saintigny, P.; Darido, C. mTOR Signalling in Head and Neck Cancer: Heads Up. *Cells* **2019**, *8*, 333. [CrossRef]
3. Bray, F.; Ferlay, J.; Soerjomataram, I.; Siegel, R.L.; Torre, L.A.; Jemal, A. Global cancer statistics 2018: GLOBOCAN estimates of incidence and mortality worldwide for 36 cancers in 185 countries. *CA Cancer J. Clin.* **2018**, *68*, 394–424. [CrossRef] [PubMed]
4. Warnakulasuriya, S. Global epidemiology of oral and oropharyngeal cancer. *Oral Oncol.* **2009**, *45*, 309–316. [CrossRef]

5. Dutzan, N.; Abusleme, L.; Bridgeman, H.; Greenwell-Wild, T.; Zangerle-Murray, T.; Fife, M.E.; Bouladoux, N.; Linley, H.; Brenchley, L.; Wemyss, K.; et al. On-going Mechanical Damage from Mastication Drives Homeostatic Th17 Cell Responses at the Oral Barrier. *Immunity* **2017**, *46*, 133–147. [CrossRef] [PubMed]
6. Darido, C.; Georgy, S.R.; Jane, S.M. The role of barrier genes in epidermal malignancy. *Oncogene* **2016**, *35*, 5705–5712. [CrossRef] [PubMed]
7. Groeger, S.; Meyle, J. Oral Mucosal Epithelial Cells. *Front. Immunol.* **2019**, *10*, 208. [CrossRef] [PubMed]
8. Martin-Belmonte, F.; Perez-Moreno, M. Epithelial cell polarity, stem cells and cancer. *Nat. Rev. Cancer* **2011**, *12*, 23–38. [CrossRef] [PubMed]
9. Jones, K.B.; Furukawa, S.; Marangoni, P.; Ma, H.; Pinkard, H.; D'Urso, R.; Zilionis, R.; Klein, A.M.; Klein, O.D. Quantitative Clonal Analysis and Single-Cell Transcriptomics Reveal Division Kinetics, Hierarchy, and Fate of Oral Epithelial Progenitor Cells. *Cell Stem Cell* **2019**, *24*, 183–192.e8. [CrossRef]
10. Iglesias-Bartolome, R.; Gutkind, J.S. Signaling circuitries controlling stem cell fate: To be or not to be. *Curr. Opin. Cell Biol.* **2011**, *23*, 716–723. [CrossRef]
11. Varga, J.; Greten, F.R. Cell plasticity in epithelial homeostasis and tumorigenesis. *Nat. Cell Biol.* **2017**, *19*, 1133–1141. [CrossRef] [PubMed]
12. Youssef, M.; Cuddihy, A.; Darido, C. Long-Lived Epidermal Cancer-Initiating Cells. *Int. J. Mol. Sci.* **2017**, *18*, 1369. [CrossRef] [PubMed]
13. Cangkrama, M.; Ting, S.B.; Darido, C. Stem cells behind the barrier. *Int. J. Mol. Sci.* **2013**, *14*, 13670–13686. [CrossRef]
14. Leemans, C.R.; Braakhuis, B.J.; Brakenhoff, R.H. The molecular biology of head and neck cancer. *Nat. Rev. Cancer* **2011**, *11*, 9–22. [CrossRef] [PubMed]
15. Dworkin, S.; Jane, S.M.; Darido, C. The planar cell polarity pathway in vertebrate epidermal development, homeostasis and repair. *Organogenesis* **2011**, *7*, 202–208. [CrossRef]
16. Clevers, H. Stem Cells. What is an adult stem cell? *Science* **2015**, *350*, 1319–1320. [CrossRef]
17. Tanaka, T.; Komai, Y.; Tokuyama, Y.; Yanai, H.; Ohe, S.; Okazaki, K.; Ueno, H. Identification of stem cells that maintain and regenerate lingual keratinized epithelial cells. *Nat. Cell Biol.* **2013**, *15*, 511–518. [CrossRef]
18. Byrd, K.M.; Piehl, N.C.; Patel, J.H.; Huh, W.J.; Sequeira, I.; Lough, K.J.; Wagner, B.L.; Marangoni, P.; Watt, F.M.; Klein, O.D.; et al. Heterogeneity within Stratified Epithelial Stem Cell Populations Maintains the Oral Mucosa in Response to Physiological Stress. *Cell Stem Cell* **2019**, *25*, 814–829.e6. [CrossRef] [PubMed]
19. Iglesias-Bartolome, R.; Uchiyama, A.; Molinolo, A.A.; Abusleme, L.; Brooks, S.R.; Callejas-Valera, J.L.; Edwards, D.; Doci, C.; Asselin-Labat, M.L.; Onaitis, M.W.; et al. Transcriptional signature primes human oral mucosa for rapid wound healing. *Sci. Transl. Med.* **2018**, *10*, eaap8798. [CrossRef]
20. Yuan, X.; Xu, Q.; Zhang, X.; Van Brunt, L.A.; Ticha, P.; Helms, J.A. Wnt-Responsive Stem Cell Fates in the Oral Mucosa. *iScience* **2019**, *21*, 84–94. [CrossRef] [PubMed]
21. Loughran, O.; Clark, L.J.; Bond, J.; Baker, A.; Berry, I.J.; Edington, K.G.; Ly, I.S.; Simmons, R.; Haw, R.; Black, D.M.; et al. Evidence for the inactivation of multiple replicative lifespan genes in immortal human squamous cell carcinoma keratinocytes. *Oncogene* **1997**, *14*, 1955–1964. [CrossRef] [PubMed]
22. Dickson, M.A.; Hahn, W.C.; Ino, Y.; Ronfard, V.; Wu, J.Y.; Weinberg, R.A.; Louis, D.N.; Li, F.P.; Rheinwald, J.G. Human keratinocytes that express hTERT and also bypass a p16(INK4a)-enforced mechanism that limits life span become immortal yet retain normal growth and differentiation characteristics. *Mol. Cell. Biol.* **2000**, *20*, 1436–1447. [CrossRef] [PubMed]
23. Jang, D.H.; Bhawal, U.K.; Min, H.K.; Kang, H.K.; Abiko, Y.; Min, B.M. A transcriptional roadmap to the senescence and differentiation of human oral keratinocytes. *J. Gerontol. A Biol. Sci. Med. Sci.* **2015**, *70*, 20–32. [CrossRef] [PubMed]
24. Natarajan, E.; Omobono, J.D., 2nd; Guo, Z.; Hopkinson, S.; Lazar, A.J.; Brenn, T.; Jones, J.C.; Rheinwald, J.G. A keratinocyte hypermotility/growth-arrest response involving laminin 5 and p16INK4A activated in wound healing and senescence. *Am. J. Pathol.* **2006**, *168*, 1821–1837. [CrossRef]
25. Veeramachaneni, R.; Walker, T.; Revil, T.; Weck, A.D.; Badescu, D.; O'Sullivan, J.; Higgins, C.; Elliott, L.; Liloglou, T.; Risk, J.M.; et al. Analysis of head and neck carcinoma progression reveals novel and relevant stage-specific changes associated with immortalisation and malignancy. *Sci. Rep.* **2019**, *9*, 11992. [CrossRef]
26. Goldie, S.J.; Chincarini, G.; Darido, C. Targeted Therapy Against the Cell of Origin in Cutaneous Squamous Cell Carcinoma. *Int. J. Mol. Sci.* **2019**, *20*, 2201. [CrossRef]
27. Wang, Y.; Xu, Q.; Sack, L.; Kang, C.; Elledge, S.J. A gain-of-function senescence bypass screen identifies the homeobox transcription factor DLX2 as a regulator of ATM-p53 signaling. *Genes Dev.* **2016**, *30*, 293–306. [CrossRef]
28. Chan, K.T.; Blake, S.; Zhu, H.; Kang, J.; Trigos, A.S.; Madhamshettiwar, P.B.; Diesch, J.; Paavolainen, L.; Horvath, P.; Hannan, R.D.; et al. A functional genetic screen defines the AKT-induced senescence signaling network. *Cell Death Differ.* **2020**, *27*, 725–741. [CrossRef]
29. Zhang, Z.; Filho, M.S.; Nör, J.E. The biology of head and neck cancer stem cells. *Oral Oncol.* **2012**, *48*, 1–9. [CrossRef]
30. Milanovic, M.; Fan, D.N.Y.; Belenki, D.; Däbritz, J.H.M.; Zhao, Z.; Yu, Y.; Dörr, J.R.; Dimitrova, L.; Lenze, D.; Monteiro Barbosa, I.A.; et al. Senescence-associated reprogramming promotes cancer stemness. *Nature* **2018**, *553*, 96–100. [CrossRef]

31. Prince, M.E.; Sivanandan, R.; Kaczorowski, A.; Wolf, G.T.; Kaplan, M.J.; Dalerba, P.; Weissman, I.L.; Clarke, M.F.; Ailles, L.E. Identification of a subpopulation of cells with cancer stem cell properties in head and neck squamous cell carcinoma. *Proc. Natl. Acad. Sci. USA* **2007**, *104*, 973–978. [CrossRef]
32. Dalley, A.J.; AbdulMajeed, A.A.; Upton, Z.; Farah, C.S. Organotypic culture of normal, dysplastic and squamous cell carcinoma-derived oral cell lines reveals loss of spatial regulation of CD44 and p75 NTR in malignancy. *J. Oral Pathol. Med.* **2013**, *42*, 37–46. [CrossRef] [PubMed]
33. Baillie, R.; Tan, S.T.; Itinteang, T. Cancer Stem Cells in Oral Cavity Squamous Cell Carcinoma: A Review. *Front. Oncol.* **2017**, *7*, 112. [CrossRef] [PubMed]
34. Chen, D.; Wu, M.; Li, Y.; Chang, I.; Yuan, Q.; Ekimyan-Salvo, M.; Deng, P.; Yu, B.; Yu, Y.; Dong, J.; et al. Targeting BMI1(+) Cancer Stem Cells Overcomes Chemoresistance and Inhibits Metastases in Squamous Cell Carcinoma. *Cell Stem Cell* **2017**, *20*, 621–634.e6. [CrossRef] [PubMed]
35. Dalley, A.J.; Pitty, L.P.; Major, A.G.; Abdulmajeed, A.A.; Farah, C.S. Expression of ABCG2 and Bmi-1 in oral potentially malignant lesions and oral squamous cell carcinoma. *Cancer Med.* **2014**, *3*, 273–283. [CrossRef]
36. Sakamoto, K.; Fujii, T.; Kawachi, H.; Miki, Y.; Omura, K.; Morita, K.; Kayamori, K.; Katsube, K.; Yamaguchi, A. Reduction of NOTCH1 expression pertains to maturation abnormalities of keratinocytes in squamous neoplasms. *Lab. Investig.* **2012**, *92*, 688–702. [CrossRef] [PubMed]
37. Nyman, P.E.; Buehler, D.; Lambert, P.F. Loss of Function of Canonical Notch Signaling Drives Head and Neck Carcinogenesis. *Clin. Cancer Res.* **2018**, *24*, 6308–6318. [CrossRef]
38. Zhong, R.; Bao, R.; Faber, P.W.; Bindokas, V.P.; Bechill, J.; Lingen, M.W.; Spiotto, M.T. Notch1 Activation or Loss Promotes HPV-Induced Oral Tumorigenesis. *Cancer Res.* **2015**, *75*, 3958–3969. [CrossRef]
39. Blanpain, C.; Lowry, W.E.; Pasolli, H.A.; Fuchs, E. Canonical notch signaling functions as a commitment switch in the epidermal lineage. *Genes Dev.* **2006**, *20*, 3022–3035. [CrossRef]
40. Loganathan, S.K.; Schleicher, K.; Malik, A.; Quevedo, R.; Langille, E.; Teng, K.; Oh, R.H.; Rathod, B.; Tsai, R.; Samavarchi-Tehrani, P.; et al. Rare driver mutations in head and neck squamous cell carcinomas converge on NOTCH signaling. *Science* **2020**, *367*, 1264–1269. [CrossRef]
41. Demehri, S.; Turkoz, A.; Kopan, R. Epidermal Notch1 loss promotes skin tumorigenesis by impacting the stromal microenvironment. *Cancer Cell* **2009**, *16*, 55–66. [CrossRef]
42. Nowell, C.S.; Radtke, F. Notch as a tumour suppressor. *Nat. Rev. Cancer* **2017**, *17*, 145–159. [CrossRef]
43. Cancer Genome Atlas Research, N.; Brat, D.J.; Verhaak, R.G.; Aldape, K.D.; Yung, W.K.; Salama, S.R.; Cooper, L.A.; Rheinbay, E.; Miller, C.R.; Vitucci, M.; et al. Comprehensive, Integrative Genomic Analysis of Diffuse Lower-Grade Gliomas. *N. Engl. J. Med.* **2015**, *372*, 2481–2498. [CrossRef]
44. Swanson, M.S.; Kokot, N.; Sinha, U.K. The Role of HPV in Head and Neck Cancer Stem Cell Formation and Tumorigenesis. *Cancers* **2016**, *8*, 24. [CrossRef]
45. De Boer, D.V.; Brink, A.; Buijze, M.; Stigter-van Walsum, M.; Hunter, K.D.; Ylstra, B.; Bloemena, E.; Leemans, C.R.; Brakenhoff, R.H. Establishment and Genetic Landscape of Precancer Cell Model Systems from the Head and Neck Mucosal Lining. *Mol. Cancer Res.* **2019**, *17*, 120–130. [CrossRef]
46. Sun, W.; Gaykalova, D.A.; Ochs, M.F.; Mambo, E.; Arnaoutakis, D.; Liu, Y.; Loyo, M.; Agrawal, N.; Howard, J.; Li, R.; et al. Activation of the NOTCH pathway in head and neck cancer. *Cancer Res.* **2014**, *74*, 1091–1104. [CrossRef]
47. Fortini, M.E. Gamma-secretase-mediated proteolysis in cell-surface-receptor signalling. *Nat. Rev. Mol. Cell. Biol.* **2002**, *3*, 673–684. [CrossRef]
48. Ran, Y.; Hossain, F.; Pannuti, A.; Lessard, C.B.; Ladd, G.Z.; Jung, J.I.; Minter, L.M.; Osborne, B.A.; Miele, L.; Golde, T.E. gamma-Secretase inhibitors in cancer clinical trials are pharmacologically and functionally distinct. *EMBO Mol. Med.* **2017**, *9*, 950–966. [CrossRef] [PubMed]
49. Zhao, B.; Tumaneng, K.; Guan, K.L. The Hippo pathway in organ size control, tissue regeneration and stem cell self-renewal. *Nat. Cell Biol.* **2011**, *13*, 877–883. [CrossRef] [PubMed]
50. Zheng, Y.; Pan, D. The Hippo Signaling Pathway in Development and Disease. *Dev. Cell* **2019**, *50*, 264–282. [CrossRef] [PubMed]
51. Zhang, H.; Pasolli, H.A.; Fuchs, E. Yes-associated protein (YAP) transcriptional coactivator functions in balancing growth and differentiation in skin. *Proc. Natl. Acad. Sci. USA* **2011**, *108*, 2270–2275. [CrossRef]
52. Omori, H.; Nishio, M.; Masuda, M.; Miyachi, Y.; Ueda, F.; Nakano, T.; Sato, K.; Mimori, K.; Taguchi, K.; Hikasa, H.; et al. YAP1 is a potent driver of the onset and progression of oral squamous cell carcinoma. *Sci. Adv.* **2020**, *6*, eaay3324. [CrossRef] [PubMed]
53. Lin, S.C.; Lin, L.H.; Yu, S.Y.; Kao, S.Y.; Chang, K.W.; Cheng, H.W.; Liu, C.J. FAT1 somatic mutations in head and neck carcinoma are associated with tumor progression and survival. *Carcinogenesis* **2018**, *39*, 1320–1330. [CrossRef] [PubMed]
54. Martin, D.; Degese, M.S.; Vitale-Cross, L.; Iglesias-Bartolome, R.; Valera, J.L.C.; Wang, Z.; Feng, X.; Yeerna, H.; Vadmal, V.; Moroishi, T.; et al. Assembly and activation of the Hippo signalome by FAT1 tumor suppressor. *Nat. Commun.* **2018**, *9*, 2372. [CrossRef]
55. Wang, Y.; Xu, X.; Maglic, D.; Dill, M.T.; Mojumdar, K.; Ng, P.K.; Jeong, K.J.; Tsang, Y.H.; Moreno, D.; Bhavana, V.H.; et al. Comprehensive Molecular Characterization of the Hippo Signaling Pathway in Cancer. *Cell Rep.* **2018**, *25*, 1304–1317.e5. [CrossRef]

56. Jerhammar, F.; Johansson, A.C.; Ceder, R.; Welander, J.; Jansson, A.; Grafstrom, R.C.; Soderkvist, P.; Roberg, K. YAP1 is a potential biomarker for cetuximab resistance in head and neck cancer. *Oral Oncol.* **2014**, *50*, 832–839. [CrossRef]
57. Laurikkala, J.; Mikkola, M.L.; James, M.; Tummers, M.; Mills, A.A.; Thesleff, I. p63 regulates multiple signalling pathways required for ectodermal organogenesis and differentiation. *Development* **2006**, *133*, 1553–1563. [CrossRef] [PubMed]
58. Romano, R.A.; Smalley, K.; Magraw, C.; Serna, V.A.; Kurita, T.; Raghavan, S.; Sinha, S. DeltaNp63 knockout mice reveal its indispensable role as a master regulator of epithelial development and differentiation. *Development* **2012**, *139*, 772–782. [CrossRef]
59. Soares, E.; Zhou, H. Master regulatory role of p63 in epidermal development and disease. *Cell Mol. Life Sci.* **2018**, *75*, 1179–1190. [CrossRef]
60. Devos, M.; Gilbert, B.; Denecker, G.; Leurs, K.; Mc Guire, C.; Lemeire, K.; Hochepied, T.; Vuylsteke, M.; Lambert, J.; Van Den Broecke, C.; et al. Elevated DeltaNp63alpha Levels Facilitate Epidermal and Biliary Oncogenic Transformation. *J. Investig. Dermatol.* **2017**, *137*, 494–505. [CrossRef]
61. Lo Muzio, L.; Santarelli, A.; Caltabiano, R.; Rubini, C.; Pieramici, T.; Trevisiol, L.; Carinci, F.; Leonardi, R.; De Lillo, A.; Lanzafame, S.; et al. p63 overexpression associates with poor prognosis in head and neck squamous cell carcinoma. *Hum. Pathol.* **2005**, *36*, 187–194. [CrossRef] [PubMed]
62. Atlasi, Y.; Stunnenberg, H.G. The interplay of epigenetic marks during stem cell differentiation and development. *Nat. Rev. Genet.* **2017**, *18*, 643–658. [CrossRef]
63. Ezhkova, E.; Pasolli, H.A.; Parker, J.S.; Stokes, N.; Su, I.H.; Hannon, G.; Tarakhovsky, A.; Fuchs, E. Ezh2 orchestrates gene expression for the stepwise differentiation of tissue-specific stem cells. *Cell* **2009**, *136*, 1122–1135. [CrossRef]
64. Gannon, O.M.; Merida de Long, L.; Endo-Munoz, L.; Hazar-Rethinam, M.; Saunders, N.A. Dysregulation of the repressive H3K27 trimethylation mark in head and neck squamous cell carcinoma contributes to dysregulated squamous differentiation. *Clin. Cancer Res.* **2013**, *19*, 428–441. [CrossRef]
65. Chua, B.A.; Van Der Werf, I.; Jamieson, C.; Signer, R.A.J. Post-Transcriptional Regulation of Homeostatic, Stressed, and Malignant Stem Cells. *Cell Stem Cell* **2020**, *26*, 138–159. [CrossRef] [PubMed]
66. Darido, C.; Georgy, S.R.; Cullinane, C.; Partridge, D.D.; Walker, R.; Srivastava, S.; Roslan, S.; Carpinelli, M.R.; Dworkin, S.; Pearson, R.B.; et al. Stage-dependent therapeutic efficacy in PI3K/mTOR-driven squamous cell carcinoma of the skin. *Cell Death Differ.* **2018**, *25*, 1146–1159. [CrossRef]
67. Goldie, S.J.; Cottle, D.L.; Tan, F.H.; Roslan, S.; Srivastava, S.; Brady, R.; Partridge, D.D.; Auden, A.; Smyth, I.M.; Jane, S.M.; et al. Loss of GRHL3 leads to TARC/CCL17-mediated keratinocyte proliferation in the epidermis. *Cell Death Dis.* **2018**, *9*, 1072. [CrossRef] [PubMed]
68. Darido, C.; Georgy, S.R.; Wilanowski, T.; Dworkin, S.; Auden, A.; Zhao, Q.; Rank, G.; Srivastava, S.; Finlay, M.J.; Papenfuss, A.T.; et al. Targeting of the tumor suppressor GRHL3 by a miR-21-dependent proto-oncogenic network results in PTEN loss and tumorigenesis. *Cancer Cell* **2011**, *20*, 635–648. [CrossRef] [PubMed]
69. Georgy, S.R.; Cangkrama, M.; Srivastava, S.; Partridge, D.; Auden, A.; Dworkin, S.; McLean, C.A.; Jane, S.M.; Darido, C. Identification of a Novel Proto-oncogenic Network in Head and Neck Squamous Cell Carcinoma. *J. Natl. Cancer Inst.* **2015**, *107*, djv152. [CrossRef]
70. Lee, A.Y. The Role of MicroRNAs in Epidermal Barrier. *Int. J. Mol. Sci.* **2020**, *21*, 5781. [CrossRef]
71. Smyth, I.; Hacking, D.F.; Hilton, A.A.; Mukhamedova, N.; Meikle, P.J.; Ellis, S.; Satterley, K.; Collinge, J.E.; de Graaf, C.A.; Bahlo, M.; et al. A mouse model of harlequin ichthyosis delineates a key role for Abca12 in lipid homeostasis. *PLoS Genet.* **2008**, *4*, e1000192. [CrossRef]
72. Kelsell, D.P.; Norgett, E.E.; Unsworth, H.; Teh, M.T.; Cullup, T.; Mein, C.A.; Dopping-Hepenstal, P.J.; Dale, B.A.; Tadini, G.; Fleckman, P.; et al. Mutations in ABCA12 underlie the severe congenital skin disease harlequin ichthyosis. *Am. J. Hum. Genet.* **2005**, *76*, 794–803. [CrossRef]
73. Quiroz, F.G.; Fiore, V.F.; Levorse, J.; Polak, L.; Wong, E.; Pasolli, H.A.; Fuchs, E. Liquid-liquid phase separation drives skin barrier formation. *Science* **2020**, *367*, eaax9554. [CrossRef] [PubMed]
74. McGrath, J.A.; Uitto, J. The filaggrin story: Novel insights into skin-barrier function and disease. *Trends Mol. Med.* **2008**, *14*, 20–27. [CrossRef]
75. Cubero, J.L.; Isidoro-Garcia, M.; Segura, N.; Benito Pescador, D.; Sanz, C.; Lorente, F.; Davila, I.; Colas, C. Filaggrin gene mutations and new SNPs in asthmatic patients: A cross-sectional study in a Spanish population. *Allergy Asthma Clin. Immunol.* **2016**, *12*, 31. [CrossRef]
76. Bai, Y.; Zhao, Z.; Boath, J.; van Denderen, B.J.; Darido, C. The functional GRHL3-filaggrin axis maintains a tumor differentiation potential and influences drug sensitivity. *Mol. Ther.* **2021**, *29*, 2571–2582. [CrossRef]
77. Wu, Z.; Meyer-Hoffert, U.; Reithmayer, K.; Paus, R.; Hansmann, B.; He, Y.; Bartels, J.; Glaser, R.; Harder, J.; Schroder, J.M. Highly complex peptide aggregates of the S100 fused-type protein hornerin are present in human skin. *J. Investig. Dermatol.* **2009**, *129*, 1446–1458. [CrossRef] [PubMed]
78. Henry, J.; Hsu, C.Y.; Haftek, M.; Nachat, R.; de Koning, H.D.; Gardinal-Galera, I.; Hitomi, K.; Balica, S.; Jean-Decoster, C.; Schmitt, A.M.; et al. Hornerin is a component of the epidermal cornified cell envelopes. *FASEB J.* **2011**, *25*, 1567–1576. [CrossRef]
79. Ribeiro, I.P.; Caramelo, F.; Esteves, L.; Menoita, J.; Marques, F.; Barroso, L.; Migueis, J.; Melo, J.B.; Carreira, I.M. Genomic predictive model for recurrence and metastasis development in head and neck squamous cell carcinoma patients. *Sci. Rep.* **2017**, *7*, 13897. [CrossRef]

80. Gonzalez-Garcia, R.; Naval-Gias, L.; Roman-Romero, L.; Sastre-Perez, J.; Rodriguez-Campo, F.J. Local recurrences and second primary tumors from squamous cell carcinoma of the oral cavity: A retrospective analytic study of 500 patients. *Head Neck* **2009**, *31*, 1168–1180. [CrossRef]
81. Curtius, K.; Wright, N.A.; Graham, T.A. An evolutionary perspective on field cancerization. *Nat. Rev. Cancer* **2018**, *18*, 19–32. [CrossRef]
82. Cramer, J.D.; Burtness, B.; Le, Q.T.; Ferris, R.L. The changing therapeutic landscape of head and neck cancer. *Nat. Rev. Clin. Oncol.* **2019**, *16*, 669–683. [CrossRef] [PubMed]
83. Ferris, R.L.; Blumenschein, G., Jr.; Fayette, J.; Guigay, J.; Colevas, A.D.; Licitra, L.; Harrington, K.; Kasper, S.; Vokes, E.E.; Even, C.; et al. Nivolumab for Recurrent Squamous-Cell Carcinoma of the Head and Neck. *N. Engl. J. Med.* **2016**, *375*, 1856–1867. [CrossRef]
84. Ock, C.Y.; Hwang, J.E.; Keam, B.; Kim, S.B.; Shim, J.J.; Jang, H.J.; Park, S.; Sohn, B.H.; Cha, M.; Ajani, J.A.; et al. Genomic landscape associated with potential response to anti-CTLA-4 treatment in cancers. *Nat. Commun.* **2017**, *8*, 1050. [CrossRef] [PubMed]
85. Koyama, S.; Akbay, E.A.; Li, Y.Y.; Herter-Sprie, G.S.; Buczkowski, K.A.; Richards, W.G.; Gandhi, L.; Redig, A.J.; Rodig, S.J.; Asahina, H.; et al. Adaptive resistance to therapeutic PD-1 blockade is associated with upregulation of alternative immune checkpoints. *Nat. Commun.* **2016**, *7*, 10501. [CrossRef]
86. Chow, L.Q.M.; Haddad, R.; Gupta, S.; Mahipal, A.; Mehra, R.; Tahara, M.; Berger, R.; Eder, J.P.; Burtness, B.; Lee, S.H.; et al. Antitumor Activity of Pembrolizumab in Biomarker-Unselected Patients with Recurrent and/or Metastatic Head and Neck Squamous Cell Carcinoma: Results from the Phase Ib KEYNOTE-012 Expansion Cohort. *J. Clin. Oncol.* **2016**, *34*, 3838–3845. [CrossRef]
87. Saada-Bouzid, E.; Defaucheux, C.; Karabajakian, A.; Coloma, V.P.; Servois, V.; Paoletti, X.; Even, C.; Fayette, J.; Guigay, J.; Loirat, D.; et al. Hyperprogression during anti-PD-1/PD-L1 therapy in patients with recurrent and/or metastatic head and neck squamous cell carcinoma. *Ann. Oncol.* **2017**, *28*, 1605–1611. [CrossRef] [PubMed]
88. Burtness, B.; Harrington, K.J.; Greil, R.; Soulieres, D.; Tahara, M.; de Castro, G., Jr.; Psyrri, A.; Baste, N.; Neupane, P.; Bratland, A.; et al. Pembrolizumab alone or with chemotherapy versus cetuximab with chemotherapy for recurrent or metastatic squamous cell carcinoma of the head and neck (KEYNOTE-048): A randomised, open-label, phase 3 study. *Lancet* **2019**, *394*, 1915–1928. [CrossRef]
89. Jiang, H.; Hegde, S.; Knolhoff, B.L.; Zhu, Y.; Herndon, J.M.; Meyer, M.A.; Nywening, T.M.; Hawkins, W.G.; Shapiro, I.M.; Weaver, D.T.; et al. Targeting focal adhesion kinase renders pancreatic cancers responsive to checkpoint immunotherapy. *Nat. Med.* **2016**, *22*, 851–860. [CrossRef]
90. Akbay, E.A.; Koyama, S.; Carretero, J.; Altabef, A.; Tchaicha, J.H.; Christensen, C.L.; Mikse, O.R.; Cherniack, A.D.; Beauchamp, E.M.; Pugh, T.J.; et al. Activation of the PD-1 pathway contributes to immune escape in EGFR-driven lung tumors. *Cancer Discov.* **2013**, *3*, 1355–1363. [CrossRef]
91. Wellenstein, M.D.; de Visser, K.E. Cancer-Cell-Intrinsic Mechanisms Shaping the Tumor Immune Landscape. *Immunity* **2018**, *48*, 399–416. [CrossRef] [PubMed]
92. Sobol, R.E.; Menander, K.B.; Chada, S.; Wiederhold, D.; Sellman, B.; Talbott, M.; Nemunaitis, J.J. Analysis of Adenoviral p53 Gene Therapy Clinical Trials in Recurrent Head and Neck Squamous Cell Carcinoma. *Front. Oncol.* **2021**, *11*, 645745. [CrossRef]
93. Slamon, D.; Eiermann, W.; Robert, N.; Pienkowski, T.; Martin, M.; Press, M.; Mackey, J.; Glaspy, J.; Chan, A.; Pawlicki, M.; et al. Adjuvant trastuzumab in HER2-positive breast cancer. *N. Engl. J. Med.* **2011**, *365*, 1273–1283. [CrossRef] [PubMed]
94. Flaherty, K.T.; Infante, J.R.; Daud, A.; Gonzalez, R.; Kefford, R.F.; Sosman, J.; Hamid, O.; Schuchter, L.; Cebon, J.; Ibrahim, N.; et al. Combined BRAF and MEK inhibition in melanoma with BRAF V600 mutations. *N. Engl. J. Med.* **2012**, *367*, 1694–1703. [CrossRef] [PubMed]
95. Shaw, A.T.; Kim, D.W.; Nakagawa, K.; Seto, T.; Crino, L.; Ahn, M.J.; De Pas, T.; Besse, B.; Solomon, B.J.; Blackhall, F.; et al. Crizotinib versus chemotherapy in advanced ALK-positive lung cancer. *N. Engl. J. Med.* **2013**, *368*, 2385–2394. [CrossRef]
96. Hata, A.N.; Niederst, M.J.; Archibald, H.L.; Gomez-Caraballo, M.; Siddiqui, F.M.; Mulvey, H.E.; Maruvka, Y.E.; Ji, F.; Bhang, H.E.; Krishnamurthy Radhakrishna, V.; et al. Tumor cells can follow distinct evolutionary paths to become resistant to epidermal growth factor receptor inhibition. *Nat. Med.* **2016**, *22*, 262–269. [CrossRef]
97. Magnani, L.; Frige, G.; Gadaleta, R.M.; Corleone, G.; Fabris, S.; Kempe, M.H.; Verschure, P.J.; Barozzi, I.; Vircillo, V.; Hong, S.P.; et al. Acquired CYP19A1 amplification is an early specific mechanism of aromatase inhibitor resistance in ERalpha metastatic breast cancer. *Nat. Genet.* **2017**, *49*, 444–450. [CrossRef]
98. Lheureux, S.; Bruce, J.P.; Burnier, J.V.; Karakasis, K.; Shaw, P.A.; Clarke, B.A.; Yang, S.Y.; Quevedo, R.; Li, T.; Dowar, M.; et al. Somatic BRCA1/2 Recovery as a Resistance Mechanism After Exceptional Response to Poly (ADP-ribose) Polymerase Inhibition. *J. Clin. Oncol.* **2017**, *35*, 1240–1249. [CrossRef]
99. Hammerman, P.S.; Hayes, D.N.; Grandis, J.R. Therapeutic insights from genomic studies of head and neck squamous cell carcinomas. *Cancer Discov.* **2015**, *5*, 239–244. [CrossRef]
100. Seiwert, T.Y.; Zuo, Z.; Keck, M.K.; Khattri, A.; Pedamallu, C.S.; Stricker, T.; Brown, C.; Pugh, T.J.; Stojanov, P.; Cho, J.; et al. Integrative and comparative genomic analysis of HPV-positive and HPV-negative head and neck squamous cell carcinomas. *Clin. Cancer Res.* **2015**, *21*, 632–641. [CrossRef]
101. Cassell, A.; Grandis, J.R. Investigational EGFR-targeted therapy in head and neck squamous cell carcinoma. *Expert Opin. Investig. Drugs* **2010**, *19*, 709–722. [CrossRef]

102. Bonner, J.A.; Harari, P.M.; Giralt, J.; Azarnia, N.; Shin, D.M.; Cohen, R.B.; Jones, C.U.; Sur, R.; Raben, D.; Jassem, J.; et al. Radiotherapy plus cetuximab for squamous-cell carcinoma of the head and neck. *N. Engl. J. Med.* **2006**, *354*, 567–578. [CrossRef] [PubMed]
103. Driehuis, E.; Kolders, S.; Spelier, S.; Lohmussaar, K.; Willems, S.M.; Devriese, L.A.; de Bree, R.; de Ruiter, E.J.; Korving, J.; Begthel, H.; et al. Oral Mucosal Organoids as a Potential Platform for Personalized Cancer Therapy. *Cancer Discov.* **2019**, *9*, 852–871. [CrossRef]
104. Pickering, C.R.; Zhang, J.; Yoo, S.Y.; Bengtsson, L.; Moorthy, S.; Neskey, D.M.; Zhao, M.; Ortega Alves, M.V.; Chang, K.; Drummond, J.; et al. Integrative genomic characterization of oral squamous cell carcinoma identifies frequent somatic drivers. *Cancer Discov.* **2013**, *3*, 770–781. [CrossRef]
105. Kang, H.; Kiess, A.; Chung, C.H. Emerging biomarkers in head and neck cancer in the era of genomics. *Nat. Rev. Clin. Oncol.* **2015**, *12*, 11–26. [CrossRef]
106. Cancer Genome Atlas, N. Comprehensive genomic characterization of head and neck squamous cell carcinomas. *Nature* **2015**, *517*, 576–582. [CrossRef]
107. Stransky, N.; Egloff, A.M.; Tward, A.D.; Kostic, A.D.; Cibulskis, K.; Sivachenko, A.; Kryukov, G.V.; Lawrence, M.S.; Sougnez, C.; McKenna, A.; et al. The mutational landscape of head and neck squamous cell carcinoma. *Science* **2011**, *333*, 1157–1160. [CrossRef] [PubMed]
108. Agrawal, N.; Frederick, M.J.; Pickering, C.R.; Bettegowda, C.; Chang, K.; Li, R.J.; Fakhry, C.; Xie, T.X.; Zhang, J.; Wang, J.; et al. Exome sequencing of head and neck squamous cell carcinoma reveals inactivating mutations in NOTCH1. *Science* **2011**, *333*, 1154–1157. [CrossRef]
109. Siegel, R.; Ward, E.; Brawley, O.; Jemal, A. Cancer statistics, 2011: The impact of eliminating socioeconomic and racial disparities on premature cancer deaths. *CA Cancer J. Clin.* **2011**, *61*, 212–236. [CrossRef] [PubMed]
110. Li, Y.; Li, L.J.; Wang, L.J.; Zhang, Z.; Gao, N.; Liang, C.Y.; Huang, Y.D.; Han, B. Selective intra-arterial infusion of rAd-p53 with chemotherapy for advanced oral cancer: A randomized clinical trial. *BMC Med.* **2014**, *12*, 16. [CrossRef] [PubMed]
111. Zhang, W.W.; Li, L.; Li, D.; Liu, J.; Li, X.; Li, W.; Xu, X.; Zhang, M.J.; Chandler, L.A.; Lin, H.; et al. The First Approved Gene Therapy Product for Cancer Ad-p53 (Gendicine): 12 Years in the Clinic. *Hum. Gene Ther.* **2018**, *29*, 160–179. [CrossRef]
112. Xue, W.; Zender, L.; Miething, C.; Dickins, R.A.; Hernando, E.; Krizhanovsky, V.; Cordon-Cardo, C.; Lowe, S.W. Senescence and tumour clearance is triggered by p53 restoration in murine liver carcinomas. *Nature* **2007**, *8*, 656–660. [CrossRef]
113. Farah, C.S. Molecular landscape of head and neck cancer and implications for therapy. *Ann. Transl. Med.* **2021**, *9*, 915. [CrossRef]
114. Keck, M.K.; Zuo, Z.; Khattri, A.; Stricker, T.P.; Brown, C.D.; Imanguli, M.; Rieke, D.; Endhardt, K.; Fang, P.; Bragelmann, J.; et al. Integrative analysis of head and neck cancer identifies two biologically distinct HPV and three non-HPV subtypes. *Clin. Cancer Res.* **2015**, *21*, 870–881. [CrossRef] [PubMed]
115. Moon, S.; Um, S.J.; Kim, E.J. Role of Asxl1 in kidney podocyte development via its interaction with Wtip. *Biochem. Biophys. Res. Commun.* **2015**, *466*, 560–566. [CrossRef]
116. Nechiporuk, T.; Fernandez, T.E.; Vasioukhin, V. Failure of epithelial tube maintenance causes hydrocephalus and renal cysts in Dlg5-/- mice. *Dev. Cell* **2007**, *13*, 338–350. [CrossRef] [PubMed]
117. Takito, J.; Al-Awqati, Q. Conversion of ES cells to columnar epithelia by hensin and to squamous epithelia by laminin. *J. Cell Biol.* **2004**, *166*, 1093–1102. [CrossRef]
118. Muraoka-Cook, R.S.; Sandahl, M.; Husted, C.; Hunter, D.; Miraglia, L.; Feng, S.M.; Elenius, K.; Earp, H.S. 3rd, The intracellular domain of ErbB4 induces differentiation of mammary epithelial cells. *Mol. Biol. Cell* **2006**, *17*, 4118–4129. [CrossRef] [PubMed]
119. Bosse, T.; Piaseckyj, C.M.; Burghard, E.; Fialkovich, J.J.; Rajagopal, S.; Pu, W.T.; Krasinski, S.D. Gata4 is essential for the maintenance of jejunal-ileal identities in the adult mouse small intestine. *Mol. Biol. Cell* **2006**, *26*, 9060–9070. [CrossRef]
120. Xia, S.; Li, X.; Johnson, T.; Seidel, C.; Wallace, D.P.; Li, R. Polycystin-dependent fluid flow sensing targets histone deacetylase 5 to prevent the development of renal cysts. *Development* **2010**, *137*, 1075–1084. [CrossRef]
121. Abouhamed, M.; Grobe, K.; San, I.V.; Thelen, S.; Honnert, U.; Balda, M.S.; Matter, K.; Bähler, M. Myosin IXa regulates epithelial differentiation and its deficiency results in hydrocephalus. *Mol. Biol. Cell* **2009**, *20*, 5074–5085. [CrossRef] [PubMed]
122. El-Hashash, A.H.; Turcatel, G.; Al Alam, D.; Buckley, S.; Tokumitsu, H.; Bellusci, S.; Warburton, D. Eya1 controls cell polarity, spindle orientation, cell fate and Notch signaling in distal embryonic lung epithelium. *Development* **2011**, *138*, 1395–1407. [CrossRef]
123. Pierreux, C.E.; Poll, A.V.; Kemp, C.R.; Clotman, F.; Maestro, M.A.; Cordi, S.; Ferrer, J.; Leyns, L.; Rousseau, G.G.; Lemaigre, F.P. The transcription factor hepatocyte nuclear factor-6 controls the development of pancreatic ducts in the mouse. *Gastroenterology* **2006**, *130*, 532–541. [CrossRef]
124. Adolphe, C.; Nieuwenhuis, E.; Villani, R.; Li, Z.J.; Kaur, P.; Hui, C.C.; Wainwright, B.J. Patched 1 and patched 2 redundancy has a key role in regulating epidermal differentiation. *J. Investig. Dermatol.* **2014**, *134*, 1981–1990. [CrossRef]
125. Lohnes, D.; Mark, M.; Mendelsohn, C.; Dollé, P.; Dierich, A.; Gorry, P.; Gansmuller, A.; Chambon, P. Function of the retinoic acid receptors (RARs) during development (I). Craniofacial and skeletal abnormalities in RAR double mutants. *Development* **1994**, *120*, 2723–2748. [CrossRef] [PubMed]
126. Darido, C.; Jane, S.M. Grhl3 and GEF19 in the front rho. *Small GTPases* **2010**, *1*, 104–107. [CrossRef]
127. Ishiuchi, T.; Takeichi, M. Willin and Par3 cooperatively regulate epithelial apical constriction through aPKC-mediated ROCK phosphorylation. *Nat. Cell Biol.* **2011**, *13*, 860–866. [CrossRef] [PubMed]

128. Lock, F.E.; Hotchin, N.A. Distinct roles for ROCK1 and ROCK2 in the regulation of keratinocyte differentiation. *PLoS ONE* **2009**, *4*, e8190. [CrossRef]
129. Sonnenberg-Riethmacher, E.; Walter, B.; Riethmacher, D.; Gödecke, S.; Birchmeier, C. The c-ros tyrosine kinase receptor controls regionalization and differentiation of epithelial cells in the epididymis. *Genes Dev.* **1996**, *10*, 1184–1193. [CrossRef]
130. Sugiyama, Y.; Shelley, E.J.; Badouel, C.; McNeill, H.; McAvoy, J.W. Atypical Cadherin Fat1 Is Required for Lens Epithelial Cell Polarity and Proliferation but Not for Fiber Differentiation. *Investig. Ophthalmol. Vis. Sci.* **2015**, *56*, 4099–4107. [CrossRef]
131. Wansleeben, C.; Feitsma, H.; Montcouquiol, M.; Kroon, C.; Cuppen, E.; Meijlink, F. Planar cell polarity defects and defective Vangl2 trafficking in mutants for the COPII gene Sec24b. *Development* **2010**, *137*, 1067–1073. [CrossRef]
132. Moskowitz, I.P.; Wang, J.; Peterson, M.A.; Pu, W.T.; Mackinnon, A.C.; Oxburgh, L.; Chu, G.C.; Sarkar, M.; Berul, C.; Smoot, L.; et al. Transcription factor genes Smad4 and Gata4 cooperatively regulate cardiac valve development. [corrected]. *Proc. Natl. Acad. Sci. USA* **2011**, *108*, 4006–4011. [CrossRef] [PubMed]
133. Gaudet, P.; Livstone, M.S.; Lewis, S.E.; Thomas, P.D. Phylogenetic-based propagation of functional annotations within the Gene Ontology consortium. *Brief. Bioinform.* **2011**, *12*, 449–462. [CrossRef] [PubMed]
134. Kitajiri, S.; Sakamoto, T.; Belyantseva, I.A.; Goodyear, R.J.; Stepanyan, R.; Fujiwara, I.; Bird, J.E.; Riazuddin, S.; Riazuddin, S.; Ahmed, Z.M.; et al. Actin-bundling protein TRIOBP forms resilient rootlets of hair cell stereocilia essential for hearing. *Cell* **2010**, *141*, 786–798. [CrossRef] [PubMed]
135. Li, S.; Wang, Y.; Zhang, Y.; Lu, M.M.; DeMayo, F.J.; Dekker, J.D.; Tucker, P.W.; Morrisey, E.E. Foxp1/4 control epithelial cell fate during lung development and regeneration through regulation of anterior gradient 2. *Development* **2012**, *139*, 2500–2509. [CrossRef] [PubMed]
136. Suzuki, K.; Haraguchi, R.; Ogata, T.; Barbieri, O.; Alegria, O.; Vieux-Rochas, M.; Nakagata, N.; Ito, M.; Mills, A.A.; Kurita, T.; et al. Abnormal urethra formation in mouse models of split-hand/split-foot malformation type 1 and type 4. *Eur. J. Hum. Genet.* **2008**, *16*, 36–44. [CrossRef]
137. Albino, D.; Longoni, N.; Curti, L.; Mello-Grand, M.; Pinton, S.; Civenni, G.; Thalmann, G.; D'Ambrosio, G.; Sarti, M.; Sessa, F.; et al. ESE3/EHF controls epithelial cell differentiation and its loss leads to prostate tumors with mesenchymal and stem-like features. *Cancer Res.* **2012**, *72*, 2889–2900. [CrossRef]
138. Harris, J.; Stanford, P.M.; Sutherland, K.; Oakes, S.R.; Naylor, M.J.; Robertson, F.G.; Blazek, K.D.; Kazlauskas, M.; Hilton, H.N.; Wittlin, S.; et al. Socs2 and elf5 mediate prolactin-induced mammary gland development. *Mol. Endocrinol.* **2006**, *20*, 1177–1187. [CrossRef]
139. Rohacek, A.M.; Bebee, T.W.; Tilton, R.K.; Radens, C.M.; McDermott-Roe, C.; Peart, N.; Kaur, M.; Zaykaner, M.; Cieply, B.; Musunuru, K.; et al. ESRP1 Mutations Cause Hearing Loss due to Defects in Alternative Splicing that Disrupt Cochlear Development. *Dev. Cell* **2017**, *43*, 318–331.e5. [CrossRef]
140. Huang, M.; He, H.; Belenkaya, T.; Lin, X. Multiple roles of epithelial heparan sulfate in stomach morphogenesis. *J. Cell Sci.* **2018**, *131*, jcs210781. [CrossRef]
141. Hao, J.; Narayanan, K.; Muni, T.; Ramachandran, A.; George, A. Dentin matrix protein 4, a novel secretory calcium-binding protein that modulates odontoblast differentiation. *J. Biol. Chem.* **2007**, *282*, 15357–15365. [CrossRef]
142. Schmidt, D.; Ovitt, C.E.; Anlag, K.; Fehsenfeld, S.; Gredsted, L.; Treier, A.C.; Treier, M. The murine winged-helix transcription factor Foxl2 is required for granulosa cell differentiation and ovary maintenance. *Development* **2004**, *131*, 933–942. [CrossRef] [PubMed]
143. Saunders, N.; Dahler, A.; Jones, S.; Smith, R.; Jetten, A. Interferon-gamma as a regulator of squamous differentiation. *J. Dermatol. Sci.* **1996**, *13*, 98–106. [CrossRef]
144. Bell, S.M.; Zhang, L.; Xu, Y.; Besnard, V.; Wert, S.E.; Shroyer, N.; Whitsett, J.A. Kruppel-like factor 5 controls villus formation and initiation of cytodifferentiation in the embryonic intestinal epithelium. *Dev. Biol.* **2013**, *375*, 128–139. [CrossRef] [PubMed]
145. Hsu, Y.C.; Osinski, J.; Campbell, C.E.; Litwack, E.D.; Wang, D.; Liu, S.; Bachurski, C.J.; Gronostajski, R.M. Mesenchymal nuclear factor I B regulates cell proliferation and epithelial differentiation during lung maturation. *Dev. Biol.* **2011**, *354*, 242–252. [CrossRef]
146. Zhang, Y.; Rath, N.; Hannenhalli, S.; Wang, Z.; Cappola, T.; Kimura, S.; Atochina-Vasserman, E.; Lu, M.M.; Beers, M.F.; Morrisey, E.E. GATA and Nkx factors synergistically regulate tissue-specific gene expression and development in vivo. *Development* **2007**, *134*, 189–198. [CrossRef]
147. Ismail, P.M.; DeMayo, F.J.; Amato, P.; Lydon, J.P. Progesterone induction of calcitonin expression in the murine mammary gland. *J. Endocrinol.* **2004**, *180*, 287–295. [CrossRef]
148. Ait-Lounis, A.; Bonal, C.; Seguín-Estévez, Q.; Schmid, C.D.; Bucher, P.; Herrera, P.L.; Durand, B.; Meda, P.; Reith, W. The transcription factor Rfx3 regulates beta-cell differentiation, function, and glucokinase expression. *Diabetes* **2010**, *59*, 1674–1685. [CrossRef]
149. Sakamoto, Y.; Hara, K.; Kanai-Azuma, M.; Matsui, T.; Miura, Y.; Tsunekawa, N.; Kurohmaru, M.; Saijoh, Y.; Koopman, P.; Kanai, Y. Redundant roles of Sox17 and Sox18 in early cardiovascular development of mouse embryos. *Biochem. Biophys. Res. Commun.* **2007**, *360*, 539–544. [CrossRef]
150. Cao, H.; Florez, S.; Amen, M.; Huynh, T.; Skobe, Z.; Baldini, A.; Amendt, B.A. Tbx1 regulates progenitor cell proliferation in the dental epithelium by modulating Pitx2 activation of p21. *Dev. Biol.* **2010**, *347*, 289–300. [CrossRef]
151. Kros, C.J.; Marcotti, W.; van Netten, S.M.; Self, T.J.; Libby, R.T.; Brown, S.D.; Richardson, G.P.; Steel, K.P. Reduced climbing and increased slipping adaptation in cochlear hair cells of mice with Myo7a mutations. *Nat. Neurosci.* **2002**, *5*, 41–47. [CrossRef] [PubMed]

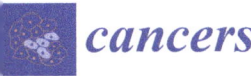

Review

Overcoming Resistance to Immunotherapy in Advanced Cutaneous Squamous Cell Carcinoma

Natalia García-Sancha [1,2,†], Roberto Corchado-Cobos [1,2,†], Lorena Bellido-Hernández [2,3], Concepción Román-Curto [2,4], Esther Cardeñoso-Álvarez [4], Jesús Pérez-Losada [1,2], Alberto Orfao [2,5,6,7] and Javier Cañueto [1,2,4,*]

1. IBMCC-CSIC, Laboratory 7, Campus Miguel de Unamuno s/n, 37007 Salamanca, Spain; nataliagarciasancha@usal.es (N.G.-S.); rober.corchado@usal.es (R.C.-C.); jperezlosada@usal.es (J.P.-L.)
2. Instituto de Investigación Biomédica de Salamanca (IBSAL), Hospital Universitario de Salamanca, Paseo de San Vicente 58-182, 37007 Salamanca, Spain; lbellido@saludcastillayleon.es (L.B.-H.); cromancurto@gmail.com (C.R.-C.); orfao@usal.es (A.O.)
3. Department of Medical Oncology, Hospital Universitario de Salamanca, Paseo de San Vicente 58-182, 37007 Salamanca, Spain
4. Departamento de Dermatología, Hospital Universitario de Salamanca, Paseo de San Vicente 58-182, 37007 Salamanca, Spain; mesthercardenoso@gmail.com
5. IBMCC-CSIC, Laboratory 11, Campus Miguel de Unamuno s/n, 37007 Salamanca, Spain
6. Cytometry Service (NUCLEUS) and Department of Medicine, University of Salamanca, 37007 Salamanca, Spain
7. Centro de Investigación Biomédica en Red de Cáncer (CIBERONC) (CB16/12/00400, CB16/12/00233, CB16/12/00369, CB16/12/00489 and CB16/12/00480), Instituto Carlos III, 28029 Madrid, Spain
* Correspondence: jcanueto@usal.es
† These authors contributed equally to this manuscript.

Simple Summary: Cutaneous squamous cell carcinoma (CSCC) is the second most frequent cancer in humans. The therapeutic landscape of CSCC has change in recent years, after the approval of immune checkpoint inhibitors (ICI) in advanced CSCC. However, not all patients will respond to ICI, and those who respond may develop resistance over time. Understanding the predictors of response to immunotherapy and the mechanisms underlying primary and acquired resistance to ICIs may help identify which patients could best benefit from these therapies. Many treatment strategies are under development to overcome resistance to immunotherapy, such as immune checkpoint inhibitors plus vaccines, oncolytic virus, radiotherapy, chemotherapy, or tumor microenvironment modulators.

Abstract: Cutaneous squamous cell carcinoma (CSCC) is the second most frequent cancer in humans, and is now responsible for as many deaths as melanoma. Immunotherapy has changed the therapeutic landscape of advanced CSCC after the FDA approval of anti-PD1 molecules for the treatment of locally advanced and metastatic CSCC. However, roughly 50% of patients will not respond to this systemic treatment and even those who do respond can develop resistance over time. The etiologies of primary and secondary resistance to immunotherapy involve changes in the neoplastic cells and the tumor microenvironment. Indirect modulation of immune system activation with new therapies, such as vaccines, oncolytic viruses, and new immunotherapeutic agents, and direct modulation of tumor immunogenicity using other systemic treatments or radiotherapy are now under evaluation in combined regimens. The identification of predictors of response is an important area of research. In this review, we focus on the features associated with the response to immunotherapy, and the evaluation of combination treatments and new molecules, a more thorough knowledge of which is likely to improve the survival of patients with advanced CSCC.

Keywords: cutaneous squamous cell carcinoma; immunotherapy; anti-PD1; biomarkers; predictive medicine; personalized medicine; cancer; immune system

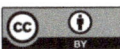

1. Introduction

Cutaneous squamous cell carcinoma (CSCC) is the second most frequent cancer in humans, with an estimated annual incidence of one million cases in the US and the cause of as many as 9000 deaths each year [1,2]. Its incidence is increasing by 3–8% per year in most countries [3] and, by 2030, the rate in Europe is expected to have doubled [4]. Although CSCC generally exhibits a benign clinical behavior, some cases may entail a poor prognosis. Local recurrence is estimated to occur in 5% of patients, lymph node metastasis in 3.7 to 5.8% and disease-specific death in 1.5 to 2.1% of cases [5,6]. CSCC is already a public health concern worldwide, and as life expectancy lengthens in general, it will become an even greater health problem.

CSCC is especially common in elderly fair-skin men. It is associated with chronic sun exposure, and immunosuppression represents a major risk factor. Actinic keratosis is the most significant independent risk factor for CSCC development. Human papillomavirus infection [7], long-term scars, and inflammatory skin conditions are other well-known risk factors [8].

Ultraviolet exposure induces *P53* mutations and genomic instability. Consequently, mutations occur in tumor suppressor genes (such as *CDKN2A* and *NOTCH*) and oncogenes (such as *RAS*). The accumulation of mutations causes deregulation of relevant oncogenic pathways (EGFR overexpression and activation of MAPK and PI3K/mTOR pathways), which results in CSCC development. Epigenetic factors, such as the methylation status and the role of miRNAs, also contribute to CSCC development [9,10]. CSCC is the solid tumor with the highest mutational burden [11], which is part of the rationale that led to immunotherapy.

Immunotherapy has changed the therapeutic landscape of CSCC in recent years. Patients with locally advanced or metastatic CSCC who would not benefit from surgery are now candidates for immune checkpoint inhibitors (only two anti-PD1 drugs are currently FDA-approved) [12]. However, not all patients respond to immunotherapy, and some begin to respond but develop resistance over time. Reasons underlying this primary and acquired resistance to immunotherapy are a matter of intensive research [13,14]. It is also important to identify which patients would most benefit from these treatments, which is why research on biomarker signatures has become a priority. Finally, novel therapies to overcome resistance to immunotherapy and to increase the response rate and maintain remission once it has been achieved are being evaluated. Combinations of immune checkpoint inhibitors (ICIs) and of ICIs with other therapies (such as radiotherapy, chemotherapy and targeted therapy), together with cancer vaccines and oncolytic viruses make up the new treatment options under evaluation in clinical trials, many of which are yielding promising results [15].

In this review, we first describe the current evidence about immunotherapy in CSCC. We then summarize the predictors of response to immunotherapy. Finally, we discuss the state-of-the-art of the known mechanisms of resistance to immunotherapy and several therapies for overcoming resistance that are under investigation, paying particular attention to novel therapies in CSCC.

2. Immunotherapy in Cutaneous Squamous Cell Carcinoma

2.1. Immune Checkpoint Inhibitors in Cutaneous Squamous Cell Carcinoma

2.1.1. Cancer Immunotherapy and Tumor Immunology

Immunotherapy has become an established mainstream treatment for in cancer and has improved the prognosis and survival of many patients, including those with hematological dyscrasias and solid malignancies. Tumor cells produce neoantigens that are recognized and targeted by the immune system as foreign molecules, thereby preventing carcinogenesis.

Antigen-presenting cells (APCs) offer tumor neoantigens to the T-cell receptor (TCR) in naïve T cells through the major histocompatibility complex (MHC) (human leucocyte antigen, HLA). To complete T-cell activation, other co-stimulatory molecules are necessary.

CD28 and B7 (CD80/CD86) are two such molecules that are required for full T-cell activation. However, co-inhibitory molecules that act as immune checkpoints are important for avoiding hyperstimulation and autoimmunity. For example, the CTLA-4 receptor is expressed in activated and regulatory T cells and competes with CD28 for B7, thereby preventing T-cell hyperactivation [16–18]. PD-1 also acts as a co-inhibitory receptor. It is expressed in T cells and binds to its ligand PD-L1, which is mainly expressed in tumor cells, thus preventing T-cell activation and inducing immunological exhaustion [19–21] (Figure 1).

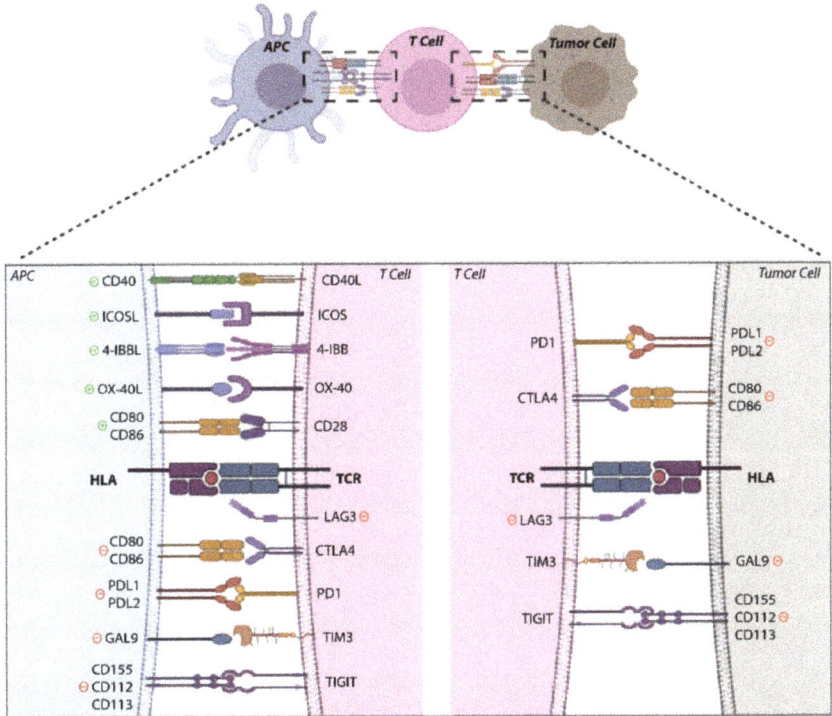

Figure 1. Scheme of co-stimulatory and co-inhibitory receptors implicated in the immune response. Created using BioRender.

In this context, the immune system can recognize the tumor and fight against it (immunosurveillance). However, if this process is not successful, tumor cells may enter into an equilibrium phase, with incomplete tumor destruction and finally, the tumor may escape to immune control. This dynamic process is known as immunoediting. The cancer immunoediting hypothesis postulates a dual role of the immune system: first, it protects the host by eliminating tumor cells, and second, it promotes tumor development by selecting tumor variants with reduced immunogenicity [22,23].

One of the ways in which tumor cells actively evade their destruction by the immune system is expressing these molecules that inhibit T-cell activation and response. The study of these mechanisms has allowed important advances to develop antibodies against CTLA-4, PD-1 and PD-L1, which have revolutionized oncology in recent years. Seven immune checkpoints inhibitors have so far received FDA approval for use with different types of cancer: one CTLA-4 inhibitor (ipilimumab), three PD-1 inhibitors (nivolumab, pembrolizumab, and cemiplimab) and three PD-L1 inhibitors (atezolizumab, durvalumab, and avelumab). However, many molecules (e.g., 4-1BB, OX40, LAG3, ICOS) are involved in T-cell activation [24] (Figure 1), and other drugs against them are being evaluated and developed.

2.1.2. Immunotherapy in CSCC

CSCC exhibits the greatest tumor mutational burden, which results in higher levels of tumor neoantigens that may be targeted by the immune system [11]. Immunocompromised patients have a higher risk of developing CSCC because their immune system is less efficient detecting and destroying cancer cells [8]. Both these factors underpin the rationale for testing immunotherapy for CSCC.

The FDA (2018) and EMA (2019) approved cemiplimab (Libtayo) as the first immunotherapeutic drug for the treatment of locally advanced or metastatic CSCC in patients who are not candidates for curative surgery or radiotherapy [25,26]. Cemiplimab is a high-affinity human monoclonal antibody directed against PD-1. The robust responsiveness of CSCCs to cemiplimab was demonstrated in expanded phase 1 and phase 2 trials (NCT02383212 and NCT02760498). In these clinical trials, the response rates were between 41% and 53% and the rates of durable disease control were between 57% and 65%. The efficacy of the treatment of metastatic and of locally advanced cutaneous squamous cell carcinoma was similar [27–30]. The second anti-PD-1 approved by the FDA, in 2020, is pembrolizumab (Keytruda). This drug has been accepted for use in patients with recurrent or metastatic CSCC that cannot be cured with surgery or radiation [31]. Its antitumor activity and durable response were established in the KEYNOTE-629 and CARSKIN clinical trials (NCT03284424 and NCT02883556) in which the response rates were 34.3% and 42% and the disease control rates were 52.4% and 60%, respectively [32,33].

The other ICIs, such as nivolumab and ipilimumab, have also been studied in clinical trials and have proved their efficacy in monotherapy in some case reports [34–36]. The greatest advantages of immune checkpoint blockers have been impressive durable response rates and manageable treatment-related adverse events compared with conventional therapies [37].

2.2. Predictors of Response to Immunotherapy

About 50% of cancers will not respond to immunotherapy, so identifying predictors of response for checkpoint blockade-based immunotherapy has become a research priority. This will identify the patients who would respond best to the treatment, and thereby help maximize the therapeutic benefit. In recent years, numerous response predictors based on the gene expression status of the tumor (PD-L1 and IFN-γ expression), genomic changes (tumor mutational burden, T cell receptor clonality, neoantigen load and tumor aneuploidy) and immune cell infiltration have been found [38]. Biomarkers in peripheral blood are also being explored as non-invasive techniques (Table 1 and Figure 2).

2.2.1. Tumor-Associated Markers
PD-L1 Status

High levels of PD-L1, detected by immunohistochemistry, are associated with the response to immunotherapy in melanoma, non-small cell lung carcinoma (NSCLC), renal cell carcinoma, colorectal carcinoma, and castration-resistant prostate cancer [39–42]. However, some studies have shown that the association with response varies over time and with the tumor type, and a sizable proportion of responses occur in PD-L1-low/negative tumors [43]. In CSCC, response to cemiplimab is independent of PD-L1 status, and durable disease control is similar in patients with <1% of PD-L1 expression and those with >50% PD-L1 expression [30]. Expression levels of PD-L1 are intratumorally heterogeneous and dynamic. The variety of antibody clones and platforms used the multiple scoring criteria and the variations in methodology make it difficult to interpret PD-L1 levels [44].

Table 1. Predictors of response to immunotherapy.

Category	Predictors	Correlation	Advantages (and Approved Tests by FDA)	Disadvantages	References
Tumor-associated markers	PD-L1 status	High levels of PD-L1 are correlated with response to anti-PD-L1/PD-1 inhibitors	Immunohistochemistry detection is easy, cheap and automated Approved in NSCLC to treat with pembrolizumab, cemiplimab, atezolizumab or nivolumab in combination with ipilimumab Approved in urothelial carcinoma to treat with pembrolizumab, cemiplimab or atezolizumab Approved in triple-negative breast cancer to treat with pembrolizumab, cemiplimab, or atezolizumab Approved in gastric carcinoma, cervical cancer, HNSCC and ESCC to treat with pembrolizumab or cemiplimab	PD-L1-negative tumors also respond to anti-PD-L1 therapy PD-L1 expression is intratumorally heterogeneous and dynamic Different antibody clones and platforms used Multiple score criteria Methodological variabilities	[39–45]
	IFN-γ expression	High levels of IFN-γ expression are correlated with response to anti-PD-1 therapies	Higher capacity to detect patients who will respond to immunotherapy than PD-L1 immunohistochemistry	No standardized commercially available gene panel Expensive	[46–50]
	Tumor mutational burden	High levels of TMB are correlated with response to anti-CTLA-4 and anti PD-1/PD-L1 therapy (except glioma)	Applicable to most solid tumors and anti-CTLA4, anti-PD-L1 and anti-PD-1 therapies Approved for treating high-TMB solid tumors with pembrolizumab	Low-TMB tumors also respond to immunotherapy Whole-exome sequencing or sequencing of 300–400 genes panels is expensive Difficult to establish a threshold for all types of cancer	[51–63]
	Neoantigen load	High levels of neoantigen load are correlated with response to immunotherapy	Knowledge of the landscape of neoantigens to use a precision medicine approach	Complex technology High mutation load is not always correlated with response	[64–67]
	Tumor-infiltrating lymphocytes	High levels of CD8+ T cells, high ratio of CD8+/CD4+ T cells and high levels of CD8+/PD-L1+/CTLA-4+ lymphocytes are correlated with response to pembrolizumab and nivolumab	Easily detected by immunohistochemistry or hematoxylin-eosin staining	Inter- and intra-observer variability in hematoxylin-eosin and immunohistochemistry samples Score criteria not validated	[68–72]
	Immunophenotypic profile	High levels of CD4+ and CD8+ T lymphocytes and low levels of neutrophils, myeloid and monocyte precursor and Treg/FoxP3+ lymphocytes are correlated with response to ipilimumab High levels of eosinophils and high total lymphocyte count are correlated with response to pembrolizumab Low levels of LDH are correlated with response to ipilimumab and pembrolizumab	Ease of sample collection, non-invasive Possibility of collecting samples at different times during treatment Cheap	Not validated in clinical practice	[73–78]
Liquid biopsy markers	Cytokines and chemokines	High levels of IL-6 reduce the probability of responding to ipilimumab Early decrease in IL-8 is associated with best response to nivolumab or pembrolizumab	Ease of sample collection, non-invasive Possibility of collecting samples at different times during treatment Cheap	Not validated in clinical practice	[79–82]
	Circulating tumor DNA and circulating tumor cells	Low basal levels of ctDNA are correlated with good prognosis and best clinical response to immunotherapy High blood-based TMB measured in circulating tumor DNA are correlated with response to ICIs A reduction of circulating tumor cells improves progression-free survival during pembrolizumab or ipilimumab treatment Patients with CTCs/PD-L1+ have better progression-free survival when receiving pembrolizumab	Ease of sample collection, non-invasive Possibility of collecting samples at different times during treatment Cheap Test approved to measure TMB in liquid biopsy samples	Not validated in clinical practice	[45,83–90]
	Soluble markers	Higher sPD-L1 plasma level is associated with poor prognosis and lower nivolumab efficacy	Ease of sample collection, non-invasive Possibility of collecting samples at different times during treatment Cheap	Not validated in clinical practice	[91,92]

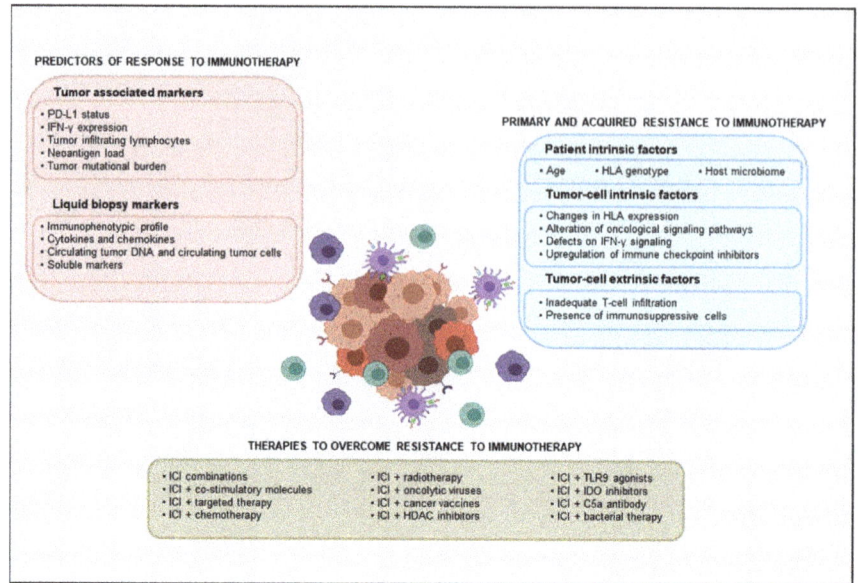

Figure 2. Representative scheme of the predictors of response to immunotherapy, the factors implicated in primary and acquired resistance to immunotherapy and the strategies to overcome these resistances.

PD-L1 is one of the biomarkers currently approved for clinical use, but only to identify PD-L1 tumor expression in certain tumor types, specifically in: NSCLC for treatment with pembrolizumab, cemiplimab, atezolizumab or nivolumab in combination with ipilimumab; urothelial carcinoma and triple-negative breast cancer (TNBC) for treatment with pembrolizumab, cemiplimab or atezolizumab; and gastric adenocarcinoma, cervical cancer, head and neck squamous cell carcinoma (HNSCC) and esophageal squamous cell carcinoma for treatment with pembrolizumab or cemiplimab [45].

Interferon-Gamma Expression

PD-L1 expression may be upregulated via interferon-gamma (IFN-γ). IFN-γ produced from CD8+ T cells drives IL-12 production by tumor-infiltrating dendritic cells, which are necessary to a successful anti-PD-1 therapy [46]. In NSCLC and melanoma, patients with a high level of mRNA expression of *IFNG* (the gene that encodes IFN-γ) exhibit longer progression-free and overall survival and have higher disease control rates with anti-PD-1 therapies [47]. In several solid tumors, responders and non-responders to pembrolizumab can be distinguished on the basis of the different levels of expression of genes associated with IFN-γ [48]. The 18-gene IFN-γ characterized by this group is better than PD-L1 immunohistochemistry at identifying patients who will respond to immunotherapy [48]. However, more experiments, currently being carried out [49,50], are needed to make clinical implementation possible.

Tumor Mutational Burden

A high tumor mutational burden (TMB) is also associated with response to ICI and improved overall survival in melanoma [51,52], NSCLC [53], urothelial carcinoma [54], among other cancers [55,56]. CSCC displays the greatest tumor mutational burden, and a large TMB has been linked to a good clinical response to immunotherapy [11,57,58]. Nevertheless, some patients with a large TMB may not respond to ICI therapy [30,59]. In some tumors, such as glioma, TMB is associated with shorter overall survival [60,61]. One advantage of TMB is that it can predict responses to CTLA-4 antibodies and PD-1/PD-1 inhibitors, but measuring TMB by whole exome sequencing or by sequencing 300–400-gene panels is an expensive and not routinely available option. Moreover, it is difficult to establish a threshold for all cancer types, hampering standardization of the technique [60,62]. Nonetheless, FDA approved FoundationOne CDx to identify patients with unresectable or metastatic solid tumors with a high mutational burden ($\geq$10 mutations/megabase) for whom treatment with pembrolizumab may be appropriate [63].

Neoantigen Load

High TMB increases the capacity of the tumor to generate new neoantigens. Tumors loaded with more neoantigens are more likely to respond to immunotherapy [64–66]. Knowledge of the neoantigen landscape, derived from proteomic experiments and computational predictive algorithms [43,67], may enable us to adopt a precision-medicine approach, although the technology required is complex.

Tumor-Infiltrating Lymphocytes

Tumor-infiltrating lymphocytes (TILs) play an important role in the response to immunotherapy. TILs comprise primarily CD8+ cytotoxic T cells and CD4+ helper T cells, including regulatory T cells (Tregs), which are exemplified by the expression of FOXP3 and CD25. TILs also encompass a smaller proportion of B and natural killer cells. In melanoma, preexisting CD8+ T cells at the invasive front (the edge of the tumor) are essential for tumor regression following pembrolizumab therapy [68]. In melanoma, patients treated with PD-1 antibodies have a response rate of 78.6% when pretreatment tumor biopsies contain more than 20% of tumor-infiltrating CD8+ T cells that express high levels of PD-1 and CTLA-4, in contrast to non-responders, who feature fewer than 20% of these cells and a 0% response rate [69]. In metastatic NSCLC and melanoma treated with pembrolizumab or nivolumab, the response rates are low (13.3 and 0%, respectively) when the pretreatment CD8+/CD4+ TIL ratio is less than 2, whereas they are high (50.0 and 81.3%, respectively) when the ratio is greater than 2 in NSCLC and greater than 2.7 in melanoma [70]. The customary evaluation of TILs using hematoxylin-eosin and immunohistochemistry has revealed notable inter- and intra-observer variability. New tools based on flow cytometry, RNA-sequencing and digitalization of images are being developed to validate and promote an immunoscore-based method [71,72].

2.2.2. Liquid Biopsy Markers

Most of the data on prediction of response to immunotherapy have focused on tumor features. Nevertheless, tumors are sometimes less accessible, and the role of the host immune system is a critical consideration. Determining the host immunological profile in blood samples allows assessment of the tumor immunovigilance state, the risk of tumor progression, and the response to treatment, which can help in establishing a panel of biomarkers that predict response.

Immunophenotypic Profile

We currently know little about the immunological profile of patients receiving treatment with cemiplimab and pembrolizumab in CSCC, and most of the information available comes from studies in melanoma. In this disease, some baseline laboratory markers have been linked to the response to ipilimumab (such as high levels of CD4+ and CD8+ T lymphocytes [73], low levels of neutrophils and LDH [74], myeloid and monocyte precursors [75]) and to the response to pembrolizumab (such as high eosinophil levels, low LDH levels, and high total lymphocyte count [76]). Furthermore, changes in the immune profile during treatment have implications for the prognosis of the disease, such as a reduction in Treg/FoxP3+ lymphocyte levels and an increase in the overall lymphocyte count [77], or an increase in the total lymphocyte and eosinophil counts [78].

Cytokines and Chemokines

The profile of peripheral blood cytokines and chemokines, which is related to the immune cell populations, offers an opportunity to define the prognosis of the disease. The level of expression of certain cytokines is known to be associated with better responses [79]. In melanoma, high levels of IL-6 reduce the likelihood of response to ipilimumab [80]. In melanoma and NSCLC patients, an early decrease in IL-8 is associated with the best response to nivolumab and pembrolizumab [81]. IL-8 is a powerful chemoattractant for neutrophils and other immune-suppressive cells and elevated baseline levels of serum IL-8 correlate with reduced clinical benefit of ICI in different advancer cancer [82].

Circulating Tumor DNA and Circulating Tumor Cells

Circulating tumor DNA (ctDNA) is one of the most reliable biomarkers available in liquid biopsy. Low basal levels of ctDNA are correlated with good prognosis and best clinical response in melanoma [83,84] and other solid tumors [85]. The TMB can be measured in ctDNA [86] and the FDA recently approved FoundationOne Liquid CDx and Guardant360 CDx [45] for comprehensive tumor mutation profiling through liquid biopsy sampling. Patients with high levels of blood-based TMB respond better to ICIs [87,88], although this is not well established for all types of cancer; the concordance of blood-TMB and tissue-TMB is currently being examined.

Circulating tumor cells (CTCs) also identify responders and non-responders. A reduction in CTC frequency during pembrolizumab or ipilimumab treatment improves progression-free survival and high quantities of CTCs are related to a higher risk of relapse [89]. In CTCs, PD-L1 expression can be determined and patients with CTCs/PD-L1+ have better progression-free survival than CTCs/PD-L1- patients when they receive pembrolizumab [90].

Soluble Markers

Soluble forms of many immune regulatory molecules, both co-stimulatory and co-inhibitory molecules, including sCTLA4 and sPD-L1, are detected in plasma of cancer patients. Higher sPD-L1 plasma levels are associated with poor prognosis in melanoma [91] and with lower nivolumab efficacy in NSCLC [92].

The combination of biomarkers may have greater predictive power than the individual markers [93,94]. A recent meta-analysis published reveals a model that combines 11 factors to predict sensitization to ICI. The multivariable model includes clonal, frameshift insertion/deletion and nonsense-mediated decay-escaping TMB, signatures associated with tobacco, UV, APOBEC and T cell-related inflammation, sex, and gene expression values for CD8A, CXCL9, and PD-L1, with better predictive value than one factor alone [95]. An integrated approach with new bioinformatic tools can help us stratify patients and select the best treatment. This will tell us which patients will, or will not, respond to ICI monotherapy. Some of those who do not respond may benefit from new therapies that are being developed to overcome resistance to immunotherapy. We discuss these therapies below.

3. Mechanisms of Resistance to Immunotherapy

Despite the success of immune checkpoint inhibitors, some patients treated with ICIs do not benefit from treatment (primary resistance), and some of those who initially do, become resistant over time (acquired resistance) (Table 2 and Figure 2). Primary and acquired resistance are both a result of complex and constant interactions between cancer cells and the tumor microenvironment. Understanding the mechanisms by which this resistance occurs is essential for developing strategies to overcome resistance.

Table 2. Mechanisms of resistance to immunotherapy.

Type of resistance	Category	Factor	Relation	References
Primary resistance to immunotherapy	Patient-intrinsic factor	Immunosenescence	Aging limits immune response	[96–100]
		HLA genotype	Homozygosity in at least one HLA-I locus is associated with poor response to ICIs	[101,102]
		Host microbiome	Changes in diversity and abundance of host microbiome modify the response to ICIs	[103–105]
	Tumor cell-intrinsic factor	Downregulation of HLA expression	Loss of HLA-I expression reduces T-cell response	[106,107]
		Alteration of oncological signaling pathways	Abnormal expression of MAPK pathway, loss of PTEN, constitutive WNT/β-catenin expression, JAK1/2 mutations and loss of IFN-γ are involved in resistance to ICIs	[108–115]
	Tumor cell-extrinsic factor	Inadequate T-cell infiltration	Absence of T cells near the tumor reduces T cell response	[116]
		Presence of immunosuppressive cells	High level of infiltration of Treg, MDSCs and TAM suppress T-cell activation and is correlated with poor prognosis and resistance to ICIs	[117–125]
Acquired resistance to immunotherapy	Tumor cell-intrinsic factor	Changes in HLA expression	Mutations in β2-microglobulin are associated with acquired resistance to ICIs	[126–131]
		Defects of IFN-γ signaling	Escape mutations in IFN-γ pathway result in loss of HLA-I and PD-L1 expression and ICI resistance	[128,132]
		Mutations in genes that encode tumor neoantigens	Mutations in genes that encode tumor neoantigens reduce tumor recognition by immune system, leading to immune evasion and clinical progression	[133,134]
		Upregulation of other immune checkpoint receptors	Upregulation of TIM3 and LAG	[135]
		Alteration of oncological signaling pathways	Loss of PTEN and increase in WNT/β-catenin expression are linked to acquired resistance	[136]

3.1. Primary Resistance to Immune Checkpoint Inhibitors

In primary resistance, patients do not respond at all to ICIs, facilitating the progress of the disease. The response rate to single-agent immune checkpoint blockade ranges from 40 to 70% in different types of cancer. Patient-intrinsic factors (such as age, HLA genotype and gut microbiome), tumor cell-intrinsic factors (such as insufficient tumor antigenicity, loss of HLA expression and alterations of several signaling pathways) and tumor cell-extrinsic factors (such as changes in tumor-associated stroma) are involved in primary resistance to immunotherapy [13,14,137].

3.1.1. Patient-Intrinsic Factors

Immunosenescence

As patients age, their immune system function becomes increasingly limited. This process, known as immunosenescence, is characterized by significant effects upon innate and adaptive immune responses.

With respect to innate immunity, aging produces changes in monocytes and macrophages (reduced phagocytic activity, HLA II expression and ROS production), dendritic cells (slower maturation and reduced antigen presentation, defective TLR expression and signaling) and neutrophils (reduced chemotaxis and altered TLR expression).

The adaptive response is limited by a drop in the frequencies of naïve B and T cells and a rise in those of senescent and exhausted T cells, Treg and myeloid-derived suppressor cells (MDSCs) [96–98]. All these changes compromise clonal expansion and cytokine and antibody production, weakening the immune response.

The results of clinical trials in this area are variable. The elderly group is underrepresented because their co-morbidities are sometimes exclusion criteria. However, in patients older than 75 years, resistance to anti-PD-1/anti-PD-L1 therapy has been observed in squamous cell carcinoma and adenocarcinoma of the lung, renal cell carcinoma and squamous cell carcinoma of the digestive tract. Nevertheless, two other studies in NSCLC reported the same benefit in the elderly as that seen in younger individuals [99,100].

HLA Haplotypes

The human leukocyte antigen class I (HLA-I) genotype is linked to differential immune responses, including different responses to ICIs. Homozygosity in at least one HLA-I locus in patients treated with anti-CTLA-4, anti-PD-1, anti-PD-L1 or with a combination of ICIs for different types of cancer (mostly melanoma and NSCLC) is associated with shorter overall survival. Conversely, maximal heterozygosity at HLA-I loci with a high TMB is associated with extended survival after ICI treatment [101]. Moreover, HLA-I genotype with two alleles with more divergent sequences, measured as HLA-I evolutionary divergence (HED), enables presentation of more diverse immunopeptidomes and is correlated with better survival after treatment with ICIs [102].

Host Microbiome

Links between the host microbiome and the response to ICIs have emerged in recent years [103]. In melanoma, patients treated with anti-PD-1 with highly diverse and abundant Faecalibacterium have enhanced systemic and anti-tumor responses mediated by increased antigen presentation. In contrast, patients with low Bacteroidales diversity have impaired anti-tumor immune responses mediated by limited intratumoral lymphoid and myeloid infiltration and higher frequencies of Treg cells and MDSCs in blood [104]. Other bacterial species found to be more abundant in responders include Bifidobacterium longum, Collinsella aerofaciens, and Enterococcus faecium [105].

3.1.2. Tumor-Associated Factors

Tumor Cell-Intrinsic Factors

Tumor cell-intrinsic factors are involved in primary resistance. The loss of HLA expression, the alteration in antigen processing machinery, the lack of antigenic mutations, the constitutive PD-L1 expression and the alteration in particular signaling pathways are the most significant tumor-intrinsic factors [137].

Tumor cells can avoid being attacked by T cells by downregulating HLA expression. An HLA-low phenotype has been observed in NSCLC, breast, prostate and colorectal cancers, HNSCC, hepatocellular carcinoma and melanoma. Several genes, such as *TAP1*, *TAP2*, *B2M*, *TAPBPR*, *ERAP1*, are involved in the synthesis, assembly, transport and surface expression of HLA I molecules, and defects in the HLA I pathways may result in the loss of 0 to 93% of HLA I expression in different types of cancer [106]. Losing HLA I antigen presentation machinery makes CD8 T cells unable to identify tumor cells, thereby making it possible for cancers to evade immune control. Loss of antigenicity is also associated with a loss of immunogenicity, due to low tumor mutational burden [107].

Alternation in oncological signaling pathways may result in resistance to ICIs. Abnormal expression of the mitogen-activated protein kinase (MAPK) pathway is associated with impaired recruitment and function of tumor infiltrate lymphocytes through expression of VEGF and other inhibitory cytokines [108,109]. In this context, it has been shown that melanomas become resistant to immunotherapy when they have previously acquired resistance to MAPK targeted therapy, in a process knowing as cross-resistance. It is due to a reactivated MAPK pathway and the induction of an immunosuppressive tumor microenvironment that lacks functional CD103+ dendritic cells, precluding an effective T cell response [110]. Similarly, loss of PTEN, which enhances PI3K signaling, is associated with resistance to immune checkpoint therapy [111]. The resistance due to PTEN deficiency is associated with high levels of VEGFA and STAT3 [112], stronger PD-L1 expression [113] and lower CD8+ T-cell density [112]. Constitutive WNT/β-catenin expression reduces expression of the cytokine CCL4 necessary to recruit CD103+ dendritic cells, which are involved in T-cell priming [114]. The occurrence of somatic JAK1/2 mutations in cancer cells leads to loss of IFN-γ signaling, making it another mechanism producing primary resistance to PD-1 blockade therapy [115].

Tumor Cell Extrinsic Factors

Tumor cells do not work alone but in conjunction with their environment, interacting with the extracellular matrix within the stroma and with the immune cells of the tumor microenvironment. The absence of T cells near the tumor, the presence of immunosuppressive cells and the expression of different inhibitory immune checkpoints have all been implicated in primary resistance.

Inadequate T-cell infiltration may be due to a variety of factors such as poor immunogenicity, downregulation of chemokines required for T-cell recruitment (CXCR3, CXCL9, CXCL10) by epigenetic silencing and upregulation of the endothelin B receptor or VEGF overexpression [116]. T-cell function may be hindered by the presence of immunosuppressive cells in the tumor microenvironment. Tregs are known to suppress effector T-cell responses by secreting certain inhibitory cytokines such as IL-10, IL-35 and TGF-B, or by direct cell contact [117]. Greater infiltration of Tregs in the tumor is correlated with poor prognosis [118] and primary resistance to anti-PD-1 therapy [119]. MDSCs, a group of immature myeloid cells with suppressive competence in the tumor microenvironment, have been implicated in angiogenesis, tumor cell invasion, and metastasis [120]. Accumulation of circulating MDSCs is negatively associated with ICI efficacy [75,121,122] and eradicating them could enhance clinical responses to immunotherapy. Tumor-associated macrophages (TAMs) also suppress T-cell activation and promote angiogenesis, contributing to immunotherapy resistance by overexpressing PD-1/PD-L1, TGF-β, VEGF, EGF, and MMP [123,124]. All these immune cells can express other co-inhibitors such as TIM-3, CTLA-4 and TIGHT to mediate tumor immune resistance. Moreover, peritumoral fibroblast that express TGFβ are also implicated in poor response and resistance to atezolizumab prohibiting infiltration of effector CD8+ T cells into the tumor parenchyma [125].

3.2. Acquired Resistance to Immune Checkpoint Inhibitors

Numerous patients respond to immunotherapy but develop resistance over time. For example, in melanoma patients treated with ipilimumab and nivolumab, 38% of those who responded developed resistance [138]. In patients with NSCLC who were treated with nivolumab, up to 65% of responders progressed after 4 years of follow-up [139]. Across tumor types, there is an inverse correlation between overall response rate to PD-1 blockade and the frequency of acquired resistance [140]. Mechanisms of acquired resistance also lead to changes in HLA expression, altered IFN-γ signaling and poor neoantigen recognition [140].

Defective HLA class I antigen processing due to mutations in β2-microglobulin (B2M), which is required for HLA class I folding and transport to the cell surface [126,127], has been observed in patients with melanoma [128,129], lung cancer [130] and mismatch repair-deficient tumors [131] whose tumor initially regressed in response to ICIs but whose disease progressed some years later. Alterations in the IFN-γ pathway have also been implicated in the loss of HLA class I [128]. Defects in the IFN-γ pathway are produced by inactivating mutations in Janus kinases (*JAK1* or *JAK2*) or in interferon-gamma receptor 1 (*IFNGR1*) [128,132]. Lack of IFN responsiveness also results in the loss of PD-L1 expression [128]. Dysfunctional tumor antigen-presenting machinery reduces tumor visibility, leading to acquired ICI resistance. Tumor recognition can also be hampered by the loss of somatic mutations encoding tumor neoantigens through clonal selection, epigenetic repression or copy-number loss, leading to immune evasion and clinical progression [133]. In NSCLC, tumors with acquired immunotherapy resistance show genomic changes in genes encoding tumor neoantigens that can be recognized by T cells [134].

Additional changes known to influence acquired resistance are the upregulation of other T-cell checkpoints (TIM3 and LAG) [135], the loss of PTEN and the increase in WNT-β-catenin activity, which is linked to the promotion of Treg and changes in the priming of dendritic cells [136].

4. Overcoming Resistance to Immune Checkpoint Inhibitors

To overcome the resistance to ICIs, it is necessary to enhance the anti-tumor activity of the immune system. Combined treatment regimens and new therapies based upon synergistic effects of targeting different immune escape pathways are emerging (Figure 2). The therapies to overcome immunotherapy resistance in CSCC currently being studied are summarized in Table 3.

Table 3. Combination therapies to overcome resistance to immunotherapy in cutaneous squamous cell carcinoma.

Type of combination	Drugs	Condition	NCT code
Combination of immune checkpoint inhibitors	Ipilimumab + nivolumab	In advanced CSCC prior to surgery	NCT04620200
	Ipilimumab + nivolumab + tacrolimus	Metastatic CSCC in treating kidney recipients	NCT03816332
Combination with co-stimulatory molecules	SL-279252 (binds to PD-L1 and OX-40)	Advanced CSCC	NCT03894618
Combination with chemotherapy	Currently not clinically trialed in CSCC		
Combination with radiotherapy	Pembrolizumab + radiotherapy (IMRT 60–66 Gy)	High risk CSCC of the head and neck	NCT03057613
	Pembrolizumab + quad-shot radiotherapy	Stage III and IV CSCC of the head and neck	NCT04454489
	Avelumab + radical radiotherapy	Unresectable CSCC	NCT03737721
Combination with targeted therapies	Pembrolizumab + cetuximab	Recurrent/metastatic CSCC	NCT03082534
	Pembrolizumab + cetuximab	Advanced/metastatic CSCC	NCT03666325
	Avelumab + cetuximab	Advanced/metastatic CSCC	NCT03944941
	Pembrolizumab/cemiplimab + ASP-1929 (EGFR antibody-dye conjugate)	Locally advanced or metastatic CSCC	NCT04305795
	Atezolizumab + cobimetinib	Metastatic CSCC	NCT03108131
Combination with oncolytic viruses	Nivolumab + talimogene laherparepvec	Advanced or refractory CSCC	NCT02978625
	Cemiplimab + RP1	Locally advanced or metastatic CSCC	NCT04050436
	Nivolumab + RP1	Locally advanced or metastatic CSCC	NCT03767348
	Pembrolizumab + ONCR-177	Advanced and/or refractory CSCC	NCT04348916
Combination with cancer vaccines	Nivolumab or pembrolizumab + CIMAVax vaccine	Stage III and IV CSCC of the head and neck	NCT02955290
	Pembrolizumab + Ad/MG1-MAGEA3	Previously treated CSCC	NCT03773744
Other combinations	Pembrolizumab + abexinostat (HDAC inhibitor)	Stage III and IV CSCC of the head and neck	NCT03590054
	Pembrolizumab or cemiplimab + cavrotolimod (TLR agonist)	Advanced/metastatic CSCC	NCT03684785
	Pembrolizumab + IFX-1 (C5a antibody)	Locally advanced or metastatic CSCC	NCT04812535

4.1. ICI Combinations

One of the first strategies used to bypass resistance is the use of a combination of immune checkpoint inhibitors. Anti-CTLA-4 (ipilimumab) plus anti-PD-1 (nivolumab) treatments are combinations approved for the treatment of melanoma [141,142], renal cell carcinoma [143,144], colorectal cancer [145], non-small cell lung cancer [146], hepatocellular carcinoma [147] and pleural mesothelioma [148]. The regulatory roles of CTLA-4 and PD-1 pathways are distinct, and simultaneously blocking the two receptors produces a synergistic effect [149,150].

In CSCC, ipilimumab is currently being tested in combination with nivolumab in a comparison with neo-adjuvant nivolumab monotherapy (NCT04620200), and combined with nivolumab and tacrolimus in treating kidney transplant recipients with metastatic CSCC (NCT03816332). However, combination therapy increases the incidence and severity of side effects. The median time to onset of a fatal adverse event tends to be earlier for a combination treatment than for monotherapy, and ICI-related deaths in combination therapies are attributed to colitis and myocarditis [151,152].

Numerous co-inhibitory molecules on the T-cell surface have been characterized in the context of T-cell activation [24]. LAG-3, TIM-3 and TIGIT are co-inhibitory molecules that regulate T-cell response and promote T-cell inhibition [153,154]. Resistance to PD-1 blockade has sometimes been associated with upregulation of these molecules [135], which has led to antibodies towards these molecules being developed and combined with traditional ICIs [155–157]. The combination of the anti-LAG-3 BMS-986016 (relatlimab) plus nivolumab strengthens the response in melanoma patients who are resistant to anti-PD-1/anti-PD-L1 therapy [158] (NCT01968109). Other anti-LAG3 agents, such as IMP-321 and LAG525, are under evaluation in a variety of cancer types [155] (NCT02676869, NCT03625323 and NCT03499899). Anti-Tim-3 and anti-TIGIT antibodies, in combination with anti-PD-1, have shown their efficacy in advanced cancers in mouse models [156,157,159]. The efficacy of these new drugs in CSCC has not yet been studied, but their combinations might be attractive options for fighting anti-PD1 resistance in this tumor.

4.2. Combination with Co-Stimulatory Molecules of T-Cell Response

OX40, ICOS and CD27 are co-stimulatory receptors present in T cells and natural killer cells that induce cellular activation. Specific agonist antibodies to these molecules have been developed to boost the immune response [160]. Anti-OX40 monotherapy suppressed tumor growth in preclinical models and enhanced anti-tumor T-cell activity when combined with ICIs [161]. In CSCC, triggering OX40 with an agonist antibody overcame the suppression exerted by Treg, increasing T-cell effector proliferation in vitro [162]. However, when the agonist BMS-986178 has been evaluated in patients with advanced cancer in monotherapy or in combination with nivolumab and/or ipilimumab (NCT02737475), no clear advantage was observed [163]. SL-279252, a bi-functional fusion protein that binds simultaneously to PD-L1 and OX-40 stimulating anti-tumor T-cell activity, is currently being tested in a clinical trial in several types of solid cancer, including CSCC (NCT03894618).

4.3. Combination with Chemotherapy

Although cancer chemotherapy has customarily been considered immunosuppressive, it is now accepted that certain cytotoxic agents can boost tumor immunity. Chemotherapy induces immunogenic cell death and changes in the tumor microenvironment. On the one hand, cytotoxic drugs attack cells, promoting their death. Dead cells release tumor antigens that bind to their receptors, activating the effector lymphocytes. Moreover, cytotoxic drugs abrogate Treg and MDSC activity, enhance dendritic cell activity, promote anti-tumor CD4+ T-cell phenotype and cell recognition [164]. FDA approved pembrolizumab in combination with chemotherapy (carboplatin and either paclitaxel or nab-paclitaxel) for treating metastatic squamous NSCLC [165] and nivolumab plus ipilimumab and chemotherapy (platinum) for metastatic NSCLC with no EGFR or ALK aberrations [166]. Recently, pembrolizumab plus paclitaxel or pembrolizumab plus gemcitabine and carboplatin have been approved for the treatment of recurrent inoperable or metastatic triple-negative breast cancer [167], and in HNSCC pembrolizumab in combination with platinum and 5-FU [168]

(NCT02358031). However, these combinations have not yet been explored in the context of CSCC.

4.4. Combination with Radiotherapy

Radiotherapy is thought to function similarly to chemotherapy, inducing immunogenic cell death and increasing tumor antigens and damage-associated molecular patterns (DAMPs), which prompt antigen presentation activity and T-cell priming. Radiotherapy also enhances infiltration of CD4+, CD8+ T cells and cytotoxic NK into the tumor microenvironment [169]. The combination of radiotherapy and ICIs is being evaluated in different tumors types and stages, in preclinical settings and in clinical trials [170–172]. In CSCC, a case report showed complete remission in a patient treated concurrently with radiotherapy and pembrolizumab [173]. A clinical trial in patients with high-risk CSCC of the head and neck (NCT03057613), and another employing quad-shot palliative radiotherapy (NCT04454489), are underway. In the UNSCARRed study, avelumab, and radical radiotherapy are combined to treat unresectable CSCC (NCT03737721). When combining radiotherapy and immunotherapy, radiotherapy doses must be optimized. Otherwise, the radiation has an immunosuppressive effect [169].

4.5. Combination with Targeted Therapies

Combining anti-PD-L1/PD1 immunotherapy with targeted therapy could improve therapeutic outcomes. MYC overexpression, EGFR and KRAS mutations, PTEN deletions and MEK/ERK alterations are known to induce PD-L1 expression [174]. In melanoma, the combination of vemurafenib (BRAF inhibitor), cobimetinib (MEK inhibitor), and atezolizumab showed an objective response rate of 71.8% [175] and longer median progression-free survival [176]. In CSCC, EGFR overexpression is associated with poor prognosis [177]. The combinations of cetuximab, an EGFR inhibitor, with pembrolizumab (NCT03082534 and NCT03666325), and with avelumab (NCT03944941), other anti-PD-L1, are currently under evaluation. ASP-1929, an antibody conjugate of cetuximab and IRDye 700DX that can be photoactivated, is being combined with pembrolizumab or cemiplimab to treat recurrent/metastatic head and neck squamous cell carcinoma and locally advanced/metastatic CSCC with EGFR overexpression (NCT04305795). Cobimetinib, in combination with atezolizumab, is also being tested in CSCC (NCT03108131).

4.6. Combination with Oncolytic Viruses and Cancer Vaccines

Oncolytic viruses (OVs) are emerging as important biological agents in cancer treatment. Native or genetically modified, they have the ability to kill cancer cells and induce systemic anti-tumor immunity, transforming "cold" into "hot" tumors [178,179]. To date, one OV therapy has been approved by the FDA for treating advanced melanoma: talimogene laherparepvec (T-VEC), a modified herpes simplex virus (HSV) that includes a gene that codes for granulocyte macrophage colony-stimulating factor (GM-CSF) to enhance durable systemic anti-tumor immune responses [180,181]. Intralesional T-VEC has been associated with an increase in melanoma-specific CD8 T cells and a corresponding decrease in suppressive immune cells, such as CD4+ FoxP3+ regulatory T cells and MDSCs within the tumor microenvironment [182]. The combination of T-VEC with ipilimumab [183,184] or pembrolizumab [185] has been explored in melanoma too, revealing a response rate double that achieved with ICI monotherapy. In CSCC, T-VEC is currently tested in monotherapy (NCT03714828), in combination with nivolumab (NCT02978625) and with panitumumab, an EGFR antibody (NCT04163952). RP1 is another modified HSV, which encodes a fusogenic glycoprotein derived from gibbon ape leukemia virus (GALV-GP-R) protein and GM-CSF. The efficacy of RP1 is being tested in the context of CSCC in adult hepatic and renal transplant recipients delivered by intratumoral injection (NCT04349436) and in combination with cemiplimab or nivolumab in immunocompetent patients (NCT04050436 and NCT03767348). Two other modified HSV-1s have been tested in CSCC: HF10 (NCT01017185) and ONCR-177, alone and in combination with pembrolizumab (NCT04348916).

A wide range of viruses has been investigated to determine their potential value as cancer therapeutic agents. In addition to those of herpesvirus, modifications of adenoviruses, vaccinia viruses, measles viruses, coxsackieviruses, polioviruses, retroviruses, reoviruses, parvoviruses and vesicular stomatitis viruses have been examined and some are currently the subject of clinical trials [178,179,186].

Immune responses may also be boosted by methods involving cancer vaccines that are designed to induce or amplify pre-existing cellular and humoral immune responses against target tumor-associated antigens (TAAs) or tumor-specific antigens (TSAs). TAAs are self-antigens that are preferentially or abnormally expressed in tumor cells, although they may also be expressed in normal cells. TSAs comprise antigens expressed by oncoviruses and neoantigens encoded by cancer mutations and are characterized by high immunogenicity. The majority of neoantigens are unique to individual patients and can be detected by computational algorithms for the purpose of designing personalized therapies [187–189]. Several therapeutic vaccine strategies have been developed, including whole tumor cell-based vaccines, protein- and peptide-based vaccines, RNA and DNA vaccines, viral vectors engineered to express tumor antigens and dendritic cell-based vaccines [187,190]. In 2010, the FDA approved the clinical use of Sipuleucel-T, the first cancer vaccine for treating castration-resistant prostate cancer based on enriched ex vivo dendritic cells of each patient [191]. IFx Hu2.0, a whole-cell cancer vaccine, is currently under trial in monotherapy in Merkel cell carcinoma and CSCC (NCT04160065). CIMAvax, a recombinant human EGF-rP64K/montanide ISA 51 vaccine, is being tested in advanced CSCC of the head and neck and NSCLC in combination with nivolumab or pembrolizumab (NCT02955290). In CSCC and metastatic melanoma, Ad/MG1-MAGEA3 is currently being assayed alone or in combination with pembrolizumab (NCT03773744). This is an innovative strategy that combines cancer vaccination with oncolytic virotherapy. It involves two viruses —a replication-deficient adenovirus type 5 (Ad) and a modified Maraba virus as an oncolytic rhabdovirus (MG1)—expressing the same TMA (Melanoma-associated antigen 3, MAGEA3) [192].

4.7. Other Combinations

Supplementing immunotherapy with epigenetic modulators, such as histone deacetylase inhibitors (HDACis), may decrease tumor progression [193,194]. HDACis reduce the expression of various inflammatory cytokines (IL-6, IL-2, IL-10 and IFN-γ), enhance infiltration of immune cells, increase central and effector T-cell memory and reduce pro-tumorigenic M2 macrophages [195,196]. Currently, in CSCC, pembrolizumab is combined with abexinostat, an HDACi (NCT03590054).

Toll-like receptors (TLRs) are a family of molecules capable of recognizing pathogen-associated molecular patterns (PAMPs) and of inducing adaptive immune responses [197]. TLR agonists and antagonists have been designed to enhance immunity and are currently being clinically trialed in monotherapy and in combination with anti-PD-1 therapy [198]. The TLR9 agonist cavrotolimod (AST-008) is being tested in combination with pembrolizumab or cemiplimab in Merkel cell carcinoma, CSCC and melanoma (NCT03684785).

Indoleamine-2,3-dioxygenase (IDO) is an enzyme that lowers the level of tryptophan, induces cell-cycle arrest and effector T-cell apoptosis, and promotes Treg activity [199]. The presence of IDO in the tumor microenvironment is considered a possible mechanism of resistance to immunotherapy and IDO inhibitors (epacadostat and indoximod) have been combined with ipilimumab, nivolumab, or pembrolizumab in melanoma [200], but not so far in CSCC.

Levels of TAM and MDSCs can be reduced using colony-stimulating factor 1 receptor (CSF1R) inhibitors. For example, CSF1R blockade combined with anti-PD-1 or anti-CTLA-1 treatment is associated with enhanced tumor regression in a mouse model of pancreatic ductal adenocarcinoma [201]. In melanoma, numerous clinical trials are underway that combine antagonists of CSF1R or M-CSF, or GM-CSF agonists with ICI [202].

C5a is a potent anaphylatoxin that modulates inflammation, tumor formation and progression by suppressing the anti-tumor CD8+T-cell-mediated response and immunosuppression by recruiting MDSCs [203]. C5a antibody (vilobelimab/IFX-1) is currently tested alone or in combination with pembrolizumab in locally advanced or metastatic CSCC (NCT04812535).

Finally, since the gut microbiome has been implicated in resistance to ICIs, combined therapies with bacteria plus immunotherapy have been developed. In mice with melanoma, a combination regimen of orally administered Bifidobacterium and anti-PD-L1 therapy abolishes tumor outgrowth [204]. Bifidobacterium species, being immunomodulators of the immune response, increase the infiltration of CD8+ effector T cells and enhance the production of IFN-γ. Moreover, the microbiota composition could predict the efficacy of immunotherapy agents (see above) [205]. A better understanding of the role of the microbiome will open up new avenues for developing new therapies [206].

5. Conclusions

The therapeutic landscape of cutaneous squamous cell carcinoma has changed since the approval of anti-PD-1 therapies. However, not all patients respond, and those who do can develop resistance over time. Therefore, it is important to develop good predictors of response to immunotherapy to be able to identify which patients could benefit from it, and to investigate new treatment regimens for overcoming immunotherapy resistance.

Author Contributions: Writing-original draft: N.G.-S and R.C.-C.; Methodology: N.G.-S, R.C.-C. and J.C.; Conceptualization: N.G.-S. and J.C.; Funding acquisition: J.C. and J.P.-L.; Supervision: J.C.; Writing-review and editing: J.C., L.B.-H., J.P.-L., C.R.-C., E.C.-A. and A.O. All authors have read and agreed to the published version of the manuscript.

Funding: Javier Cañueto is partially supported by the grants GRS2139/A/20 (Gerencia Regional de Salud de Castilla y León), by the PI18/00587 and PI21/01207 (Instituto de Salud Carlos III, cofinanciado con fondos FEDER) and by the "Programa de Intensificación" of the ISCIII, grant number INT20/00074. Sponsors and funders did not influence the design and conduct of the study, the collection, management, analysis, and interpretation of the data, the preparation, review, or approval of the manuscript, or the decision to submit the manuscript for publication.

Conflicts of Interest: The authors declare no conflict of interest.

References

1. Rogers, H.W.; Weinstock, M.A.; Feldman, S.R.; Coldiron, B.M. Incidence Estimate of Nonmelanoma Skin Cancer (Keratinocyte Carcinomas) in the U.S. Population, 2012. *JAMA Dermatol.* **2015**, *151*, 1081–1086. [CrossRef]
2. Karia, P.S.; Han, J.; Schmults, C.D. Cutaneous squamous cell carcinoma: Estimated incidence of disease, nodal metastasis, and deaths from disease in the United States, 2012. *J. Am. Acad. Dermatol.* **2013**, *68*, 957–966. [CrossRef]
3. Leiter, U.; Keim, U.; Garbe, C. Epidemiology of Skin Cancer: Update 2019. *Adv. Exp. Med. Biol.* **2020**, *1268*, 123–139. [CrossRef] [PubMed]
4. Leiter, U.; Keim, U.; Eigentler, T.; Katalinic, A.; Holleczek, B.; Martus, P.; Garbe, C. Incidence, Mortality, and Trends of Nonmelanoma Skin Cancer in Germany. *J. Investig. Dermatol.* **2017**, *137*, 1860–1867. [CrossRef] [PubMed]
5. Schmults, C.D.; Karia, P.S.; Carter, J.B.; Han, J.; Qureshi, A.A. Factors predictive of recurrence and death from cutaneous squamous cell carcinoma: A 10-year, single-institution cohort study. *JAMA Dermatol.* **2013**, *149*, 541–547. [CrossRef] [PubMed]
6. Brantsch, K.D.; Meisner, C.; Schonfisch, B.; Trilling, B.; Wehner-Caroli, J.; Rocken, M.; Breuninger, H. Analysis of risk factors determining prognosis of cutaneous squamous-cell carcinoma: A prospective study. *Lancet. Oncol.* **2008**, *9*, 713–720. [CrossRef]
7. Becerril, S.; Corchado-Cobos, R.; Garcia-Sancha, N.; Revelles, L.; Revilla, D.; Ugalde, T.; Roman-Curto, C.; Perez-Losada, J.; Canueto, J. Viruses and Skin Cancer. *Int. J. Mol. Sci.* **2021**, *22*, 5399. [CrossRef]
8. Que, S.K.T.; Zwald, F.O.; Schmults, C.D. Cutaneous squamous cell carcinoma: Incidence, risk factors, diagnosis, and staging. *J. Am. Acad. Dermatol.* **2018**, *78*, 237–247. [CrossRef]
9. Corchado-Cobos, R.; Garcia-Sancha, N.; Gonzalez-Sarmiento, R.; Perez-Losada, J.; Canueto, J. Cutaneous Squamous Cell Carcinoma: From Biology to Therapy. *Int. J. Mol. Sci.* **2020**, *21*, 2956. [CrossRef]
10. Garcia-Sancha, N.; Corchado-Cobos, R.; Perez-Losada, J.; Canueto, J. MicroRNA Dysregulation in Cutaneous Squamous Cell Carcinoma. *Int. J. Mol. Sci.* **2019**, *20*, 2181. [CrossRef]

11. Pickering, C.R.; Zhou, J.H.; Lee, J.J.; Drummond, J.A.; Peng, S.A.; Saade, R.E.; Tsai, K.Y.; Curry, J.L.; Tetzlaff, M.T.; Lai, S.Y.; et al. Mutational landscape of aggressive cutaneous squamous cell carcinoma. *Clin. Cancer Res. Off. J. Am. Assoc. Cancer Res.* **2014**, *20*, 6582–6592. [CrossRef]
12. Wessely, A.; Steeb, T.; Leiter, U.; Garbe, C.; Berking, C.; Heppt, M.V. Immune Checkpoint Blockade in Advanced Cutaneous Squamous Cell Carcinoma: What Do We Currently Know in 2020? *Int. J. Mol. Sci.* **2020**, *21*, 9300. [CrossRef]
13. Kalbasi, A.; Ribas, A. Tumour-intrinsic resistance to immune checkpoint blockade. *Nat. Rev. Immunol.* **2020**, *20*, 25–39. [CrossRef] [PubMed]
14. Van Elsas, M.J.; van Hall, T.; van der Burg, S.H. Future Challenges in Cancer Resistance to Immunotherapy. *Cancers* **2020**, *12*, 935. [CrossRef]
15. Fares, C.M.; Van Allen, E.M.; Drake, C.G.; Allison, J.P.; Hu-Lieskovan, S. Mechanisms of Resistance to Immune Checkpoint Blockade: Why Does Checkpoint Inhibitor Immunotherapy Not Work for All Patients? *Am. Soc. Clin. Oncol. Educ. Book. Am. Soc. Clin. Oncol. Annu. Meet.* **2019**, *39*, 147–164. [CrossRef]
16. Brunet, J.F.; Denizot, F.; Luciani, M.F.; Roux-Dosseto, M.; Suzan, M.; Mattei, M.G.; Golstein, P. A new member of the immunoglobulin superfamily–CTLA-4. *Nature* **1987**, *328*, 267–270. [CrossRef] [PubMed]
17. Krummel, M.F.; Allison, J.P. CD28 and CTLA-4 have opposing effects on the response of T cells to stimulation. *J. Exp. Med.* **1995**, *182*, 459–465. [CrossRef]
18. Walunas, T.L.; Lenschow, D.J.; Bakker, C.Y.; Linsley, P.S.; Freeman, G.J.; Green, J.M.; Thompson, C.B.; Bluestone, J.A. CTLA-4 can function as a negative regulator of T cell activation. *Immunity* **1994**, *1*, 405–413. [CrossRef]
19. Ishida, Y.; Agata, Y.; Shibahara, K.; Honjo, T. Induced expression of PD-1, a novel member of the immunoglobulin gene superfamily, upon programmed cell death. *EMBO J.* **1992**, *11*, 3887–3895. [CrossRef]
20. Freeman, G.J.; Long, A.J.; Iwai, Y.; Bourque, K.; Chernova, T.; Nishimura, H.; Fitz, L.J.; Malenkovich, N.; Okazaki, T.; Byrne, M.C.; et al. Engagement of the PD-1 immunoinhibitory receptor by a novel B7 family member leads to negative regulation of lymphocyte activation. *J. Exp. Med.* **2000**, *192*, 1027–1034. [CrossRef]
21. Barber, D.L.; Wherry, E.J.; Masopust, D.; Zhu, B.; Allison, J.P.; Sharpe, A.H.; Freeman, G.J.; Ahmed, R. Restoring function in exhausted CD8 T cells during chronic viral infection. *Nature* **2006**, *439*, 682–687. [CrossRef]
22. Schreiber, R.D.; Old, L.J.; Smyth, M.J. Cancer immunoediting: Integrating immunity's roles in cancer suppression and promotion. *Science* **2011**, *331*, 1565–1570. [CrossRef]
23. Dunn, G.P.; Old, L.J.; Schreiber, R.D. The immunobiology of cancer immunosurveillance and immunoediting. *Immunity* **2004**, *21*, 137–148. [CrossRef] [PubMed]
24. Chen, L.; Flies, D.B. Molecular mechanisms of T cell co-stimulation and co-inhibition. *Nat. Rev. Immunol.* **2013**, *13*, 227–242. [CrossRef]
25. Regeneron Pharmaceuticals. LIBTAYO [cemiplimab-rwlc] Injection Full US Prescribing Information. 2018. Available online: www.accessdata.fda.gov/drugsatfda_docs/label/2018/761097s000lbl.pdf (accessed on 1 September 2021).
26. European Medicines Agency. LIBTAYO EPAR. 2019. Available online: www.ema.europa.eu/en/medicines/human/EPAR/libtayo (accessed on 1 September 2021).
27. Falchook, G.S.; Leidner, R.; Stankevich, E.; Piening, B.; Bifulco, C.; Lowy, I.; Fury, M.G. Responses of metastatic basal cell and cutaneous squamous cell carcinomas to anti-PD1 monoclonal antibody REGN2810. *J. Immunother. Cancer* **2016**, *4*, 70. [CrossRef] [PubMed]
28. Migden, M.R.; Rischin, D.; Schmults, C.D.; Guminski, A.; Hauschild, A.; Lewis, K.D.; Chung, C.H.; Hernandez-Aya, L.; Lim, A.M.; Chang, A.L.S.; et al. PD-1 Blockade with Cemiplimab in Advanced Cutaneous Squamous-Cell Carcinoma. *N. Engl. J. Med.* **2018**, *379*, 341–351. [CrossRef]
29. Rischin, D.; Migden, M.R.; Lim, A.M.; Schmults, C.D.; Khushalani, N.I.; Hughes, B.G.M.; Schadendorf, D.; Dunn, L.A.; Hernandez-Aya, L.; Chang, A.L.S.; et al. Phase 2 study of cemiplimab in patients with metastatic cutaneous squamous cell carcinoma: Primary analysis of fixed-dosing, long-term outcome of weight-based dosing. *J. Immunother. Cancer* **2020**, *8*, e000775. [CrossRef] [PubMed]
30. Migden, M.R.; Khushalani, N.I.; Chang, A.L.S.; Lewis, K.D.; Schmults, C.D.; Hernandez-Aya, L.; Meier, F.; Schadendorf, D.; Guminski, A.; Hauschild, A.; et al. Cemiplimab in locally advanced cutaneous squamous cell carcinoma: Results from an open-label, phase 2, single-arm trial. *Lancet. Oncol.* **2020**, *21*, 294–305. [CrossRef]
31. Merck and Company. Keytruda (pembrolizumab) Injection US Prescribing Information. 2020. Available online: www.accessdata.fda.gov/drugsatfda_docs/label/2020/125514s088lbl.pdf (accessed on 1 September 2021).
32. Grob, J.J.; Gonzalez, R.; Basset-Seguin, N.; Vornicova, O.; Schachter, J.; Joshi, A.; Meyer, N.; Grange, F.; Piulats, J.M.; Bauman, J.R.; et al. Pembrolizumab Monotherapy for Recurrent or Metastatic Cutaneous Squamous Cell Carcinoma: A Single-Arm Phase II Trial (KEYNOTE-629). *J. Clin. Oncol. Off. J. Am. Soc. Clin. Oncol.* **2020**, *38*, 2916–2925. [CrossRef]
33. Maubec, E.; Boubaya, M.; Petrow, P.; Beylot-Barry, M.; Basset-Seguin, N.; Deschamps, L.; Grob, J.J.; Dreno, B.; Scheer-Senyarich, I.; Bloch-Queyrat, C.; et al. Phase II Study of Pembrolizumab As First-Line, Single-Drug Therapy for Patients With Unresectable Cutaneous Squamous Cell Carcinomas. *J. Clin. Oncol. Off. J. Am. Soc. Clin. Oncol.* **2020**, *38*, 3051–3061. [CrossRef]
34. Oro-Ayude, M.; Suh-Oh, H.J.; Sacristan-Santos, V.; Vazquez-Bartolome, P.; Florez, A. Nivolumab for Metastatic Cutaneous Squamous Cell Carcinoma. *Case Rep. Dermatol.* **2020**, *12*, 37–41. [CrossRef]
35. Blum, V.; Muller, B.; Hofer, S.; Pardo, E.; Zeidler, K.; Diebold, J.; Strobel, K.; Brand, C.; Aebi, S.; Gautschi, O. Nivolumab for recurrent cutaneous squamous cell carcinoma: Three cases. *Eur. J. Dermatol. EJD* **2018**, *28*, 78–81. [CrossRef]

36. Day, F.; Kumar, M.; Fenton, L.; Gedye, C. Durable Response of Metastatic Squamous Cell Carcinoma of the Skin to Ipilimumab Immunotherapy. *J. Immunother.* **2017**, *40*, 36–38. [CrossRef]
37. Michot, J.M.; Bigenwald, C.; Champiat, S.; Collins, M.; Carbonnel, F.; Postel-Vinay, S.; Berdelou, A.; Varga, A.; Bahleda, R.; Hollebecque, A.; et al. Immune-related adverse events with immune checkpoint blockade: A comprehensive review. *Eur. J. Cancer* **2016**, *54*, 139–148. [CrossRef] [PubMed]
38. Li, X.; Song, W.; Shao, C.; Shi, Y.; Han, W. Emerging predictors of the response to the blockade of immune checkpoints in cancer therapy. *Cell. Mol. Immunol.* **2019**, *16*, 28–39. [CrossRef] [PubMed]
39. Topalian, S.L.; Hodi, F.S.; Brahmer, J.R.; Gettinger, S.N.; Smith, D.C.; McDermott, D.F.; Powderly, J.D.; Carvajal, R.D.; Sosman, J.A.; Atkins, M.B.; et al. Safety, activity, and immune correlates of anti-PD-1 antibody in cancer. *N. Engl. J. Med.* **2012**, *366*, 2443–2454. [CrossRef] [PubMed]
40. Gibney, G.T.; Weiner, L.M.; Atkins, M.B. Predictive biomarkers for checkpoint inhibitor-based immunotherapy. *Lancet Oncol.* **2016**, *17*, e542–e551. [CrossRef]
41. Duffy, M.J.; Crown, J. Biomarkers for Predicting Response to Immunotherapy with Immune Checkpoint Inhibitors in Cancer Patients. *Clin. Chem.* **2019**, *65*, 1228–1238. [CrossRef]
42. Shen, X.; Zhao, B. Efficacy of PD-1 or PD-L1 inhibitors and PD-L1 expression status in cancer: Meta-analysis. *BMJ* **2018**, *362*, k3529. [CrossRef]
43. Keenan, T.E.; Burke, K.P.; Van Allen, E.M. Genomic correlates of response to immune checkpoint blockade. *Nat. Med.* **2019**, *25*, 389–402. [CrossRef]
44. Cottrell, T.R.; Taube, J.M. PD-L1 and Emerging Biomarkers in Immune Checkpoint Blockade Therapy. *Cancer J.* **2018**, *24*, 41–46. [CrossRef]
45. US FDA. List of Cleared or Approved Companion Diagnostic Devices (In Vitro and Imaging Tools). Update: April 8, 2021. Available online: https://www.fda.gov/medical-devices/vitro-diagnostics/list-cleared-or-approved-companion-diagnostic-devices-vitro-and-imaging-tools (accessed on 1 September 2021).
46. Garris, C.S.; Arlauckas, S.P.; Kohler, R.H.; Trefny, M.P.; Garren, S.; Piot, C.; Engblom, C.; Pfirschke, C.; Siwicki, M.; Gungabeesoon, J.; et al. Successful Anti-PD-1 Cancer Immunotherapy Requires T Cell-Dendritic Cell Crosstalk Involving the Cytokines IFN-gamma and IL-12. *Immunity* **2018**, *49*, 1148–1161.e7. [CrossRef]
47. Karachaliou, N.; Gonzalez-Cao, M.; Crespo, G.; Drozdowskyj, A.; Aldeguer, E.; Gimenez-Capitan, A.; Teixido, C.; Molina-Vila, M.A.; Viteri, S.; De Los Llanos Gil, M.; et al. Interferon gamma, an important marker of response to immune checkpoint blockade in non-small cell lung cancer and melanoma patients. *Ther. Adv. Med. Oncol.* **2018**, *10*, 1758834017749748. [CrossRef]
48. Ayers, M.; Lunceford, J.; Nebozhyn, M.; Murphy, E.; Loboda, A.; Kaufman, D.R.; Albright, A.; Cheng, J.D.; Kang, S.P.; Shankaran, V.; et al. IFN-gamma-related mRNA profile predicts clinical response to PD-1 blockade. *J. Clin. Investig.* **2017**, *127*, 2930–2940. [CrossRef]
49. Lu, S.; Stein, J.E.; Rimm, D.L.; Wang, D.W.; Bell, J.M.; Johnson, D.B.; Sosman, J.A.; Schalper, K.A.; Anders, R.A.; Wang, H.; et al. Comparison of Biomarker Modalities for Predicting Response to PD-1/PD-L1 Checkpoint Blockade: A Systematic Review and Meta-analysis. *JAMA Oncol.* **2019**, *5*, 1195–1204. [CrossRef]
50. Cui, C.; Xu, C.; Yang, W.; Chi, Z.; Sheng, X.; Si, L.; Xie, Y.; Yu, J.; Wang, S.; Yu, R.; et al. Ratio of the interferon-gamma signature to the immunosuppression signature predicts anti-PD-1 therapy response in melanoma. *NPJ Genom. Med.* **2021**, *6*, 7. [CrossRef]
51. Van Allen, E.M.; Miao, D.; Schilling, B.; Shukla, S.A.; Blank, C.; Zimmer, L.; Sucker, A.; Hillen, U.; Foppen, M.H.G.; Goldinger, S.M.; et al. Genomic correlates of response to CTLA-4 blockade in metastatic melanoma. *Science* **2015**, *350*, 207–211. [CrossRef]
52. Snyder, A.; Makarov, V.; Merghoub, T.; Yuan, J.; Zaretsky, J.M.; Desrichard, A.; Walsh, L.A.; Postow, M.A.; Wong, P.; Ho, T.S.; et al. Genetic basis for clinical response to CTLA-4 blockade in melanoma. *N. Engl. J. Med.* **2014**, *371*, 2189–2199. [CrossRef]
53. Rizvi, N.A.; Hellmann, M.D.; Snyder, A.; Kvistborg, P.; Makarov, V.; Havel, J.J.; Lee, W.; Yuan, J.; Wong, P.; Ho, T.S.; et al. Cancer immunology. Mutational landscape determines sensitivity to PD-1 blockade in non-small cell lung cancer. *Science* **2015**, *348*, 124–128. [CrossRef]
54. Rosenberg, J.E.; Hoffman-Censits, J.; Powles, T.; van der Heijden, M.S.; Balar, A.V.; Necchi, A.; Dawson, N.; O'Donnell, P.H.; Balmanoukian, A.; Loriot, Y.; et al. Atezolizumab in patients with locally advanced and metastatic urothelial carcinoma who have progressed following treatment with platinum-based chemotherapy: A single-arm, multicentre, phase 2 trial. *Lancet* **2016**, *387*, 1909–1920. [CrossRef]
55. Yarchoan, M.; Hopkins, A.; Jaffee, E.M. Tumor Mutational Burden and Response Rate to PD-1 Inhibition. *N. Engl. J. Med.* **2017**, *377*, 2500–2501. [CrossRef]
56. Goodman, A.M.; Kato, S.; Bazhenova, L.; Patel, S.P.; Frampton, G.M.; Miller, V.; Stephens, P.J.; Daniels, G.A.; Kurzrock, R. Tumor Mutational Burden as an Independent Predictor of Response to Immunotherapy in Diverse Cancers. *Mol. Cancer Ther.* **2017**, *16*, 2598–2608. [CrossRef]
57. Inman, G.J.; Wang, J.; Nagano, A.; Alexandrov, L.B.; Purdie, K.J.; Taylor, R.G.; Sherwood, V.; Thomson, J.; Hogan, S.; Spender, L.C.; et al. The genomic landscape of cutaneous SCC reveals drivers and a novel azathioprine associated mutational signature. *Nat. Commun.* **2018**, *9*, 3667. [CrossRef]
58. Goodman, A.M.; Kato, S.; Chattopadhyay, R.; Okamura, R.; Saunders, I.M.; Montesion, M.; Frampton, G.M.; Miller, V.A.; Daniels, G.A.; Kurzrock, R. Phenotypic and Genomic Determinants of Immunotherapy Response Associated with Squamousness. *Cancer Immunol. Res.* **2019**, *7*, 866–873. [CrossRef]

59. Hanna, G.J.; Ruiz, E.S.; LeBoeuf, N.R.; Thakuria, M.; Schmults, C.D.; Decaprio, J.A.; Silk, A.W. Real-world outcomes treating patients with advanced cutaneous squamous cell carcinoma with immune checkpoint inhibitors (CPI). *Br. J. Cancer* **2020**, *123*, 1535–1542. [CrossRef]
60. Samstein, R.M.; Lee, C.H.; Shoushtari, A.N.; Hellmann, M.D.; Shen, R.; Janjigian, Y.Y.; Barron, D.A.; Zehir, A.; Jordan, E.J.; Omuro, A.; et al. Tumor mutational load predicts survival after immunotherapy across multiple cancer types. *Nat. Genet.* **2019**, *51*, 202–206. [CrossRef]
61. Gromeier, M.; Brown, M.C.; Zhang, G.; Lin, X.; Chen, Y.; Wei, Z.; Beaubier, N.; Yan, H.; He, Y.; Desjardins, A.; et al. Very low mutation burden is a feature of inflamed recurrent glioblastomas responsive to cancer immunotherapy. *Nat. Commun.* **2021**, *12*, 352. [CrossRef]
62. Strickler, J.H.; Hanks, B.A.; Khasraw, M. Tumor Mutational Burden as a Predictor of Immunotherapy Response: Is More Always Better? *Clin. Cancer Res. Off. J. Am. Assoc. Cancer Res.* **2021**, *27*, 1236–1241. [CrossRef]
63. FDA Approves Pembrolizumab for Adults and Children with TMB-H Solid Tumors. Available online: https://www.fda.gov/drugs/drug-approvals-and-databases/fda-approves-pembrolizumab-adults-and-children-tmb-h-solid-tumors (accessed on 1 September 2021).
64. Schumacher, T.N.; Schreiber, R.D. Neoantigens in cancer immunotherapy. *Science* **2015**, *348*, 69–74. [CrossRef]
65. McGranahan, N.; Furness, A.J.; Rosenthal, R.; Ramskov, S.; Lyngaa, R.; Saini, S.K.; Jamal-Hanjani, M.; Wilson, G.A.; Birkbak, N.J.; Hiley, C.T.; et al. Clonal neoantigens elicit T cell immunoreactivity and sensitivity to immune checkpoint blockade. *Science* **2016**, *351*, 1463–1469. [CrossRef]
66. Alspach, E.; Lussier, D.M.; Miceli, A.P.; Kizhvatov, I.; DuPage, M.; Luoma, A.M.; Meng, W.; Lichti, C.F.; Esaulova, E.; Vomund, A.N.; et al. MHC-II neoantigens shape tumour immunity and response to immunotherapy. *Nature* **2019**, *574*, 696–701. [CrossRef]
67. Kim, K.; Kim, H.S.; Kim, J.Y.; Jung, H.; Sun, J.M.; Ahn, J.S.; Ahn, M.J.; Park, K.; Lee, S.H.; Choi, J.K. Predicting clinical benefit of immunotherapy by antigenic or functional mutations affecting tumour immunogenicity. *Nat. Commun.* **2020**, *11*, 951. [CrossRef]
68. Tumeh, P.C.; Harview, C.L.; Yearley, J.H.; Shintaku, I.P.; Taylor, E.J.; Robert, L.; Chmielowski, B.; Spasic, M.; Henry, G.; Ciobanu, V.; et al. PD-1 blockade induces responses by inhibiting adaptive immune resistance. *Nature* **2014**, *515*, 568–571. [CrossRef]
69. Daud, A.I.; Loo, K.; Pauli, M.L.; Sanchez-Rodriguez, R.; Sandoval, P.M.; Taravati, K.; Tsai, K.; Nosrati, A.; Nardo, L.; Alvarado, M.D.; et al. Tumor immune profiling predicts response to anti-PD-1 therapy in human melanoma. *J. Clin. Investig.* **2016**, *126*, 3447–3452. [CrossRef]
70. Uryvaev, A.; Passhak, M.; Hershkovits, D.; Sabo, E.; Bar-Sela, G. The role of tumor-infiltrating lymphocytes (TILs) as a predictive biomarker of response to anti-PD1 therapy in patients with metastatic non-small cell lung cancer or metastatic melanoma. *Med. Oncol.* **2018**, *35*, 25. [CrossRef]
71. Shaban, M.; Khurram, S.A.; Fraz, M.M.; Alsubaie, N.; Masood, I.; Mushtaq, S.; Hassan, M.; Loya, A.; Rajpoot, N.M. A Novel Digital Score for Abundance of Tumour Infiltrating Lymphocytes Predicts Disease Free Survival in Oral Squamous Cell Carcinoma. *Sci. Rep.* **2019**, *9*, 13341. [CrossRef]
72. Zhang, L.; Zhang, Z. Recharacterizing Tumor-Infiltrating Lymphocytes by Single-Cell RNA Sequencing. *Cancer Immunol. Res.* **2019**, *7*, 1040–1046. [CrossRef]
73. Martens, A.; Wistuba-Hamprecht, K.; Yuan, J.; Postow, M.A.; Wong, P.; Capone, M.; Madonna, G.; Khammari, A.; Schilling, B.; Sucker, A.; et al. Increases in Absolute Lymphocytes and Circulating CD4+ and CD8+ T Cells Are Associated with Positive Clinical Outcome of Melanoma Patients Treated with Ipilimumab. *Clin. Cancer Res. Off. J. Am. Assoc. Cancer Res.* **2016**, *22*, 4848–4858. [CrossRef]
74. Valpione, S.; Martinoli, C.; Fava, P.; Mocellin, S.; Campana, L.G.; Quaglino, P.; Ferrucci, P.F.; Pigozzo, J.; Astrua, C.; Testori, A.; et al. Personalised medicine: Development and external validation of a prognostic model for metastatic melanoma patients treated with ipilimumab. *Eur. J. Cancer* **2015**, *51*, 2086–2094. [CrossRef]
75. Gebhardt, C.; Sevko, A.; Jiang, H.; Lichtenberger, R.; Reith, M.; Tarnanidis, K.; Holland-Letz, T.; Umansky, L.; Beckhove, P.; Sucker, A.; et al. Myeloid Cells and Related Chronic Inflammatory Factors as Novel Predictive Markers in Melanoma Treatment with Ipilimumab. *Clin. Cancer Res. Off. J. Am. Assoc. Cancer Res.* **2015**, *21*, 5453–5459. [CrossRef]
76. Weide, B.; Martens, A.; Hassel, J.C.; Berking, C.; Postow, M.A.; Bisschop, K.; Simeone, E.; Mangana, J.; Schilling, B.; Di Giacomo, A.M.; et al. Baseline Biomarkers for Outcome of Melanoma Patients Treated with Pembrolizumab. *Clin. Cancer Res. Off. J. Am. Assoc. Cancer Res.* **2016**, *22*, 5487–5496. [CrossRef]
77. Simeone, E.; Gentilcore, G.; Giannarelli, D.; Grimaldi, A.M.; Caraco, C.; Curvietto, M.; Esposito, A.; Paone, M.; Palla, M.; Cavalcanti, E.; et al. Immunological and biological changes during ipilimumab treatment and their potential correlation with clinical response and survival in patients with advanced melanoma. *Cancer Immunol. Immunother. CII* **2014**, *63*, 675–683. [CrossRef]
78. Delyon, J.; Mateus, C.; Lefeuvre, D.; Lanoy, E.; Zitvogel, L.; Chaput, N.; Roy, S.; Eggermont, A.M.; Routier, E.; Robert, C. Experience in daily practice with ipilimumab for the treatment of patients with metastatic melanoma: An early increase in lymphocyte and eosinophil counts is associated with improved survival. *Ann. Oncol. Off. J. Eur. Soc. Med Oncol.* **2013**, *24*, 1697–1703. [CrossRef]
79. Bridge, J.A.; Lee, J.C.; Daud, A.; Wells, J.W.; Bluestone, J.A. Cytokines, Chemokines, and Other Biomarkers of Response for Checkpoint Inhibitor Therapy in Skin Cancer. *Front. Med.* **2018**, *5*, 351. [CrossRef]

80. Bjoern, J.; Juul Nitschke, N.; Zeeberg Iversen, T.; Schmidt, H.; Fode, K.; Svane, I.M. Immunological correlates of treatment and response in stage IV malignant melanoma patients treated with Ipilimumab. *Oncoimmunology* **2016**, *5*, e1100788. [CrossRef]
81. Sanmamed, M.F.; Perez-Gracia, J.L.; Schalper, K.A.; Fusco, J.P.; Gonzalez, A.; Rodriguez-Ruiz, M.E.; Onate, C.; Perez, G.; Alfaro, C.; Martin-Algarra, S.; et al. Changes in serum interleukin-8 (IL-8) levels reflect and predict response to anti-PD-1 treatment in melanoma and non-small-cell lung cancer patients. *Ann. Oncol. Off. J. Eur. Soc. Med Oncol.* **2017**, *28*, 1988–1995. [CrossRef]
82. Schalper, K.A.; Carleton, M.; Zhou, M.; Chen, T.; Feng, Y.; Huang, S.P.; Walsh, A.M.; Baxi, V.; Pandya, D.; Baradet, T.; et al. Elevated serum interleukin-8 is associated with enhanced intratumor neutrophils and reduced clinical benefit of immune-checkpoint inhibitors. *Nat. Med.* **2020**, *26*, 688–692. [CrossRef]
83. Seremet, T.; Jansen, Y.; Planken, S.; Njimi, H.; Delaunoy, M.; El Housni, H.; Awada, G.; Schwarze, J.K.; Keyaerts, M.; Everaert, H.; et al. Undetectable circulating tumor DNA (ctDNA) levels correlate with favorable outcome in metastatic melanoma patients treated with anti-PD1 therapy. *J. Transl. Med.* **2019**, *17*, 303. [CrossRef]
84. Lee, J.H.; Long, G.V.; Boyd, S.; Lo, S.; Menzies, A.M.; Tembe, V.; Guminski, A.; Jakrot, V.; Scolyer, R.A.; Mann, G.J.; et al. Circulating tumour DNA predicts response to anti-PD1 antibodies in metastatic melanoma. *Ann. Oncol. Off. J. Eur. Soc. Med. Oncol.* **2017**, *28*, 1130–1136. [CrossRef]
85. Bratman, S.V.; Yang, S.Y.C.; Lafolla, M.A.J.; Liu, Z.; Hansen, A.R.; Bedard, P.L.; Lheureux, S.; Spreafico, A.; Razak, A.R.A.; Shchegrova, S.; et al. Personalized circulating tumor DNA analysis as a predictive biomarker in solid tumor patients treated with pembrolizumab. *Nat. Cancer* **2020**, *1*, 873–881. [CrossRef]
86. Wang, Z.; Duan, J.; Cai, S.; Han, M.; Dong, H.; Zhao, J.; Zhu, B.; Wang, S.; Zhuo, M.; Sun, J.; et al. Assessment of Blood Tumor Mutational Burden as a Potential Biomarker for Immunotherapy in Patients With Non-Small Cell Lung Cancer With Use of a Next-Generation Sequencing Cancer Gene Panel. *JAMA Oncol.* **2019**, *5*, 696–702. [CrossRef]
87. Gandara, D.R.; Paul, S.M.; Kowanetz, M.; Schleifman, E.; Zou, W.; Li, Y.; Rittmeyer, A.; Fehrenbacher, L.; Otto, G.; Malboeuf, C.; et al. Blood-based tumor mutational burden as a predictor of clinical benefit in non-small-cell lung cancer patients treated with atezolizumab. *Nat. Med.* **2018**, *24*, 1441–1448. [CrossRef]
88. Si, H.; Kuziora, M.; Quinn, K.J.; Helman, E.; Ye, J.; Liu, F.; Scheuring, U.; Peters, S.; Rizvi, N.A.; Brohawn, P.Z.; et al. A Blood-based Assay for Assessment of Tumor Mutational Burden in First-line Metastatic NSCLC Treatment: Results from the MYSTIC Study. *Clin. Cancer Res. Off. J. Am. Assoc. Cancer Res.* **2021**, *27*, 1631–1640. [CrossRef]
89. Hong, X.; Sullivan, R.J.; Kalinich, M.; Kwan, T.T.; Giobbie-Hurder, A.; Pan, S.; LiCausi, J.A.; Milner, J.D.; Nieman, L.T.; Wittner, B.S.; et al. Molecular signatures of circulating melanoma cells for monitoring early response to immune checkpoint therapy. *Proc. Natl. Acad. Sci. USA* **2018**, *115*, 2467–2472. [CrossRef]
90. Khattak, M.A.; Reid, A.; Freeman, J.; Pereira, M.; McEvoy, A.; Lo, J.; Frank, M.H.; Meniawy, T.; Didan, A.; Spencer, I.; et al. PD-L1 Expression on Circulating Tumor Cells May Be Predictive of Response to Pembrolizumab in Advanced Melanoma: Results from a Pilot Study. *Oncologist* **2019**, *25*, e520–e527. [CrossRef]
91. Zhou, J.; Mahoney, K.M.; Giobbie-Hurder, A.; Zhao, F.; Lee, S.; Liao, X.; Rodig, S.; Li, J.; Wu, X.; Butterfield, L.H.; et al. Soluble PD-L1 as a Biomarker in Malignant Melanoma Treated with Checkpoint Blockade. *Cancer Immunol. Res.* **2017**, *5*, 480–492. [CrossRef]
92. Okuma, Y.; Wakui, H.; Utsumi, H.; Sagawa, Y.; Hosomi, Y.; Kuwano, K.; Homma, S. Soluble Programmed Cell Death Ligand 1 as a Novel Biomarker for Nivolumab Therapy for Non-Small-cell Lung Cancer. *Clin. Lung Cancer* **2018**, *19*, 410–417.e1. [CrossRef]
93. Yu, Y.; Zeng, D.; Ou, Q.; Liu, S.; Li, A.; Chen, Y.; Lin, D.; Gao, Q.; Zhou, H.; Liao, W.; et al. Association of Survival and Immune-Related Biomarkers With Immunotherapy in Patients With Non-Small Cell Lung Cancer: A Meta-analysis and Individual Patient-Level Analysis. *JAMA Netw. Open* **2019**, *2*, e196879. [CrossRef]
94. Jiang, P.; Gu, S.; Pan, D.; Fu, J.; Sahu, A.; Hu, X.; Li, Z.; Traugh, N.; Bu, X.; Li, B.; et al. Signatures of T cell dysfunction and exclusion predict cancer immunotherapy response. *Nat. Med.* **2018**, *24*, 1550–1558. [CrossRef]
95. Litchfield, K.; Reading, J.L.; Puttick, C.; Thakkar, K.; Abbosh, C.; Bentham, R.; Watkins, T.B.K.; Rosenthal, R.; Biswas, D.; Rowan, A.; et al. Meta-analysis of tumor- and T cell-intrinsic mechanisms of sensitization to checkpoint inhibition. *Cell* **2021**, *184*, 596–614.e14. [CrossRef]
96. Oh, S.J.; Lee, J.K.; Shin, O.S. Aging and the Immune System: The Impact of Immunosenescence on Viral Infection, Immunity and Vaccine Immunogenicity. *Immune Netw.* **2019**, *19*, e37. [CrossRef] [PubMed]
97. Aw, D.; Silva, A.B.; Palmer, D.B. Immunosenescence: Emerging challenges for an ageing population. *Immunology* **2007**, *120*, 435–446. [CrossRef] [PubMed]
98. Bueno, V.; Sant'Anna, O.A.; Lord, J.M. Ageing and myeloid-derived suppressor cells: Possible involvement in immunosenescence and age-related disease. *Age* **2014**, *36*, 9729. [CrossRef] [PubMed]
99. Granier, C.; Gey, A.; Roncelin, S.; Weiss, L.; Paillaud, E.; Tartour, E. Immunotherapy in older patients with cancer. *Biomed. J.* **2020**, *44*, 260–271. [CrossRef] [PubMed]
100. Daste, A.; Domblides, C.; Gross-Goupil, M.; Chakiba, C.; Quivy, A.; Cochin, V.; de Mones, E.; Larmonier, N.; Soubeyran, P.; Ravaud, A. Immune checkpoint inhibitors and elderly people: A review. *Eur. J. Cancer* **2017**, *82*, 155–166. [CrossRef] [PubMed]
101. Chowell, D.; Morris, L.G.T.; Grigg, C.M.; Weber, J.K.; Samstein, R.M.; Makarov, V.; Kuo, F.; Kendall, S.M.; Requena, D.; Riaz, N.; et al. Patient HLA class I genotype influences cancer response to checkpoint blockade immunotherapy. *Science* **2018**, *359*, 582–587. [CrossRef] [PubMed]

102. Chowell, D.; Krishna, C.; Pierini, F.; Makarov, V.; Rizvi, N.A.; Kuo, F.; Morris, L.G.T.; Riaz, N.; Lenz, T.L.; Chan, T.A. Evolutionary divergence of HLA class I genotype impacts efficacy of cancer immunotherapy. *Nat. Med.* **2019**, *25*, 1715–1720. [CrossRef] [PubMed]
103. Qiu, Q.; Lin, Y.; Ma, Y.; Li, X.; Liang, J.; Chen, Z.; Liu, K.; Huang, Y.; Luo, H.; Huang, R.; et al. Exploring the Emerging Role of the Gut Microbiota and Tumor Microenvironment in Cancer Immunotherapy. *Front. Immunol.* **2020**, *11*, 612202. [CrossRef] [PubMed]
104. Gopalakrishnan, V.; Spencer, C.N.; Nezi, L.; Reuben, A.; Andrews, M.C.; Karpinets, T.V.; Prieto, P.A.; Vicente, D.; Hoffman, K.; Wei, S.C.; et al. Gut microbiome modulates response to anti-PD-1 immunotherapy in melanoma patients. *Science* **2018**, *359*, 97–103. [CrossRef] [PubMed]
105. Matson, V.; Fessler, J.; Bao, R.; Chongsuwat, T.; Zha, Y.; Alegre, M.L.; Luke, J.J.; Gajewski, T.F. The commensal microbiome is associated with anti-PD-1 efficacy in metastatic melanoma patients. *Science* **2018**, *359*, 104–108. [CrossRef] [PubMed]
106. Dhatchinamoorthy, K.; Colbert, J.D.; Rock, K.L. Cancer Immune Evasion Through Loss of MHC Class I Antigen Presentation. *Front. Immunol.* **2021**, *12*, 636568. [CrossRef] [PubMed]
107. Beatty, G.L.; Gladney, W.L. Immune escape mechanisms as a guide for cancer immunotherapy. *Clin. Cancer Res. Off. J. Am. Assoc. Cancer Res.* **2015**, *21*, 687–692. [CrossRef]
108. Liu, C.; Peng, W.; Xu, C.; Lou, Y.; Zhang, M.; Wargo, J.A.; Chen, J.Q.; Li, H.S.; Watowich, S.S.; Yang, Y.; et al. BRAF inhibition increases tumor infiltration by T cells and enhances the antitumor activity of adoptive immunotherapy in mice. *Clin. Cancer Res. Off. J. Am. Assoc. Cancer Res.* **2013**, *19*, 393–403. [CrossRef]
109. Khalili, J.S.; Liu, S.; Rodriguez-Cruz, T.G.; Whittington, M.; Wardell, S.; Liu, C.; Zhang, M.; Cooper, Z.A.; Frederick, D.T.; Li, Y.; et al. Oncogenic BRAF(V600E) promotes stromal cell-mediated immunosuppression via induction of interleukin-1 in melanoma. *Clin. Cancer Res. Off. J. Am. Assoc. Cancer Res.* **2012**, *18*, 5329–5340. [CrossRef] [PubMed]
110. Haas, L.; Elewaut, A.; Gerard, C.L.; Umkehrer, C.; Leiendecker, L.; Pedersen, M.; Krecioch, I.; Hoffmann, D.; Novatchkova, M.; Kuttke, M.; et al. Acquired resistance to anti-MAPK targeted therapy confers an immune-evasive tumor microenvironment and cross-resistance to immunotherapy in melanoma. *Nat. Cancer* **2021**, *2*, 693–708. [CrossRef]
111. Peng, W.; Chen, J.Q.; Liu, C.; Malu, S.; Creasy, C.; Tetzlaff, M.T.; Xu, C.; McKenzie, J.A.; Zhang, C.; Liang, X.; et al. Loss of PTEN Promotes Resistance to T Cell-Mediated Immunotherapy. *Cancer Discov.* **2016**, *6*, 202–216. [CrossRef]
112. George, S.; Miao, D.; Demetri, G.D.; Adeegbe, D.; Rodig, S.J.; Shukla, S.; Lipschitz, M.; Amin-Mansour, A.; Raut, C.P.; Carter, S.L.; et al. Loss of PTEN Is Associated with Resistance to Anti-PD-1 Checkpoint Blockade Therapy in Metastatic Uterine Leiomyosarcoma. *Immunity* **2017**, *46*, 197–204. [CrossRef]
113. Lastwika, K.J.; Wilson, W., 3rd; Li, Q.K.; Norris, J.; Xu, H.; Ghazarian, S.R.; Kitagawa, H.; Kawabata, S.; Taube, J.M.; Yao, S.; et al. Control of PD-L1 Expression by Oncogenic Activation of the AKT-mTOR Pathway in Non-Small Cell Lung Cancer. *Cancer Res.* **2016**, *76*, 227–238. [CrossRef]
114. Spranger, S.; Bao, R.; Gajewski, T.F. Melanoma-intrinsic beta-catenin signalling prevents anti-tumour immunity. *Nature* **2015**, *523*, 231–235. [CrossRef]
115. Shin, D.S.; Zaretsky, J.M.; Escuin-Ordinas, H.; Garcia-Diaz, A.; Hu-Lieskovan, S.; Kalbasi, A.; Grasso, C.S.; Hugo, W.; Sandoval, S.; Torrejon, D.Y.; et al. Primary Resistance to PD-1 Blockade Mediated by JAK1/2 Mutations. *Cancer Discov.* **2017**, *7*, 188–201. [CrossRef]
116. Gide, T.N.; Wilmott, J.S.; Scolyer, R.A.; Long, G.V. Primary and Acquired Resistance to Immune Checkpoint Inhibitors in Metastatic Melanoma. *Clin. Cancer Res. Off. J. Am. Assoc. Cancer Res.* **2018**, *24*, 1260–1270. [CrossRef]
117. Tanaka, A.; Sakaguchi, S. Regulatory T cells in cancer immunotherapy. *Cell Res.* **2017**, *27*, 109–118. [CrossRef]
118. Chaudhary, B.; Elkord, E. Regulatory T Cells in the Tumor Microenvironment and Cancer Progression: Role and Therapeutic Targeting. *Vaccines* **2016**, *4*, 28. [CrossRef]
119. Ngiow, S.F.; Young, A.; Jacquelot, N.; Yamazaki, T.; Enot, D.; Zitvogel, L.; Smyth, M.J. A Threshold Level of Intratumor CD8+ T-cell PD1 Expression Dictates Therapeutic Response to Anti-PD1. *Cancer Res.* **2015**, *75*, 3800–3811. [CrossRef] [PubMed]
120. Gabrilovich, D.I.; Nagaraj, S. Myeloid-derived suppressor cells as regulators of the immune system. *Nat. Rev. Immunol.* **2009**, *9*, 162–174. [CrossRef] [PubMed]
121. Weide, B.; Martens, A.; Zelba, H.; Stutz, C.; Derhovanessian, E.; Di Giacomo, A.M.; Maio, M.; Sucker, A.; Schilling, B.; Schadendorf, D.; et al. Myeloid-derived suppressor cells predict survival of patients with advanced melanoma: Comparison with regulatory T cells and NY-ESO-1- or melan-A-specific T cells. *Clin. Cancer Res. Off. J. Am. Assoc. Cancer Res.* **2014**, *20*, 1601–1609. [CrossRef] [PubMed]
122. Meyer, C.; Cagnon, L.; Costa-Nunes, C.M.; Baumgaertner, P.; Montandon, N.; Leyvraz, L.; Michielin, O.; Romano, E.; Speiser, D.E. Frequencies of circulating MDSC correlate with clinical outcome of melanoma patients treated with ipilimumab. *Cancer Immunol. Immunother. CII* **2014**, *63*, 247–257. [CrossRef] [PubMed]
123. Xiang, X.; Wang, J.; Lu, D.; Xu, X. Targeting tumor-associated macrophages to synergize tumor immunotherapy. *Signal Transduct. Target. Ther.* **2021**, *6*, 75. [CrossRef] [PubMed]
124. Noy, R.; Pollard, J.W. Tumor-associated macrophages: From mechanisms to therapy. *Immunity* **2014**, *41*, 49–61. [CrossRef]
125. Mariathasan, S.; Turley, S.J.; Nickles, D.; Castiglioni, A.; Yuen, K.; Wang, Y.; Kadel, E.E., III; Koeppen, H.; Astarita, J.L.; Cubas, R.; et al. TGFbeta attenuates tumour response to PD-L1 blockade by contributing to exclusion of T cells. *Nature* **2018**, *554*, 544–548. [CrossRef]

126. D'Urso, C.M.; Wang, Z.G.; Cao, Y.; Tatake, R.; Zeff, R.A.; Ferrone, S. Lack of HLA class I antigen expression by cultured melanoma cells FO-1 due to a defect in B2m gene expression. *J. Clin. Investig.* **1991**, *87*, 284–292. [CrossRef] [PubMed]
127. Bernier, G.M. beta 2-Microglobulin: Structure, function and significance. *Vox Sang.* **1980**, *38*, 323–327. [CrossRef] [PubMed]
128. Zaretsky, J.M.; Garcia-Diaz, A.; Shin, D.S.; Escuin-Ordinas, H.; Hugo, W.; Hu-Lieskovan, S.; Torrejon, D.Y.; Abril-Rodriguez, G.; Sandoval, S.; Barthly, L.; et al. Mutations Associated with Acquired Resistance to PD-1 Blockade in Melanoma. *N. Engl. J. Med.* **2016**, *375*, 819–829. [CrossRef] [PubMed]
129. Sade-Feldman, M.; Jiao, Y.J.; Chen, J.H.; Rooney, M.S.; Barzily-Rokni, M.; Eliane, J.P.; Bjorgaard, S.L.; Hammond, M.R.; Vitzthum, H.; Blackmon, S.M.; et al. Resistance to checkpoint blockade therapy through inactivation of antigen presentation. *Nat. Commun.* **2017**, *8*, 1136. [CrossRef] [PubMed]
130. Gettinger, S.; Choi, J.; Hastings, K.; Truini, A.; Datar, I.; Sowell, R.; Wurtz, A.; Dong, W.; Cai, G.; Melnick, M.A.; et al. Impaired HLA Class I Antigen Processing and Presentation as a Mechanism of Acquired Resistance to Immune Checkpoint Inhibitors in Lung Cancer. *Cancer Discov.* **2017**, *7*, 1420–1435. [CrossRef] [PubMed]
131. Le, D.T.; Durham, J.N.; Smith, K.N.; Wang, H.; Bartlett, B.R.; Aulakh, L.K.; Lu, S.; Kemberling, H.; Wilt, C.; Luber, B.S.; et al. Mismatch repair deficiency predicts response of solid tumors to PD-1 blockade. *Science* **2017**, *357*, 409–413. [CrossRef] [PubMed]
132. Sucker, A.; Zhao, F.; Pieper, N.; Heeke, C.; Maltaner, R.; Stadtler, N.; Real, B.; Bielefeld, N.; Howe, S.; Weide, B.; et al. Acquired IFNgamma resistance impairs anti-tumor immunity and gives rise to T-cell-resistant melanoma lesions. *Nat. Commun.* **2017**, *8*, 15440. [CrossRef] [PubMed]
133. Rosenthal, R.; Cadieux, E.L.; Salgado, R.; Bakir, M.A.; Moore, D.A.; Hiley, C.T.; Lund, T.; Tanic, M.; Reading, J.L.; Joshi, K.; et al. Neoantigen-directed immune escape in lung cancer evolution. *Nature* **2019**, *567*, 479–485. [CrossRef]
134. Anagnostou, V.; Smith, K.N.; Forde, P.M.; Niknafs, N.; Bhattacharya, R.; White, J.; Zhang, T.; Adleff, V.; Phallen, J.; Wali, N.; et al. Evolution of Neoantigen Landscape during Immune Checkpoint Blockade in Non-Small Cell Lung Cancer. *Cancer Discov.* **2017**, *7*, 264–276. [CrossRef]
135. Koyama, S.; Akbay, E.A.; Li, Y.Y.; Herter-Sprie, G.S.; Buczkowski, K.A.; Richards, W.G.; Gandhi, L.; Redig, A.J.; Rodig, S.J.; Asahina, H.; et al. Adaptive resistance to therapeutic PD-1 blockade is associated with upregulation of alternative immune checkpoints. *Nat. Commun.* **2016**, *7*, 10501. [CrossRef]
136. Trujillo, J.A.; Luke, J.J.; Zha, Y.; Segal, J.P.; Ritterhouse, L.L.; Spranger, S.; Matijevich, K.; Gajewski, T.F. Secondary resistance to immunotherapy associated with beta-catenin pathway activation or PTEN loss in metastatic melanoma. *J. Immunother. Cancer* **2019**, *7*, 295. [CrossRef]
137. Sharma, P.; Hu-Lieskovan, S.; Wargo, J.A.; Ribas, A. Primary, Adaptive, and Acquired Resistance to Cancer Immunotherapy. *Cell* **2017**, *168*, 707–723. [CrossRef]
138. Larkin, J.; Chiarion-Sileni, V.; Gonzalez, R.; Grob, J.J.; Rutkowski, P.; Lao, C.D.; Cowey, C.L.; Schadendorf, D.; Wagstaff, J.; Dummer, R.; et al. Five-Year Survival with Combined Nivolumab and Ipilimumab in Advanced Melanoma. *N. Engl. J. Med.* **2019**, *381*, 1535–1546. [CrossRef] [PubMed]
139. Antonia, S.J.; Borghaei, H.; Ramalingam, S.S.; Horn, L.; De Castro Carpeno, J.; Pluzanski, A.; Burgio, M.A.; Garassino, M.; Chow, L.Q.M.; Gettinger, S.; et al. Four-year survival with nivolumab in patients with previously treated advanced non-small-cell lung cancer: A pooled analysis. *Lancet Oncol.* **2019**, *20*, 1395–1408. [CrossRef]
140. Schoenfeld, A.J.; Hellmann, M.D. Acquired Resistance to Immune Checkpoint Inhibitors. *Cancer Cell* **2020**, *37*, 443–455. [CrossRef]
141. Postow, M.A.; Chesney, J.; Pavlick, A.C.; Robert, C.; Grossmann, K.; McDermott, D.; Linette, G.P.; Meyer, N.; Giguere, J.K.; Agarwala, S.S.; et al. Nivolumab and ipilimumab versus ipilimumab in untreated melanoma. *N. Engl. J. Med.* **2015**, *372*, 2006–2017. [CrossRef] [PubMed]
142. Hodi, F.S.; Chesney, J.; Pavlick, A.C.; Robert, C.; Grossmann, K.F.; McDermott, D.F.; Linette, G.P.; Meyer, N.; Giguere, J.K.; Agarwala, S.S.; et al. Combined nivolumab and ipilimumab versus ipilimumab alone in patients with advanced melanoma: 2-year overall survival outcomes in a multicentre, randomised, controlled, phase 2 trial. *Lancet Oncol.* **2016**, *17*, 1558–1568. [CrossRef]
143. Motzer, R.J.; Rini, B.I.; McDermott, D.F.; Aren Frontera, O.; Hammers, H.J.; Carducci, M.A.; Salman, P.; Escudier, B.; Beuselinck, B.; Amin, A.; et al. Nivolumab plus ipilimumab versus sunitinib in first-line treatment for advanced renal cell carcinoma: Extended follow-up of efficacy and safety results from a randomised, controlled, phase 3 trial. *Lancet Oncol.* **2019**, *20*, 1370–1385. [CrossRef]
144. Motzer, R.J.; Escudier, B.; McDermott, D.F.; Aren Frontera, O.; Melichar, B.; Powles, T.; Donskov, F.; Plimack, E.R.; Barthelemy, P.; Hammers, H.J.; et al. Survival outcomes and independent response assessment with nivolumab plus ipilimumab versus sunitinib in patients with advanced renal cell carcinoma: 42-month follow-up of a randomized phase 3 clinical trial. *J. Immunother. Cancer* **2020**, *8*, e000891. [CrossRef] [PubMed]
145. Overman, M.J.; Lonardi, S.; Wong, K.Y.M.; Lenz, H.J.; Gelsomino, F.; Aglietta, M.; Morse, M.A.; Van Cutsem, E.; McDermott, R.; Hill, A.; et al. Durable Clinical Benefit With Nivolumab Plus Ipilimumab in DNA Mismatch Repair-Deficient/Microsatellite Instability-High Metastatic Colorectal Cancer. *J. Clin. Oncol. Off. J. Am. Soc. Clin. Oncol.* **2018**, *36*, 773–779. [CrossRef] [PubMed]
146. Hellmann, M.D.; Paz-Ares, L.; Bernabe Caro, R.; Zurawski, B.; Kim, S.W.; Carcereny Costa, E.; Park, K.; Alexandru, A.; Lupinacci, L.; de la Mora Jimenez, E.; et al. Nivolumab plus Ipilimumab in Advanced Non-Small-Cell Lung Cancer. *N. Engl. J. Med.* **2019**, *381*, 2020–2031. [CrossRef] [PubMed]

147. El-Khoueiry, A.B.; Sangro, B.; Yau, T.; Crocenzi, T.S.; Kudo, M.; Hsu, C.; Kim, T.Y.; Choo, S.P.; Trojan, J.; Welling, T.H.R.; et al. Nivolumab in patients with advanced hepatocellular carcinoma (CheckMate 040): An open-label, non-comparative, phase 1/2 dose escalation and expansion trial. *Lancet* **2017**, *389*, 2492–2502. [CrossRef]
148. Baas, P.; Scherpereel, A.; Nowak, A.K.; Fujimoto, N.; Peters, S.; Tsao, A.S.; Mansfield, A.S.; Popat, S.; Jahan, T.; Antonia, S.; et al. First-line nivolumab plus ipilimumab in unresectable malignant pleural mesothelioma (CheckMate 743): A multicentre, randomised, open-label, phase 3 trial. *Lancet* **2021**, *397*, 375–386. [CrossRef]
149. Buchbinder, E.I.; Desai, A. CTLA-4 and PD-1 Pathways: Similarities, Differences, and Implications of Their Inhibition. *Am. J. Clin. Oncol.* **2016**, *39*, 98–106. [CrossRef] [PubMed]
150. Wei, S.C.; Duffy, C.R.; Allison, J.P. Fundamental Mechanisms of Immune Checkpoint Blockade Therapy. *Cancer Discov.* **2018**, *8*, 1069–1086. [CrossRef]
151. Martins, F.; Sofiya, L.; Sykiotis, G.P.; Lamine, F.; Maillard, M.; Fraga, M.; Shabafrouz, K.; Ribi, C.; Cairoli, A.; Guex-Crosier, Y.; et al. Adverse effects of immune-checkpoint inhibitors: Epidemiology, management and surveillance. *Nat. Rev. Clin. Oncol.* **2019**, *16*, 563–580. [CrossRef] [PubMed]
152. Wang, D.Y.; Salem, J.E.; Cohen, J.V.; Chandra, S.; Menzer, C.; Ye, F.; Zhao, S.; Das, S.; Beckermann, K.E.; Ha, L.; et al. Fatal Toxic Effects Associated With Immune Checkpoint Inhibitors: A Systematic Review and Meta-analysis. *JAMA Oncol.* **2018**, *4*, 1721–1728. [CrossRef]
153. Anderson, A.C.; Joller, N.; Kuchroo, V.K. Lag-3, Tim-3, and TIGIT: Co-inhibitory Receptors with Specialized Functions in Immune Regulation. *Immunity* **2016**, *44*, 989–1004. [CrossRef]
154. Rotte, A.; Jin, J.Y.; Lemaire, V. Mechanistic overview of immune checkpoints to support the rational design of their combinations in cancer immunotherapy. *Ann. Oncol. Off. J. Eur. Soc. Med. Oncol.* **2018**, *29*, 71–83. [CrossRef]
155. Andrews, L.P.; Marciscano, A.E.; Drake, C.G.; Vignali, D.A. LAG3 (CD223) as a cancer immunotherapy target. *Immunol. Rev.* **2017**, *276*, 80–96. [CrossRef]
156. Acharya, N.; Sabatos-Peyton, C.; Anderson, A.C. Tim-3 finds its place in the cancer immunotherapy landscape. *J. Immunother. Cancer* **2020**, *8*, e000911. [CrossRef]
157. Chauvin, J.M.; Zarour, H.M. TIGIT in cancer immunotherapy. *J. Immunother. Cancer* **2020**, *8*, e000957. [CrossRef]
158. Ascierto, P.A.B.P.; Bhatia, S.; Melero, I.; Nyakas, M.S.; Svane, I.-M.; Larkin, J.; Gomez-Roca, C.; Schadendorf, D.; Dummer, R.; Marabelle, A.; et al. Efficacy of BMS-986016, a monoclonal antibody that targets lymphocyte activation gene-3 (LAG-3), in combination with nivolumab in pts with melanoma who progressed during prior anti–PD-1/PD-L1 therapy (mel prior IO) in all-comer and biomarker-enriched populations. *Ann. Oncol.* **2017**, *28*, v611–v612. [CrossRef]
159. Wolf, Y.; Anderson, A.C.; Kuchroo, V.K. TIM3 comes of age as an inhibitory receptor. *Nat. Rev. Immunol.* **2020**, *20*, 173–185. [CrossRef]
160. Sanmamed, M.F.; Pastor, F.; Rodriguez, A.; Perez-Gracia, J.L.; Rodriguez-Ruiz, M.E.; Jure-Kunkel, M.; Melero, I. Agonists of Co-stimulation in Cancer Immunotherapy Directed Against CD137, OX40, GITR, CD27, CD28, and ICOS. *Semin. Oncol.* **2015**, *42*, 640–655. [CrossRef]
161. Redmond, W.L.; Linch, S.N.; Kasiewicz, M.J. Combined targeting of costimulatory (OX40) and coinhibitory (CTLA-4) pathways elicits potent effector T cells capable of driving robust antitumor immunity. *Cancer Immunol. Res.* **2014**, *2*, 142–153. [CrossRef]
162. Lai, C.; August, S.; Albibas, A.; Behar, R.; Cho, S.Y.; Polak, M.E.; Theaker, J.; MacLeod, A.S.; French, R.R.; Glennie, M.J.; et al. OX40+ Regulatory T Cells in Cutaneous Squamous Cell Carcinoma Suppress Effector T-Cell Responses and Associate with Metastatic Potential. *Clin. Cancer Res. Off. J. Am. Assoc. Cancer Res.* **2016**, *22*, 4236–4248. [CrossRef] [PubMed]
163. Gutierrez, M.; Moreno, V.; Heinhuis, K.M.; Olszanski, A.J.; Spreafico, A.; Ong, M.; Chu, Q.; Carvajal, R.D.; Trigo, J.; Ochoa de Olza, M.; et al. OX40 Agonist BMS-986178 Alone or in Combination With Nivolumab and/or Ipilimumab in Patients With Advanced Solid Tumors. *Clin. Cancer Res. Off. J. Am. Assoc. Cancer Res.* **2021**, *27*, 460–472. [CrossRef] [PubMed]
164. Emens, L.A.; Middleton, G. The interplay of immunotherapy and chemotherapy: Harnessing potential synergies. *Cancer Immunol. Res.* **2015**, *3*, 436–443. [CrossRef] [PubMed]
165. Paz-Ares, L.; Luft, A.; Vicente, D.; Tafreshi, A.; Gumus, M.; Mazieres, J.; Hermes, B.; Cay Senler, F.; Csoszi, T.; Fulop, A.; et al. Pembrolizumab plus Chemotherapy for Squamous Non-Small-Cell Lung Cancer. *N. Engl. J. Med.* **2018**, *379*, 2040–2051. [CrossRef]
166. Paz-Ares, L.; Ciuleanu, T.E.; Cobo, M.; Schenker, M.; Zurawski, B.; Menezes, J.; Richardet, E.; Bennouna, J.; Felip, E.; Juan-Vidal, O.; et al. First-line nivolumab plus ipilimumab combined with two cycles of chemotherapy in patients with non-small-cell lung cancer (CheckMate 9LA): An international, randomised, open-label, phase 3 trial. *Lancet Oncol.* **2021**, *22*, 198–211. [CrossRef]
167. Cortes, J.; Cescon, D.W.; Rugo, H.S.; Nowecki, Z.; Im, S.A.; Yusof, M.M.; Gallardo, C.; Lipatov, O.; Barrios, C.H.; Holgado, E.; et al. Pembrolizumab plus chemotherapy versus placebo plus chemotherapy for previously untreated locally recurrent inoperable or metastatic triple-negative breast cancer (KEYNOTE-355): A randomised, placebo-controlled, double-blind, phase 3 clinical trial. *Lancet* **2020**, *396*, 1817–1828. [CrossRef]
168. Burtness, B.; Harrington, K.J.; Greil, R.; Soulieres, D.; Tahara, M.; de Castro, G., Jr.; Psyrri, A.; Baste, N.; Neupane, P.; Bratland, A.; et al. Pembrolizumab alone or with chemotherapy versus cetuximab with chemotherapy for recurrent or metastatic squamous cell carcinoma of the head and neck (KEYNOTE-048): A randomised, open-label, phase 3 study. *Lancet* **2019**, *394*, 1915–1928. [CrossRef]
169. Wang, Y.; Deng, W.; Li, N.; Neri, S.; Sharma, A.; Jiang, W.; Lin, S.H. Combining Immunotherapy and Radiotherapy for Cancer Treatment: Current Challenges and Future Directions. *Front. Pharmacol.* **2018**, *9*, 185. [CrossRef]

170. Twyman-Saint Victor, C.; Rech, A.J.; Maity, A.; Rengan, R.; Pauken, K.E.; Stelekati, E.; Benci, J.L.; Xu, B.; Dada, H.; Odorizzi, P.M.; et al. Radiation and dual checkpoint blockade activate non-redundant immune mechanisms in cancer. *Nature* **2015**, *520*, 373–377. [CrossRef] [PubMed]
171. Dovedi, S.J.; Cheadle, E.J.; Popple, A.L.; Poon, E.; Morrow, M.; Stewart, R.; Yusko, E.C.; Sanders, C.M.; Vignali, M.; Emerson, R.O.; et al. Fractionated Radiation Therapy Stimulates Antitumor Immunity Mediated by Both Resident and Infiltrating Polyclonal T-cell Populations when Combined with PD-1 Blockade. *Clin. Cancer Res. Off. J. Am. Assoc. Cancer Res.* **2017**, *23*, 5514–5526. [CrossRef] [PubMed]
172. Yu, J.; Green, M.D.; Li, S.; Sun, Y.; Journey, S.N.; Choi, J.E.; Rizvi, S.M.; Qin, A.; Waninger, J.J.; Lang, X.; et al. Liver metastasis restrains immunotherapy efficacy via macrophage-mediated T cell elimination. *Nat. Med.* **2021**, *27*, 152–164. [CrossRef]
173. Vaidya, P.; Mehta, A.; Ragab, O.; Lin, S.; In, G.K. Concurrent radiation therapy with programmed cell death protein 1 inhibition leads to a complete response in advanced cutaneous squamous cell carcinoma. *JAAD Case Rep.* **2019**, *5*, 763–766. [CrossRef] [PubMed]
174. Ju, X.; Zhang, H.; Zhou, Z.; Wang, Q. Regulation of PD-L1 expression in cancer and clinical implications in immunotherapy. *Am. J. Cancer Res.* **2020**, *10*, 1–11.
175. Sullivan, R.J.; Hamid, O.; Gonzalez, R.; Infante, J.R.; Patel, M.R.; Hodi, F.S.; Lewis, K.D.; Tawbi, H.A.; Hernandez, G.; Wongchenko, M.J.; et al. Atezolizumab plus cobimetinib and vemurafenib in BRAF-mutated melanoma patients. *Nat. Med.* **2019**, *25*, 929–935. [CrossRef]
176. Gutzmer, R.; Stroyakovskiy, D.; Gogas, H.; Robert, C.; Lewis, K.; Protsenko, S.; Pereira, R.P.; Eigentler, T.; Rutkowski, P.; Demidov, L.; et al. Atezolizumab, vemurafenib, and cobimetinib as first-line treatment for unresectable advanced BRAF(V600) mutation-positive melanoma (IMspire150): Primary analysis of the randomised, double-blind, placebo-controlled, phase 3 trial. *Lancet* **2020**, *395*, 1835–1844. [CrossRef]
177. Canueto, J.; Cardenoso, E.; Garcia, J.L.; Santos-Briz, A.; Castellanos-Martin, A.; Fernandez-Lopez, E.; Blanco Gomez, A.; Perez-Losada, J.; Roman-Curto, C. Epidermal growth factor receptor expression is associated with poor outcome in cutaneous squamous cell carcinoma. *Br. J. Dermatol.* **2017**, *176*, 1279–1287. [CrossRef]
178. Shi, T.; Song, X.; Wang, Y.; Liu, F.; Wei, J. Combining Oncolytic Viruses With Cancer Immunotherapy: Establishing a New Generation of Cancer Treatment. *Front. Immunol.* **2020**, *11*, 683. [CrossRef]
179. Lawler, S.E.; Speranza, M.C.; Cho, C.F.; Chiocca, E.A. Oncolytic Viruses in Cancer Treatment: A Review. *JAMA Oncol.* **2017**, *3*, 841–849. [CrossRef] [PubMed]
180. Andtbacka, R.H.; Kaufman, H.L.; Collichio, F.; Amatruda, T.; Senzer, N.; Chesney, J.; Delman, K.A.; Spitler, L.E.; Puzanov, I.; Agarwala, S.S.; et al. Talimogene Laherparepvec Improves Durable Response Rate in Patients With Advanced Melanoma. *J. Clin. Oncol. Off. J. Am. Soc. Clin. Oncol.* **2015**, *33*, 2780–2788. [CrossRef]
181. Andtbacka, R.H.I.; Collichio, F.; Harrington, K.J.; Middleton, M.R.; Downey, G.; hrling, K.; Kaufman, H.L. Final analyses of OPTiM: A randomized phase III trial of talimogene laherparepvec versus granulocyte-macrophage colony-stimulating factor in unresectable stage III-IV melanoma. *J. Immunother. Cancer* **2019**, *7*, 145. [CrossRef] [PubMed]
182. Kaufman, H.L.; Kim, D.W.; DeRaffele, G.; Mitcham, J.; Coffin, R.S.; Kim-Schulze, S. Local and distant immunity induced by intralesional vaccination with an oncolytic herpes virus encoding GM-CSF in patients with stage IIIc and IV melanoma. *Ann. Surg. Oncol.* **2010**, *17*, 718–730. [CrossRef]
183. Chesney, J.; Puzanov, I.; Collichio, F.; Singh, P.; Milhem, M.M.; Glaspy, J.; Hamid, O.; Ross, M.; Friedlander, P.; Garbe, C.; et al. Randomized, Open-Label Phase II Study Evaluating the Efficacy and Safety of Talimogene Laherparepvec in Combination With Ipilimumab Versus Ipilimumab Alone in Patients With Advanced, Unresectable Melanoma. *J. Clin. Oncol. Off. J. Am. Soc. Clin. Oncol.* **2018**, *36*, 1658–1667. [CrossRef]
184. Chesney, J.; Puzanov, I.; Collichio, F.; Milhem, M.M.; Hauschild, A.; Chen, L.; Sharma, A.; Garbe, C.; Singh, P.; Mehnert, J.M. Patterns of response with talimogene laherparepvec in combination with ipilimumab or ipilimumab alone in metastatic unresectable melanoma. *Br. J. Cancer* **2019**, *121*, 417–420. [CrossRef]
185. Ribas, A.; Dummer, R.; Puzanov, I.; VanderWalde, A.; Andtbacka, R.H.I.; Michielin, O.; Olszanski, A.J.; Malvehy, J.; Cebon, J.; Fernandez, E.; et al. Oncolytic Virotherapy Promotes Intratumoral T Cell Infiltration and Improves Anti-PD-1 Immunotherapy. *Cell* **2018**, *174*, 1031–1032. [CrossRef] [PubMed]
186. Russell, L.; Peng, K.W.; Russell, S.J.; Diaz, R.M. Oncolytic Viruses: Priming Time for Cancer Immunotherapy. *BioDrugs Clin. Immunother. Biopharm. Gene Ther.* **2019**, *33*, 485–501. [CrossRef]
187. Hu, Z.; Ott, P.A.; Wu, C.J. Towards personalized, tumour-specific, therapeutic vaccines for cancer. *Nat. Reviews. Immunol.* **2018**, *18*, 168–182. [CrossRef]
188. Hollingsworth, R.E.; Jansen, K. Turning the corner on therapeutic cancer vaccines. *NPJ Vaccines* **2019**, *4*, 7. [CrossRef]
189. Sahin, U.; Tureci, O. Personalized vaccines for cancer immunotherapy. *Science* **2018**, *359*, 1355–1360. [CrossRef]
190. Mougel, A.; Terme, M.; Tanchot, C. Therapeutic Cancer Vaccine and Combinations With Antiangiogenic Therapies and Immune Checkpoint Blockade. *Front. Immunol.* **2019**, *10*, 467. [CrossRef]
191. Tanimoto, T.; Hori, A.; Kami, M. Sipuleucel-T immunotherapy for castration-resistant prostate cancer. *N. Engl. J. Med.* **2010**, *363*, 1966, author reply 1967–1968. [CrossRef] [PubMed]

192. Pol, J.G.; Acuna, S.A.; Yadollahi, B.; Tang, N.; Stephenson, K.B.; Atherton, M.J.; Hanwell, D.; El-Warrak, A.; Goldstein, A.; Moloo, B.; et al. Preclinical evaluation of a MAGE-A3 vaccination utilizing the oncolytic Maraba virus currently in first-in-human trials. *Oncoimmunology* **2019**, *8*, e1512329. [CrossRef] [PubMed]
193. Woods, D.M.; Sodre, A.L.; Villagra, A.; Sarnaik, A.; Sotomayor, E.M.; Weber, J. HDAC Inhibition Upregulates PD-1 Ligands in Melanoma and Augments Immunotherapy with PD-1 Blockade. *Cancer Immunol. Res.* **2015**, *3*, 1375–1385. [CrossRef] [PubMed]
194. Dunn, J.; Rao, S. Epigenetics and immunotherapy: The current state of play. *Mol. Immunol.* **2017**, *87*, 227–239. [CrossRef]
195. Knox, T.; Sahakian, E.; Banik, D.; Hadley, M.; Palmer, E.; Noonepalle, S.; Kim, J.; Powers, J.; Gracia-Hernandez, M.; Oliveira, V.; et al. Selective HDAC6 inhibitors improve anti-PD-1 immune checkpoint blockade therapy by decreasing the anti-inflammatory phenotype of macrophages and down-regulation of immunosuppressive proteins in tumor cells. *Sci. Rep.* **2019**, *9*, 6136. [CrossRef]
196. Banik, D.; Moufarrij, S.; Villagra, A. Immunoepigenetics Combination Therapies: An Overview of the Role of HDACs in Cancer Immunotherapy. *Int. J. Mol. Sci.* **2019**, *20*, 2241. [CrossRef] [PubMed]
197. Adams, S. Toll-like receptor agonists in cancer therapy. *Immunotherapy* **2009**, *1*, 949–964. [CrossRef]
198. Murciano-Goroff, Y.R.; Warner, A.B.; Wolchok, J.D. The future of cancer immunotherapy: Microenvironment-targeting combinations. *Cell Res.* **2020**, *30*, 507–519. [CrossRef] [PubMed]
199. Munn, D.H.; Mellor, A.L. Indoleamine 2,3 dioxygenase and metabolic control of immune responses. *Trends Immunol.* **2013**, *34*, 137–143. [CrossRef] [PubMed]
200. Trojaniello, C.; Vitale, M.G.; Scarpato, L.; Esposito, A.; Ascierto, P.A. Melanoma immunotherapy: Strategies to overcome pharmacological resistance. *Expert Rev. Anticancer. Ther.* **2020**, *20*, 289–304. [CrossRef] [PubMed]
201. Zhu, Y.; Knolhoff, B.L.; Meyer, M.A.; Nywening, T.M.; West, B.L.; Luo, J.; Wang-Gillam, A.; Goedegebuure, S.P.; Linehan, D.C.; DeNardo, D.G. CSF1/CSF1R blockade reprograms tumor-infiltrating macrophages and improves response to T-cell checkpoint immunotherapy in pancreatic cancer models. *Cancer Res.* **2014**, *74*, 5057–5069. [CrossRef] [PubMed]
202. Ceci, C.; Atzori, M.G.; Lacal, P.M.; Graziani, G. Targeting Tumor-Associated Macrophages to Increase the Efficacy of Immune Checkpoint Inhibitors: A Glimpse into Novel Therapeutic Approaches for Metastatic Melanoma. *Cancers* **2020**, *12*, 3401. [CrossRef] [PubMed]
203. Markiewski, M.M.; DeAngelis, R.A.; Benencia, F.; Ricklin-Lichtsteiner, S.K.; Koutoulaki, A.; Gerard, C.; Coukos, G.; Lambris, J.D. Modulation of the antitumor immune response by complement. *Nat. Immunol.* **2008**, *9*, 1225–1235. [CrossRef]
204. Sivan, A.; Corrales, L.; Hubert, N.; Williams, J.B.; Aquino-Michaels, K.; Earley, Z.M.; Benyamin, F.W.; Lei, Y.M.; Jabri, B.; Alegre, M.L.; et al. Commensal Bifidobacterium promotes antitumor immunity and facilitates anti-PD-L1 efficacy. *Science* **2015**, *350*, 1084–1089. [CrossRef]
205. Vetizou, M.; Pitt, J.M.; Daillere, R.; Lepage, P.; Waldschmitt, N.; Flament, C.; Rusakiewicz, S.; Routy, B.; Roberti, M.P.; Duong, C.P.; et al. Anticancer immunotherapy by CTLA-4 blockade relies on the gut microbiota. *Science* **2015**, *350*, 1079–1084. [CrossRef]
206. Dai, Z.; Zhang, J.; Wu, Q.; Fang, H.; Shi, C.; Li, Z.; Lin, C.; Tang, D.; Wang, D. Intestinal microbiota: A new force in cancer immunotherapy. *Cell Commun. Signal. CCS* **2020**, *18*, 90. [CrossRef] [PubMed]

cancers

Article

Cathepsin S Evokes PAR$_2$-Dependent Pain in Oral Squamous Cell Carcinoma Patients and Preclinical Mouse Models

Nguyen Huu Tu [1,†], Kenji Inoue [1,†], Elyssa Chen [1], Bethany M. Anderson [2], Caroline M. Sawicki [1], Nicole N. Scheff [1,3], Hung D. Tran [1], Dong H. Kim [1], Robel G. Alemu [1], Lei Yang [1], John C. Dolan [1], Cheng Z. Liu [4], Malvin N. Janal [5], Rocco Latorre [6], Dane D. Jensen [1,6], Nigel W. Bunnett [6,7], Laura E. Edgington-Mitchell [1,2,8,*,‡] and Brian L. Schmidt [1,7,*,‡]

1. Bluestone Center for Clinical Research, Department of Oral and Maxillofacial Surgery, New York University (NYU) College of Dentistry, New York, NY 10010, USA; n.h.tu@nyu.edu (N.H.T.); ki630@nyu.edu (K.I.); ec128@nyu.edu (E.C.); cs6135@nyu.edu (C.M.S.); nns18@pitt.edu (N.N.S.); hdt222@nyu.edu (H.D.T.); dhk422@nyu.edu (D.H.K.); rga283@nyu.edu (R.G.A.); ly2176@nyu.edu (L.Y.); jcd10@nyu.edu (J.C.D.); ddj3@nyu.edu (D.D.J.)
2. Department of Biochemistry and Pharmacology, Bio21 Institute, University of Melbourne, Parkville, VIC 3052, Australia; bethany@student.unimelb.edu.au
3. Hillman Cancer Research Center, Department of Neurobiology, University of Pittsburgh, Pittsburgh, PA 15232, USA
4. Pathology Department, New York University (NYU) Langone Health, New York, NY 10016, USA; cheng.liu@nyulangone.org
5. Department of Epidemiology and Health Promotion, New York University (NYU) College of Dentistry, New York, NY 10010, USA; mj62@nyu.edu
6. Department of Molecular Pathobiology, New York University (NYU) College of Dentistry, New York, NY 10010, USA; rl3423@nyu.edu (R.L.); nwb2@nyu.edu (N.W.B.)
7. Department of Neuroscience and Physiology, Neuroscience Institute, New York University (NYU) Langone Health, New York, NY 10016, USA
8. Drug Discovery Biology, Monash Institute of Pharmaceutical Sciences, Monash University, Parkville, VIC 3052, Australia
* Correspondence: laura.edgingtonmitchell@unimelb.edu.au (L.E.E.-M.); bls322@nyu.edu (B.L.S.)
† Equal contribution from first authors.
‡ Equal contribution from senior authors.

Simple Summary: Oral cancer is often deadly and severely painful. Because this form of cancer pain cannot be adequately treated with current medications including opiates, new treatment approaches are needed. Cathepsin S, a lysosomal cysteine protease may play a role in oral cancer pain through a protease-activated receptor-2 (PAR$_2$)-dependent mechanism. We undertook a series of experiments to define the role of cathepsin S in oral cancer pain. We compared cathepsin S activity in human oral cancer tumors versus patient-matched normal tissue; a human oral cancer cell line versus a benign dysplastic oral keratinocyte cell line; and in an orthotopic xenograft tongue cancer mouse model versus normal controls in mice. We localized cathepsin S in macrophages and carcinoma cells in human oral cancers. The injection of cathepsin S caused nociception in a mouse model while the injection of oral cancer cells in which the gene for cathepsin S is deleted generated less nociception. Our findings will lay the foundations for clinical trials of cathepsin S inhibitors for treating oral cancer pain.

Abstract: Oral squamous cell carcinoma (SCC) pain is more prevalent and severe than pain generated by any other form of cancer. We previously showed that protease-activated receptor-2 (PAR$_2$) contributes to oral SCC pain. Cathepsin S is a lysosomal cysteine protease released during injury and disease that can activate PAR$_2$. We report here a role for cathepsin S in PAR$_2$-dependent cancer pain. We report that cathepsin S was more active in human oral SCC than matched normal tissue, and in an orthotopic xenograft tongue cancer model than normal tongue. The multiplex immunolocalization of cathepsin S in human oral cancers suggests that carcinoma and macrophages generate cathepsin S in the oral cancer microenvironment. After cheek or paw injection, cathepsin S evoked nociception in wild-type mice but not in mice lacking PAR$_2$ in Na$_v$1.8-positive neurons (Par$_2$Na$_v$1.8), nor in mice treated with LY3000328 or an endogenous cathepsin S inhibitor (cystatin C). The human oral SCC cell line (HSC-3) with homozygous deletion of the gene for cathepsin S (*CTSS*) with CRISPR/Cas9 provoked significantly less mechanical allodynia and thermal hyperalgesia, as did those treated with LY3000328, compared to the control cancer mice. Our results indicate that cathepsin S is activated in oral SCC, and that cathepsin S contributes to cancer pain through PAR_2 on neurons.

Keywords: oral cancer; pain; cathepsin S; protease-activated receptor-2; PAR_2; cancer pain; oral squamous cell carcinoma

1. Introduction

Cathepsin S is a lysosomal cysteine protease that degrades proteins along the endocytic pathway, including the invariant chain necessary for MHC class II antigen processing and presentation [1]. Of the 11 human cathepsins, most require an acidic environment, such as the interior of lysosomes, to be active. Cathepsin S is distinct because it is active at a wide pH range of 4.5–8.0 [2]. Because of the capacity of cathepsin S to function at a neutral pH, it is active in the extracellular environment, where it degrades extracellular matrix proteins. The dysregulated expression and activity of proteases contributes to pathologic conditions including inflammation, pain and cancer. For most proteases, inhibition as a therapy is limited by the wide tissue expression of proteases and resultant side effects; for this reason, treatment with matrix metalloproteinase inhibitors is highly limited [3]. Cathepsin S, on the other hand, has limited tissue expression, primarily in antigen presenting cells in the lymph and spleen [4,5]. Thus, cathepsin S is an attractive target, and cathepsin S inhibitors have been tested in clinical trials (NCT 00425321, 01515358); the inhibitors exhibit good safety profiles [6].

Human cancers, including prostate, gastrointestinal (gastric, colorectal), lung, and brain tumors (astrocytoma, glioblastoma) upregulate cathepsin S [7–9]. Microdialysis, an extracellular fluid sampling approach originally designed to collect neurotransmitters, confirmed that cathepsin S was present in the extracellular space of brain tumors [10]. In the setting of cancer, both tumor cells and tumor-associated macrophages produce cathepsin S [11]. Cathepsin S contributes to several hallmarks of cancer including proliferation, angiogenesis, invasion and metastasis [8,12–14]. Mice in which the SV40 T antigen (Tag) transgene is controlled and driven by the rat insulin II promoter (RIP1-Tag2) spontaneously develop pancreatic beta-cell islet carcinoma. This mouse model was crossed with a cathepsin S null mouse, and cathepsin S was shown to regulate invasion and angiogenesis [11,15]. In a separate study, the combined depletion of cathepsin S in the cancer and macrophages was required to reduce the metastasis of breast cancer to the brain [16]. More recently, cathepsin S has been shown to mediate autophagy and apoptosis in human oral cancer cell lines through p38 MAPK/JNK signaling pathways [17].

In addition to carcinogenesis, cathepsin S produces pain. Cathepsin S cleaves protease-activated receptor-2 (PAR_2), a G protein-coupled receptor (GPCR) expressed on peripheral nociceptors that mediates neurogenic inflammation and pain [18]. Peripheral nerve injury leads to cathepsin S upregulation and secretion from microglia. The cathepsin S inhibitor—morpholinurea-leucine-homophenylalanine-vinyl phenyl sulfone (LHVS)—reverses neuropathic pain [19]. Although the role of cathepsin S in carcinogenesis and pain has been studied, the question of whether cathepsin S contributes to cancer pain has not been answered. We hypothesized that cathepsin S released by oral cancer and/or associated macrophages in the oral cancer microenvironment generates cancer pain through the activation of PAR_2. To test our hypothesis, we measured cathepsin S expression and activity in human and mouse oral cancers, immunolocalized cathepsin S in cancer cells and macrophages in human oral cancers, and used a series of mouse models, including a model in which the gene for PAR_2 is selectively deleted on sensory neurons, to test whether cathepsin S mediated oral cancer pain.

2. Materials and Methods

2.1. Oral SCC Patients

Patients were screened and enrolled through the NYU Oral Cancer Center after consent was obtained. Detailed demographic information (age, sex, ethnicity, cancer location, primary tumor stage, and evidence of metastasis) was collected. Self-reported oral cancer pain was measured with the University of California Oral Cancer Pain Questionnaire prior to surgery. The instrument consists of 8 questions; question 7 addresses mechanical sensitivity [20,21]. The questionnaire uses a visual analog scale for each question, which ranges from 0 to 100. During surgical resection, tumor and matched normal oral mucosa specimens were collected (normal was harvested at an anatomically matched contralateral site). Specimens were frozen in liquid nitrogen and maintained at −80 °C. For one patient with tongue cancer, a portion of the lingual nerve innervating the side of the tongue affected by cancer was harvested as part of the resection specimen. In the same patient, the contralateral lingual nerve innervating the unaffected tongue was harvested. The lingual nerves were immersed in 10% neutral buffered saline for 24 h at 4 °C. The nerves were then washed 3 times with PBS and kept in 70% ethanol. The nerves were embedded in paraffin and sectioned at 5 μm. The Committee on Human Research at NYU Langone Medical Center approved human studies (10-01261, 15 September 2020).

2.2. Mice

Female and male wild-type (WT) C57BL/6J (stock number 000664) and NU/J $Foxn1^{nu}$ athymic (stock number 002019), which were four to eight weeks old, were obtained from The Jackson Laboratory at Bar Harbor, ME. To delete Par_2 in peripheral neurons, $F2rl1$ conditional knock-out (KO) C57BL/6 mice generated by genOway in Lyon, France, as described in [22], were crossed with mice expressing Cre recombinase under the control of the $Scn10a$ gene promoter (B6.129-Scn10a$^{tm2(cre)Jnw}$/H [23]. The animals were kept and bred in specific-pathogen-free rooms in the Animal Center of NYU College of Dentistry under the following conditions: a 12 h/12 h light/dark cycle, constant temperature of 22 ± 2 °C and 60 ± 10% humidity. They received food and water ad libitum. The NYU Institutional Animal Care and Use Committee approved our studies in mice.

2.3. Tongue Xenograft Cancer Model

We generated the orthotopic xenograft tongue cancer model on the NU/J $Foxn1^{nu}$ athymic mice of 4 to 6 weeks old by injecting 1×10^5 HSC-3 (human tongue oral SCC cell line, cell number JCRB0623, from the Japanese Collection of Research Bioresources Cell Bank) into the tongue. The HSC-3 cells were suspended in 20 μL vehicle (1:1 mixture of DMEM and Matrigel; Corning, Ref. #354234). The mice were anesthetized by 1% isoflurane in 1 L per minute medical oxygen during the injection. Two weeks after inoculation, xenografted tongues were collected and snap frozen for protein analysis.

2.4. Analysis of Total and Active Cathepsin S in Human Oral Cancer and Mouse Oral Cancer Tissues

Snap frozen human and murine tissues were sonicated in PBS, pH 7.4 (10 μL/mg tissue). Solids were cleared by centrifugation and protein concentration was measured by the BCA assay (Pierce). Protein was diluted in PBS (50 μg/20 μL buffer), and the cathepsin S-selective activity-based probe, BMV157, was added from a 100× DMSO stock (1 μM final) [24]. Samples were incubated at 37 °C for 30 min and the reaction was quenched with 5× sample buffer (200 mM Tris-Cl [pH 6.8], 8% SDS, 0.04% bromophenol blue, 5% β-mercaptoethanol, and 40% glycerol). Protein was resolved on a 15% polyacrylamide gel under reducing conditions. BMV157 binding was detected by scanning the gel for Cy5 fluorescence using a Typhoon 5 (GE Healthcare, Chicago, IL, USA). Proteins were transferred to nitrocellulose membranes for immunoblotting. The following antibodies were diluted in 50% LI-COR blocking buffer and 50% PBS-T containing 0.05% Tween-20: goat anti-human cathepsin S antibody (1:500, AF1183, lot # ICO0818121, R&D, Minneapolis,

MN, USA); donkey-anti goat-HRP (1:10,000, A15999, Invitrogen, Waltham, MA, USA). Clarity Western ECL Substrate (Bio-Rad, CA, USA) was used for detection.

2.5. Quantification of Cathepsin S Activity in Oral SCC Cells and Dysplastic Oral Keratinocytes

HSC-3 or DOK cells were seeded in 6-well plates and switched to serum-free medium when 80% confluency was reached. After 17 h, cells were live labeled with the cathepsin S-selective probe BMV157 or the pan cathepsin S probe BMV109 (1 µM, 0.1% DMSO) for 7 h [25,26]. Cells were washed with PBS, lysed on ice in PBS containing 0.1% Triton X-100. Solids were cleared by centrifugation and proteins were solubilized in sample buffer. Total protein (~60 µg) was resolved by SDS-PAGE. Gels were scanned for Cy5 fluorescence and proteins were transferred to nitrocellulose membranes for cathepsin S immunoblotting as described above. The rabbit anti-actin antibody (1:10,000, A5060, lot #068M4870V, Sigma Aldrich, St. Louis, MO, USA) was detected with goat anti-Rabbit-IRDye 800CW (1:10,000, 926-32211, LI-COR) on the Typhoon 5.

2.6. Multiplex Immunostaining of Human Oral SCC Tissue and Adjacent Normal Mucosa

Five-micron paraffin-embedded human oral SCC tongue or adjacent normal sections were stained either with H&E or with Akoya Biosciences® Opal™ multiplex automation kit reagents on a Leica BondRX® autostainer, according to manufacturers' instructions. All slides underwent sequential epitope retrieval with either Leica Biosystems epitope retrieval 1 (ER1, citrate based, pH 6.0, Cat. AR9961) or epitope retrieval 2 solution (ER2, EDTA based, pH 9.0, Cat. AR9640), primary and secondary antibody incubation and tyramide signal amplification (TSA) with Opal® fluorophores Op480, Op570 and Op690. The primary antibodies against human cathepsin S (1:100, Cat # SC-74429, Santa Cruz, Dallas, TX, USA), CD68 (1:100, Cat # GA609, Agilent, Santa Clara, CA, USA) and CK5 (1:1200 dilution, Cat # PRB-160P, Biolegend, San Diego, CA, USA), and the horse radish peroxidase-coupled secondary antibodies (Cat # ARH1001, Akoya HRP Polymer) were removed during sequential heat retrieval steps while fluorophores remained covalently attached to the epitope. ER1 was used for 60 min for the epitope retrieval of the antibody against human cathepsin S. For antibodies against CD68 and CK5, epitope retrieval was performed with ER2 for 20 min. Sections were counter-stained with DAPI. Semi-automated whole slide scanning was performed on a Vectra® Polaris multispectral imaging system and the images were visualized with Akoya Phenochart software.

2.7. Measurement of F2RL1 mRNA, with RNAscope®, in Human Tongue Cancer and Contralateral Normal Tongue in the Same Patient

RNAScope® chromogenic in situ hybridization (Advanced Cell Diagnostics by Bio-Techne, MN, USA) was performed according to the manufacturer's pretreatment protocol for fresh-frozen tissue. Samples were hybridized with RNAscope® probe Hs-*F2RL1* and signals were visualized by RNAscope® 2.5 HD Assay RED and counterstained with hematoxylin. All the slides were scanned at the maximum available magnification and stored as digital high-resolution images. Chromogenic dots were quantified with NIH ImageJ software. Five randomly chosen fields at 40× magnification were counted by a blinded investigator.

2.8. Measurement of PAR_2 Protein, with Immunohistochemistry, in the Human Lingual Nerve Innervating Tongue Cancer, Compared to the Lingual Nerve Innervating Contralateral, Unaffected Tongue

After deparaffinization, we performed antigen retrieval with sodium citrate buffer at pH 6, 82 °C for 20 min. The samples were kept at room temperature for 30 min and then washed three times with PBS. The samples were treated with 0.1% Triton X-100 in PBS for 5 min, followed by a blocking step with 3% bovine serum albumin (BSA) in PBS for 1 h at room temperature. The rabbit anti-PGP9.5 antibody (concentration 2 µg/mL, PB9840, Boster Biological Technology,) and mouse anti-PAR_2 antibody (1:50 in 3% BSA in PBS, SAM11, sc-13504, Santa Cruz Biotechnology) were applied to the sections overnight at 4 °C. The samples were washed 3 times with PBS. The sections were then treated with secondary antibodies, which included goat anti-rabbit 594, (1:300 in 3% BSA in PBS, A32740, Invitrogen), and goat anti-mouse 488 (1:300 in 3% BSA in PBS, A11029, Invitrogen) for 2.5 h at room temperature. The sections were washed three times with PBS, treated with Prolong™ Diamond Antifade Mountant (P36965, Invitrogen) and coverslips were applied. Images were captured with a laser confocal microscope Carl Zeiss LSM 700 within 3 days after staining. For the negative control staining of PAR$_2$, we performed immunohistochemical staining on HSC-3 cancer cells in which *F2RL1* was deleted with CRISPR/Cas9. Deletion of *F2RL1* resulted in the lack of PAR$_2$ signal. PAR$_2$ signal intensity was quantified in the lingual nerve innervating the tongue cancer (n = 300 axons), and the lingual nerve innervating contralateral normal tongue (n = 275 axons) with NIH ImageJ software by a blinded investigator.

2.9. FLAG Imaging

HEK-FLAG-PAR$_2$ cells have previously been characterized [27]. HEK-FLAG-PAR$_2$ cells were plated on poly-D-lysine-coated 12 mm glass coverslips and treated as described previously [27]. Cells were exposed to HSC-3 supernatant and fixed with 4% paraformaldehyde. Cells were washed with PBS two times and blocked with PBS + 0.3% saponin + 3% NHS for 1 h at room temperature. Cells were incubated with mouse anti-FLAG (1:500, #8146, Cell Signaling) overnight at 4 °C. Cells were washed three times in PBS and incubated with donkey anti-mouse Alexa 488 (1:1000, A32766, Thermo Fisher Scientific) for 1 h at room temperature. Cells were incubated with DAPI for 5 min (1 µM) in saline, washed 4x with PBS, and mounted with the ProLong Glass hard-set mounting medium (Thermo Fisher Scientific, Waltham, MA, USA). Cells were imaged in a Leica SP8 laser scanning confocal microscope. Micrographs were processed using ImageJ and Adobe Illustrator.

2.10. On-Cell Westerns Assay

FLAG-PAR$_2$ cells were plated on poly-D-lysine-coated 96-well plates (30,000 cells/well) incubated for 48 h. HSC-3 supernatant was thawed and warmed to 37 °C and was pretreated for 30 min with either vehicle (DMSO), LY3000328 (1 µM) or cystatin C (1 µM) for 30 min. Cells were washed two times in HBSS (pH 7.4) and incubated with 100 µL of either $CTSS^{+/+}$ HSC-3 supernatant, $CTSS^{-/-}$ HSC-3 supernatant, trypsin (10 nM), cathepsin S (100 nM), or HSC-3 supernatant pretreated with either LY3000328 or cystatin C. Cells were incubated for 30 min at 37 °C, washed 1× in HBSS and fixed with 4% paraformaldehyde in PBS for 20 min on ice. Cells were washed two times in PBS and incubated with blocking buffer (PBS + 3% normal horse serum, NHS, Cat. # 31874 Thermo Fisher Scientific Waltham, MA, USA) for 1 h at room temperature. Cells were incubated with mouse anti-FLAG antibody (1:500, Cell Signaling, Boston, MA, USA) in PBS + 1% NHS overnight at 4° C. Cells were washed two times in PBS and incubated with donkey anti-mouse Alexa 790 (1:1000, A11371, Thermo Fisher) in PBS + 1% NHS for 1 h at room temperature. Cells were washed in PBS and incubated with SYTO™ 82 Orange (1 µM, Thermo Fisher) in saline for 30 min. Cells were washed two times in PBS and imaged on an Amersham Typhoon imaging system (GE, Pittsburg, PA, USA). FLAG immunofluorescent labeling was quantified using ImageJ and was normalized to the nuclear fluorescent intensity to correct for cell loss.

2.11. Transfection and Clonal Isolation

HSC-3 cells plated in a 6-well plate at a density of 2×10^5 cells per 3 mL of DMEM supplemented with 10% fetal bovine serum (FBS) were incubated for 24 h. To generate *CTSS* knockout cells, 1 µg of *CTSS* CRISPR/Cas9 KO plasmid (cat# sc-417407, Santa Cruz Biotechnologies, Dallas, TX, USA), 1 µg of *CTSS* HDR plasmid (cat# sc-41407-HDR, Santa Cruz Biotechnology) and modified Tat (1 mM) were combined in a 5% glucose solution with a final volume of 60 µL/well. The solution was mixed for 5 s. After the mixture was incubated at room temperature for 30 min, the cap of the sample tube was removed to expose the solution to the air. The sample was then vigorously shaken for 90 min. Eight µL of FuGENE HD transfection reagent (cat# E2311, Promega, Madison, WI, USA) was added and then the solution was incubated at room temperature for 15 min. Sixty µL complexes (containing 2 µg DNA and FuGENE) were placed in the wells of a 6-well plate. The plate was gently mixed and incubated for 48 h. Following incubation, the medium was replaced with RPMI complete medium with 500 ng/mL puromycin dihydrochloride (Santa Cruz Biotechnology) every 2 days to eliminate wild-type puromycin-sensitive cells. After puromycin selection, single-cell clones were isolated by limiting dilution into 96-well plates. Clones were expanded and transferred to larger plates as the individual clones reached confluence. Clones were genotyped by RT-PCR. Finally, cathepsin S expression was determined by ELISA assay. For controls, 1 µg of control CRISPR/Cas9 plasmid (cat# sc-4148922, Santa Cruz Biotechnology) was used.

2.12. RT-PCR

For reverse-transcription polymerase chain reaction (RT-PCR), total RNA was isolated using TRIzol reagent (Invitrogen). RNA concentration was measured by NanoDrop ND-1000 Spectrophotometer (NanoDrop Technologies, Wilmington, DE, USA) and cDNA was synthesized from a total of 1 µg RNA using QuantiTect® Quantiscript reverse-transcriptase and RT Primer Mix (Qiagen, Hilden, Germany), according to the manufacturer's protocol. RT-PCR was performed using Taq PCR Master Mix Kit (Qiagen), according to standard protocols. The sequence of beta actin (*ACTB*) and cathepsin S (*CTSS*) gene-specific primers were as follows: *ACTB* (5′-CATGTACGTTGCTATCCAGGC-3′(sense) and 5′- CTCCTTAATGTCACGCACGAT-3′(antisense); product size 250bp) and *CTSS* (5′- TGACAACGGCTTTCCAGTACA-3′(sense), 5′- GGCAGCACGATATTTTGAGTCAT-3′(antisense)]; product size 113 bp). PCR products were analyzed with 1% agarose gel electrophoresis.

2.13. Cathepsin S Quantification by ELISA

HSC-3 or OSC-20 cells were plated in a 12-well plate (2×10^5 cells/well) and were incubated for 24 h. Medium was removed, cells were washed with 3 mL PBS without Ca^{2+} and Mg^{2+}, and DMEM (500 µL) was added to each well. After 48 h, the medium was collected and centrifuged (1000 rpm, 5 min, 4 °C). The pellet was discarded. Total cellular protein was collected from HSC-3 and OSC-20 cell lines (cell number JCRB0197, was from Japanese Collection of Research Bioresources Cell Bank) using standard RIPA lysis buffer (500 µL/well). Cathepsin S concentration was quantified by enzyme-linked immunosorbent assay (ELISA) for human cathepsin S (Cat#: ab155427, Abcam, Cambridge, UK). A standard curve was constructed before each experiment. Protein samples were diluted in dilution buffer and 100 µL was added to each well. The plate was incubated overnight at 4 °C and washed four times with washing solution. The diluted biotinylated anti-human cathepsin S antibody (100 µL) was added to each well and incubated for 1 h at room temperature. Following the washing steps, 100 µL of 1× HRP–streptavidin solution was added to each well and the plate was kept in a dark environment at room temperature for 45 min. After incubation, the plate was washed and TMB substrate reagent (Cat#: ab210902, Abcam) was added to each well. Finally, the reaction was stopped by the addition of 50 µL of stop solution. The absorbance was read at 450 nm in a microtiter plate reader immediately. The absorbance was measured using a 450 nm filter on GloMax®-Multi Microplate Multimode Reader (Promega).

2.14. Facial Mechanical Nociception

The rat facial mechanical nociception assay was modified for mice [27,28]. Two weeks prior to the assay, mice were acclimated for 1 h in the testing room every other day. In ascending order, von Frey filaments ranging from 0.008 to 4 g force (11 filaments in total) were used to measure withdrawal responses to mechanical stimulation of the left cheek. Each fiber was applied once to the cheek, defined by the area between the nose and the ear, below the eye. If the mouse was moving or the response was unclear to the researcher, the same von Frey filament was reapplied to the same area of the cheek 10 s after the first stimulus or until the mouse stopped moving. A 5 min interval was set between the applications of von Frey filaments of different intensities. The facial nociception score was reported as a numerical average of the 11 responses in the response categories as we reported [22]. In some experiments, gavage treatment of LY3000328 (cathepsin S inhibitor) or the subcutaneous injection of cystatin C (endogenous cathepsin inhibitor) into the cheek was administered for 2 or 1 h, respectively, before the facial mechanical nociception assay under 1% isoflurane in 1 L per minute medical oxygen.

2.15. Paw Xenograft Cancer Model

The paw xenograft cancer model permits the measurement of mechanical and thermal nociception in the paw. Baseline mechanical and thermal withdrawal thresholds were measured prior to tumor cell inoculation. The left hind paw of NU/J $Foxn1^{nu}$ athymic mice of 4 to 6 weeks old was injected with 1×10^5 HSC-3 in 20 µL of DMEM and matrigel (1:1) [29,30]. Mechanical and thermal nociception assays were conducted at post inoculation weeks 1, 2, 3 and 4. In some experiments, on post inoculation week 4, LY3000328 (cathepsin S inhibitor, 30 mg·kg^{-1}, 100 µL) was administered by oral gavage. Mechanical and thermal nociception assays were performed at 1, 3, 6, 12, and 24 h after LY3000328 treatment. At the end of the experiments, the cancer paw was collected and processed for histological hematoxylin and eosin (H&E) staining to confirm viable carcinoma.

2.16. Mechanical and Thermal Nociception in the Hind Paw

To assess mechanical nociception, mice were placed on a platform with a metal mesh floor and acclimated for 1 h. The paw withdrawal threshold was measured with von Frey filaments (Stoelting, Wood Dale, IL, USA) according to the up–down method for rats published by Chaplan et al. in 1994 with modifications for mice [31,32]. The withdrawal threshold was defined as the gram-force sufficient to elicit left hindpaw withdrawal. A positive response was recorded if the mice showed one of the following reactions: 1—quick paw withdrawal; 2—immediate flinch when the tip of the von Frey filament is removed; 3—digit extension; 4—paw lift and licking of the paw; 5—repeated flapping of the paw to the mesh; or 6—attempt to run to escape from the stimulation. In some tests, the withdrawal threshold for each animal was determined as the mean of 3 trials for each animal. The interval between two trials was 10 s. The cut-off value was 4 g to prevent the paw from mechanical injury.

To assess thermal nociception in the paw, we used a thermal stimulator (IITC Life Sciences, Woodland Hills, CA, USA) [33]. Two weeks before the assay was performed, the mice were acclimated to the stimulator for one hour every other day. Mice were placed individually in a plastic chamber on a 25 °C glass surface. A radiant heat source was focused on the left hind paw and withdrawal latency was measured in seconds from the time the heat source started to project into the paw until the time the mice withdrew its paw. The outcome variable was the mean of 3 trials undertaken at intervals of 5 or more minutes. A 20 s cut-off latency was established to prevent heat injury of the paw.

2.17. Cancer Paw Volume Measurement

The paw xenograft model permits the measurement of cancer paw volume at the time of behavioral assessment. Prior to cancer cell inoculation and at 1, 2, 3 and 4 weeks after inoculation, a plethysmometer (cat #. II-520MR, World Precision Instruments, Sarasota, FL, USA) was used to measure the volume of cancer paw in anesthetized mice. Volumes were measured 3 times and reported as the mean.

2.18. Histologic Determination of the Area of Cancer in the Paw

Four weeks after the inoculation of cancer cells into the paw, the cancer paw was collected. The paw was defined as the area from the tip of the digits to the ankle crease.

The paw was longitudinally sectioned through the thickest area of the tumor, which generated 2 cut surfaces within the largest area of cancer. The paw was then immersed in 10% neutral buffer formalin (NBF) for 48 h at 4 °C. NBF was then replaced with 10% ethylenediaminetetraacetic acid (EDTA) for paw decalcification. The EDTA solution was changed every 2 days for 14 days and then replaced with 70% Et-OH for 3 days prior to paraffin embedding. One section was made on each cut surface of the cancer paw for H&E histological staining. The H&E image was scanned on a Hamamatsu Nanozoomer. The area of cancer was determined as the average area from the 2 sections as quantified by the NIH ImageJ® software. Two independent researchers quantified the area of cancer and the average was recorded.

2.19. Statistics

GraphPad Prism 7 and 8 (GraphPad Software, Inc., San Diego, CA, USA) was used for the statistical analysis. Results were expressed as mean ± standard error (SEM). For cell-based assays, triplicate measurements were made; differences were evaluated by one- or two-way repeated measures ANOVA and Dunnett's or Tukey's multiple comparisons test. One-way ANOVA and Tukey's or Sidak's multiple comparisons and Student's t-test were used for in vivo behavioral experiments. An independent samples Student's t-test was used to compare values between 2 groups. The relationship between participant pain scores, as measured by the University of California San Francisco Oral Cancer Pain Questionnaire, and cathepsin S activity was analyzed using Spearman correlation.

3. Results

3.1. Cathepsin S Activity and Expression in Human Oral Cancers

To determine whether cathepsin S is activated in oral SCCs, we collected oral SCC specimens and matched normal oral mucosa from seven patients (Table 1). Specimens were incubated with a fluorescently quenched activity-based probe (BMV157) selective for cathepsin S. A BMV157-labeled species of 25 kDa was activated in oral SCC versus normal tissue (Figure 1a). Oral SCC showed increased expression and activity of cathepsin S relative to matched normal tissue in all patients (Figure 1b–e). All participants reported pain. Self-reported mechanical sensitivity tended to increase with cathepsin S activity in the tumor (r_s = 0.78, p = 0.041).

Table 1. Demographic, anatomic location and tumor staging for patients for which cathepsin S activity was measured in oral SCC and matched normal tissue. Reported pain, as measured by question 7 of the University of California San Francisco Oral Cancer Pain Questionnaire, is provided for each patient.

Patient #	Sex	Age	Ethnicity	Tumor Location	Primary Tumor Stage	Nodal Status	Reported Pain (0–100)
1	F	71	Hispanic	Mandibular gingiva	pT4a	pN0	86
2	M	57	Hispanic	Mandibular gingiva	pT2	pN2a	92
3	M	66	Hispanic	Floor of mouth, Mandibular gingiva	pT4a	pN0	95
4	F	77	White/Non-Hispanic	Mandibular gingiva	pT4a	pN0	86
5	F	50	Asian	Tongue	pT1	pN0	10
6	M	93	Asian	Mandibular gingiva	pT2	pN0	5
7	F	81	White/Non-Hispanic	Maxillary gingiva	pT2	pN0	74

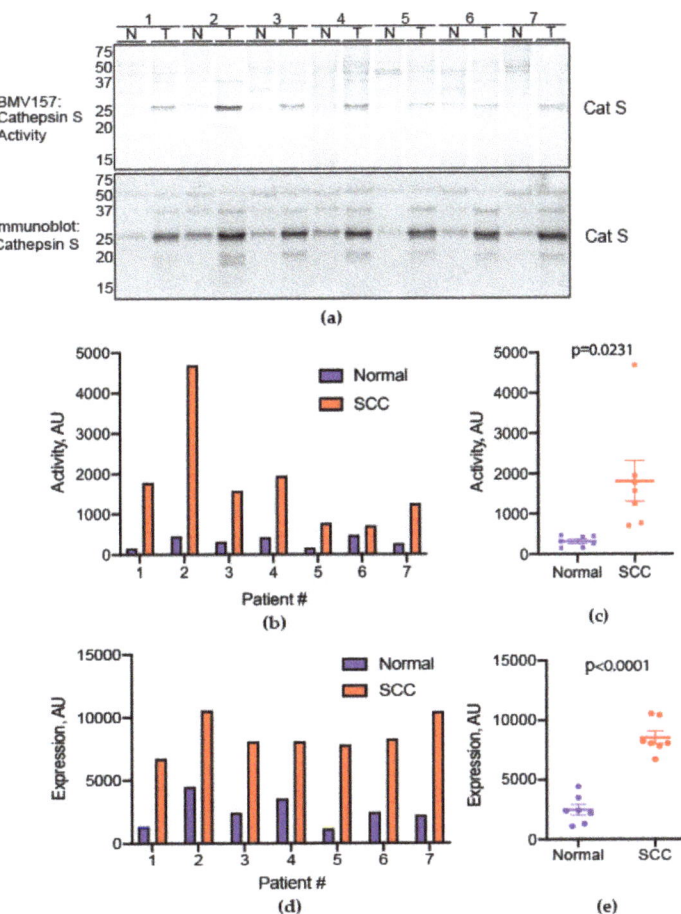

Figure 1. Cathepsin S activity is increased in human oral cancer compared to match normal tissue. (a) Active cathepsin S labeled by BMV157 (upper panel) as shown by in-gel fluorescence and total cathepsin S immunoreactivity (lower panel) in oral SCC biopsies (T) and patient-matched normal oral mucosa (N). The gel (upper panel) was transferred to nitrocellulose and immunoblotted for total cathepsin S levels (lower panel). The uncropped western blot figure is presented in Figure S1. (b) Densitometry of the 25 kDa species labeled by BMV157, displayed as individual values for all normal and oral SCC samples. (c) Average cathepsin S activity was higher in oral SCC samples (independent samples Student's t-test). (d) Densitometry of the 25 kDa species labeled by BMV157, displayed as individual values for all normal and oral SCC samples. (e) Average total cathepsin S levels were higher in oral SCC samples (independent samples Student's t-test).

We used multiplex immunostaining to localize cathepsin S in human oral SCC patients (Table 2). Adjacent normal tissue in one of the oral SCC patients (Table 2, Patient A) served as the control. Cathepsin S was expressed in CD68[+] macrophages in human oral SCC tissue (Figure 2). Cathepsin-S expression was extremely low in an adjacent normal tissue section from an oral SCC patient (Figure 2). In separate tissue sections from the same patients (Table 2), cathepsin S was identified within keratin-positive cells (CK5[+]) indicating that cathepsin S was expressed by both tumor cells and macrophages within the oral SCC microenvironment (Figure 3).

Table 2. Localization of cathepsin S in human oral cancer tissue.

Patient #	Sex	Age	Ethnicity	Tumor Location	Primary Tumor Stage	Nodal Status
A *	F	56	White/Not Hispanic	Tongue	pT4a	pN3b
B	F	75	White/Not Hispanic	Tongue	pT2	pN0
C	M	38	White/Not Hispanic	Tongue	pT2	pN0
D	F	66	White/Not Hispanic	Tongue	pT3	pN1

* The tissue evaluated for patient A includes normal mucosa adjacent to the oral SCC.

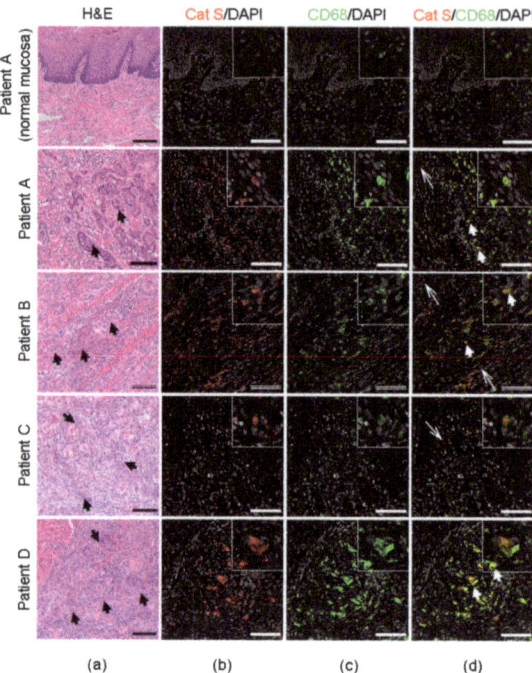

Figure 2. Localization of cathepsin S expression in macrophages associated with human oral cancers. (**a**) H&E staining of tongue tissue from four patients with tongue oral SCC, and adjacent normal tongue tissue section from one of the patients with oral SCC (Patient A) (Table 2). Black arrows in H&E sections indicate SCC. (**b**) Co-immunofluorescent staining of cathepsin S (Cat S, red) and DAPI (gray); (**c**) CD68$^+$ macrophages (green) and DAPI (gray); (**d**) Cat S (red), CD68$^+$ macrophages (green) and DAPI (gray). White thick arrows indicate cathepsin S in CD68$^+$ macrophages; white thin arrows indicate cathepsin S in cancer microenvironment, but not in macrophages. Scale bars, 100 µm.

3.2. F2RL1 mRNA in Human Tongue Cancer Compared to Contralateral Normal Tongue, and PAR$_2$ Protein Expression in the Lingual Nerve Innervating the Tongue Cancer Compared to the Lingual Nerve Innervating the Contralateral Unaffected Tongue

We measured *F2RL1* mRNA, with RNAscope® in situ hybridization, in a human tongue cancer and compared it to contralateral unaffected tongue in the same patient (i.e., matched) (Figure 4a,b). The level of *F2RL1* mRNA was five times higher in the tongue cancer than in the matched tongue tissue (3.0 ± 0.4 in cancer tongue versus 0.6 ± 0.2 in normal tongue, Figure 4b). We measured PAR$_2$ protein, with immunohistochemistry, in the lingual nerve innervating the tongue cancer (Figure 4d) and compared it to the lingual nerve innervating the contralateral unaffected tongue (Figure 4c). PAR$_2$ protein was significantly higher in the lingual nerve innervating the tongue cancer than in the lingual nerve innervating the contralateral tongue (Figure 4e).

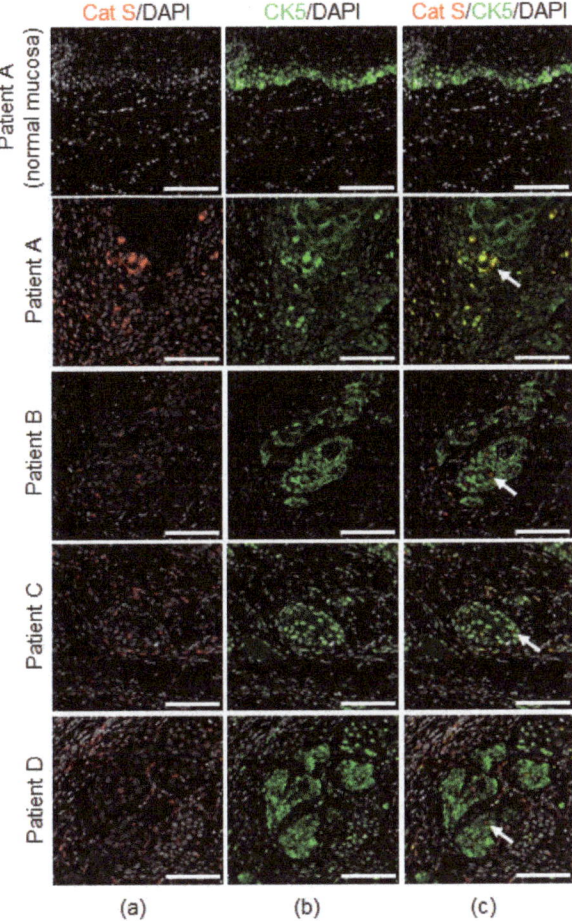

Figure 3. Localization of cathepsin S expression in human oral cancer cells. The immunofluorescent staining of four patients with oral SCC, and adjacent normal tongue tissue section from one of the patients with oral SCC (Table 2). (**a**) Co-immunofluorescent staining of cathepsin S (Cat S, red) and DAPI (gray); (**b**) cytokeratin for SCC cells (CK5, green) and DAPI (gray); (**c**) Cat S (red), CK5 (green) and DAPI (gray). White arrows indicate cathepsin S in SCC cells. Scale bars, 100 μm.

3.3. Cathepsin S Activity in Mouse Oral Cancers

Using BMV157, we measured cathepsin S activity in the mouse orthotopic xenograft model in which HSC-3 human oral SCC cells were inoculated into the tongue. Compared to normal mouse tongues, HSC-3 orthotopic xenografts exhibited increased cathepsin S activity and increased total levels of immunoreactive cathepsin S (Figure 5a–c). Thus, the xenograft model mimics our findings in human SCC.

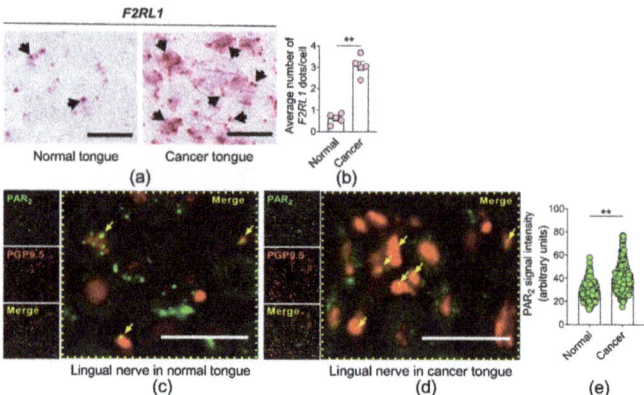

Figure 4. (**a,b**) *F2RL1* mRNA expression in a human cancer tongue is elevated compared to the contralateral unaffected normal tongue in the same patient. (**a**) Microscopy shows *F2RL1* expression in human cancer tongue (right panel) and contralateral unaffected normal tongue (left panel). Black arrows indicate *F2RL1* chromogenic dots. (**b**) The cancer tongue expressed approximately five times the amount of *F2RL1* mRNA expressed by the unaffected normal tongue. ** $p < 0.01$. One-way ANOVA. (**c**) PAR$_2$ protein in human lingual nerve innervating contralateral unaffected normal tongue compared to (**d**) cancer tongue. The lingual nerves were counterstained with PGP9.5 (a neuronal marker). (**e**) PAR$_2$ signal intensity in the lingual nerve innervating the cancer tongue ($n = 300$ axons) was higher than PAR$_2$ signal intensity from lingual nerve innervating contralateral unaffected normal tongue ($n = 275$ axons). Arrows indicate PAR$_2$ in axons. Scale bar, 10 μm. ** $p < 0.01$, Student's *t*-test.

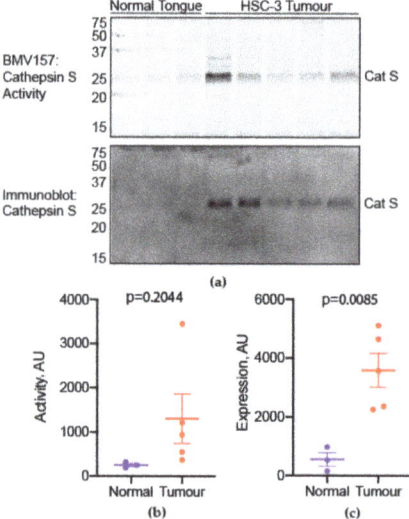

Figure 5. Cathepsin S activity is increased in the oral cancer of the mouse orthotopic xenograft model compared to mouse normal tongue. (**a**) Active cathepsin S labeled by BMV157 (upper panel) as shown by in-gel fluorescence and total cathepsin S immunoreactivity (lower panel). The gel (upper panel) was transferred to nitrocellulose and immunoblotted for total cathepsin S levels (lower panel). The uncropped western blot figure is presented in Figure S2. (**b**) Cathepsin S activity was higher in oral HSC-3 xenografts compared to normal tongues (unpaired Student's *t*-test). (**c**) Cathepsin S expression was higher in HSC-3 xenografts compared to normal tongues (unpaired Student's *t*-test).

3.4. Cathepsin S Activity in a Human Oral Cancer Cell Line Compared to a Human Dysplastic Oral Keratinocyte Line

We measured cathepsin S activity in HSC-3 cells and dysplastic oral keratinocytes (DOK, non-cancer cell line, cell number, 94122104, was from SIGMA-ALDRICH) with BMV157, the cathepsin S-selective probe, and BMV109, a pan cathepsin probe. Cathepsin S activity was higher in HSC-3 than DOK, as measured by both probes (Figure 6a–c). Likewise, total cathepsin S levels were increased in HSC-3 cells compared to DOKs (Figure 6a,d). We also used ELISA to measure the intracellular and secreted cathepsin S in HSC-3 cells as well as a second human oral cancer line, OSC-20 (Figure 6e).

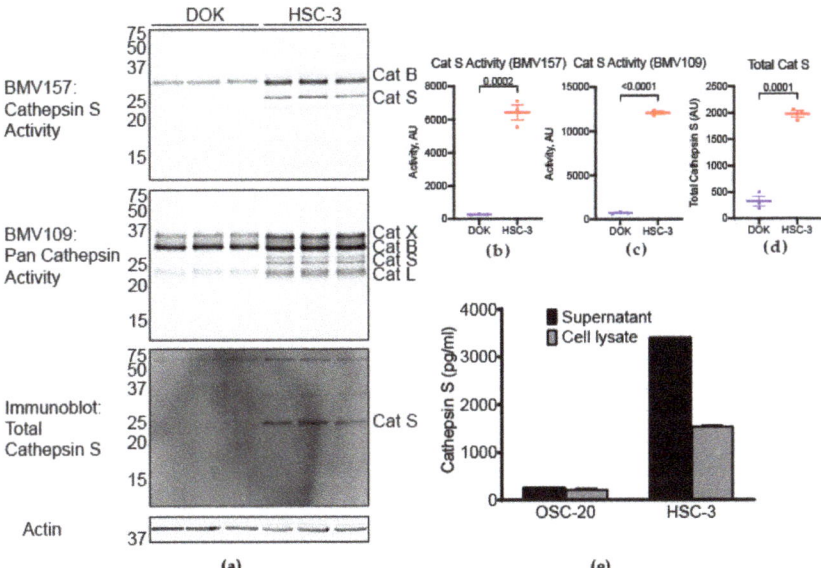

Figure 6. Cathepsin S activity and expression are increased in human oral cancer cells. Cathepsin S activity was compared between HSC-3 and the human dysplastic oral keratinocyte cell line, DOK. (**a**) Labeling of cathepsin S activity with BMV157 selective for cathepsin S in DOK and HSC-3, as shown by in-gel fluorescence; immunoblots confirmed cathepsin S. Labeling of pan cathepsin activity with BMV109 in DOK and HSC-3; immunoblots confirmed cathepsin X, B, S and L; cathepsin S activity is significantly higher in HSC-3 compared to DOK as measured by (**b**) BMV157, and (**c**) BMV 109. The uncropped western blot figure is presented in Figure S3. (**d**) Total cathepsin S activity in HSC-3 is significantly higher than in DOK. (**e**) ELISA assay to measure cathepsin S in supernatant and whole-cell lysate from HSC-3 and a second human oral squamous cell line, OSC-20.

3.5. Cathepsin S from Human Oral Cancer Cell Lines Cleaves PAR$_2$

To determine whether cathepsin S in cancer supernatant cleaves the exodomain of PAR$_2$, FLAG-PAR$_2$ plasmids were transiently transfected in HEK cells and PAR$_2$ cleavage was measured with the On-Cell Western assay. These cells expressed PAR$_2$ with an extracellular N-terminal FLAG epitope that is upstream of the site of cathepsin S cleavage (Figure 7a). In cells treated with the negative control vehicle, the FLAG epitope was intact, thus it was visualized on the plasma membrane using immunohistochemistry with anti-FLAG antibody (Figure 7b, left image, green color). In contrast, cathepsin S (100 nM for 30 min) cleaved the exodomain of PAR$_2$, and caused a loss of surface FLAG immunoreactivity (Figure 7b, right image, green color). The result indicates that cathepsin S cleaved PAR$_2$ and removed the FLAG epitope.

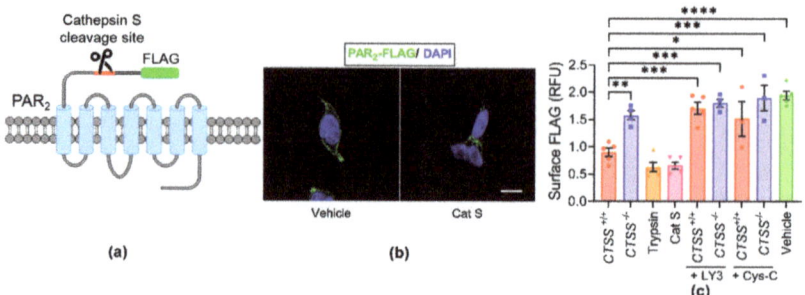

Figure 7. Cathepsin S cleavage of PAR_2. (**a**) Human PAR_2 construct showing extracellular FLAG epitope and cathepsin S cleavage site. (**b**) Localization of PAR_2 using antibodies to extracellular N-terminal FLAG in HEK-FLAG-PAR_2 cells incubated with vehicle control (vehicle, left image) or cathepsin S (Cat S, right image). Scale bar, 10 μm. (**c**) On-Cell Western assay shows that HSC-3 $CTSS^{+/+}$ supernatant, trypsin, and cathepsin S remove the extracellular N-terminal FLAG epitope from HEK-FLAG-PAR_2 cells. LY3 and cystatin C (Cys-C) inhibit PAR_2 cleavage in HEK-FLAG-PAR_2 by HSC-3 $CTSS^{+/+}$ and $CTSS^{-/-}$ supernatant. One-way ANOVA followed by Tukey's multiple comparisons test, each data point representing the mean ± S.E.M., * $p < 0.05$, ** $p < 0.01$, *** $p < 0.001$, **** $p < 0.0001$ ($n \geq 3$ cells).

The On-Cell Western assay was also used to quantify the removal of the FLAG epitope. In cathepsin S-incubated cells (Cat S, 100 nM, 30 min, 37 °C), FLAG immunoreactivity was reduced by 66.02% (1.94 ± 0.17 in vehicle-treated cells versus 0.66 ± 0.14 in Cat S-treated cells). Similarly, the FLAG immunoreactivity was reduced by 42.83% when supernatant from the HSC-3 $CTSS^{+/+}$ was applied to cells in comparison to the supernatant from the HSC-3 $CTSS^{-/-}$ (1.55 ± 0.16 in $CTSS^{-/-}$ versus 0.90 ± 0.17 in $CTSS^{+/+}$) (Figure 7c). LY3 and cystatin C inhibit PAR_2 cleavage by $CTSS^{+/+}$ cells (Figure 7c). Collectively, these results indicated that cathepsin S from human cancer cell lines cleaves membrane PAR_2.

3.6. Cathepsin S Causes Orofacial Nociception That Is Neuronal PAR_2 Dependent

We previously demonstrated that cathepsin S produces nociceptive behavior through the cleavage of PAR_2 when injected into tissue innervated by dorsal root ganglia [34]; however, the nociceptive effect of cathepsin S in the trigeminal system has not been demonstrated. To study the nociceptive effect of cathepsin S on orofacial nociception, we injected cathepsin S into the cheek that is innervated by trigeminal neurons (Figure 8a,d,g). The facial von Frey nociception assay was conducted before and at 1, 3, 6, 12 and 24 h after cathepsin S injection into the cheek to monitor the cathepsin S-evoked nociceptive behavior. We found that cathepsin S increased the facial nociception score compared to the vehicle control demonstrating that cathepsin S induces orofacial nociception (Figure 8b,e,h). To confirm that the nociceptive effect was dependent on the proteolytic activity of cathepsin S, we used a specific cathepsin S inhibitor, LY3000328, (Figure 8a–c) or an endogenous cathepsin S inhibitor, cystatin C (Figure 8d–f). Both cathepsin S inhibitors (Figure 8b,c,e,f) reversed the nociceptive effect of cathepsin S. We then questioned whether the nociceptive effect of cathepsin S was dependent on neuronal PAR_2. We injected cathepsin S into the cheek of WT C57BL/6J mice and $Par_2Na_v1.8$ KO mice which lack the gene for PAR_2 in $Na_v1.8$-positive neurons (Figure 8g). The $Par_2Na_v1.8$ KO mice exhibited a 56.0% reduction in the facial nociception score at 1 h after cathepsin S injection (Figure 8h), and a 57.3% reduction over the course of 24 h after cathepsin S injection (Figure 8i).

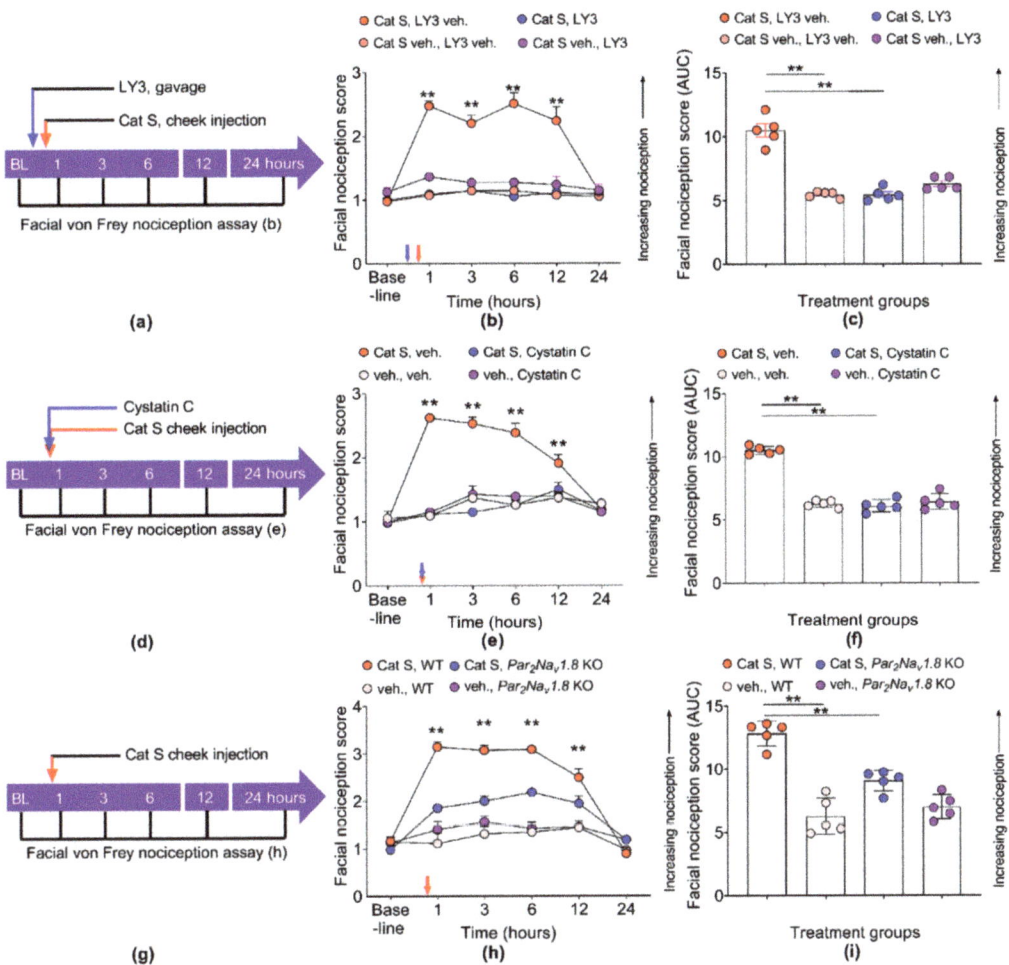

Figure 8. Cathepsin S induces facial nociception through PAR$_2$. (**a**,**d**) Experiment timeline for cathepsin S (red arrow) injection into the left cheek of WT C57BL/6J mice or (**g**) Par$_2$Na$_v$1.8 KO mice. Wild-type mice were treated with (**a**) cathepsin S inhibitor, LY3000328 (LY3) or (**d**) endogenous cathepsin S inhibitor, cystatin C. The facial von Frey nociception assay was conducted before injection (BL or baseline), 1, 3, 6, 12, and 24 h after injection. (**b**) Cathepsin S increased the facial nociception score higher than vehicle injection; the cathepsin S inhibitor LY3 reversed the nociceptive effect of cathepsin S. ** $p < 0.01$, comparison of cathepsin S, cathepsin S inhibitor vehicle to remaining groups at the indicated time point, two-way ANOVA multiple comparisons. $N = 5$ mice in each group. (**c**) Area under the curve (AUC) of each individual mouse in (**b**) was plotted. ** $p < 0.01$, one-way ANOVA. (**e**) Cathepsin S increased the facial nociception score higher than the vehicle; however, cystatin C reversed the nociceptive effect of cathepsin S. ** $p < 0.01$, comparison of cathepsin S, cystatin C vehicle to remaining groups at indicated time point, two-way ANOVA multiple comparisons. $N = 5$ mice in each group. (**f**) AUC of each individual mouse in (**e**) was plotted. ** $p < 0.01$, one-way ANOVA. (**h**) Cathepsin S increased facial nociception score higher than vehicle injection in WT mice, but not in Par$_2$Na$_v$1.8 KO mice. ** $p < 0.01$ cathepsin S, WT versus cathepsin S, Par$_2$Na$_v$1.8 KO at indicated time points, two-way ANOVA. $N = 5$ mice in each group. (**i**) The AUC of each individual mouse in (**h**) was plotted. ** $p < 0.01$, one-way ANOVA.

3.7. Deletion of CTSS with CRISPR/Cas9 in HSC-3 Reduces Nociception, but Not Tumor Volume in the Xenograft Model

Having demonstrated that purified recombinant cathepsin S can invoke facial nociception in vivo, we then investigated the ability of tumor cell-derived cathepsin S to provoke oral cancer pain. We deleted $CTSS$ in HSC-3 by CRISPR/Cas9. RT-PCR semi-quantitative analysis of $CTSS$ gene expression in HSC-3 cells confirmed the lack of $CTSS$ in HSC-3 $CTSS^{-/-}$ (Figure 9a). An ELISA assay on an HSC-3 culture supernatant and cell lysate confirmed the lack of cathepsin S protein in HSC-3 $CTSS^{-/-}$ (Figure 9b). To monitor the development of cancer-induced mechanical allodynia and thermal hyperalgesia, we used the paw von Frey nociception assay (Figure 9c,d) and the Hargreaves thermal assay (Figure 9c,e), respectively. Measurements were taken prior to the inoculation of HSC-3 cells in the paw (baseline) and weekly thereafter for four weeks. Xenografts generated from cathepsin S-deficient HSC-3 cells ($CTSS^{-/-}$CRISPR/Cas9) provoked reduced mechanical allodynia and thermal hyperalgesia relative to xenografts generated from wild-type HSC-3 cells (untreated naïve cells or cells treated with random guide RNA) (Figure 9c,d,e). Cancer mice generated with HSC-3 $CTSS^{-/-}$ showed a 58.7% reduction in mechanical allodynia (Figure 9d) and an 87.0% reduction in thermal hyperalgesia (Figure 9e) compared to cancer mice generated with HSC-3 treated with random CRISPR/Cas9 at 4 weeks after inoculation.

We tested whether the deletion of $CTSS$ in HSC-3 with CRISPR/Cas9 altered tumor proliferation as measured by tumor volume. The cancer paw volume was measured before (BL) and every week until 4 weeks after HSC-3 inoculation (Figure 9f). The cancer paw volume was not different between mice generated with HSC-3 $CTSS^{-/-}$ or HSC-3 treated with random CRISPR/Cas9 or naïve HSC-3 cells (Figure 9g). We confirmed the cancer growth in the paw by histology and H&E staining (Figure 9h). The cancer area quantified by histology showed no difference between groups (Figure 9i).

3.8. The Cathepsin S Inhibitor Reduces Cancer Nociception, but Not Tumor Volume, in Cancer Mice Generated with Two Human Tongue Oral Cancer Cell Lines, HSC-3 and OSC-20

We tested whether two human oral cancer cell lines produced nociception through cathepsin S. We generated separate groups of xenograft mice with HSC-3 and OSC-20. Prior to and following paw inoculation, the mice were tested every week for 4 weeks with the paw von Frey nociception assay and the Hargreaves thermal assay to monitor the development of mechanical allodynia and thermal hyperalgesia, respectively (Figure 10a). The HSC-3 cancer mice developed nociception at 2 and 3 weeks (Figure 10b,c) while the OSC-20 cancer mice developed cancer nociception at 3 and 4 weeks (Figure 10e,f) after the cancer cells were inoculated into the paw. When the mice developed cancer nociception, a single dose of the cathepsin S inhibitor, LY3000328, was administered. The mice were then tested with the mechanical and thermal assays at 1, 3, 6, 12 and 24 h after LY3000328 was administered (Figure 10a). LY3000328 reduced mechanical cancer allodynia in HSC-3 and OSC-20 by 55.7% and 47.7%, respectively. LY3000328 reduced thermal cancer hyperalgesia in HSC-3 and OSC-20 by 73.6% and 56.3%, respectively. We measured the cancer paw volume in the mice before and every week until 4 weeks after the HSC-3 or OSC-20 cancer cells were inoculated into the paw. The cancer paw volume was similar between treatment groups and control groups (Figure 10d,g); LY3000328 did not alter paw volume after administration to the mice.

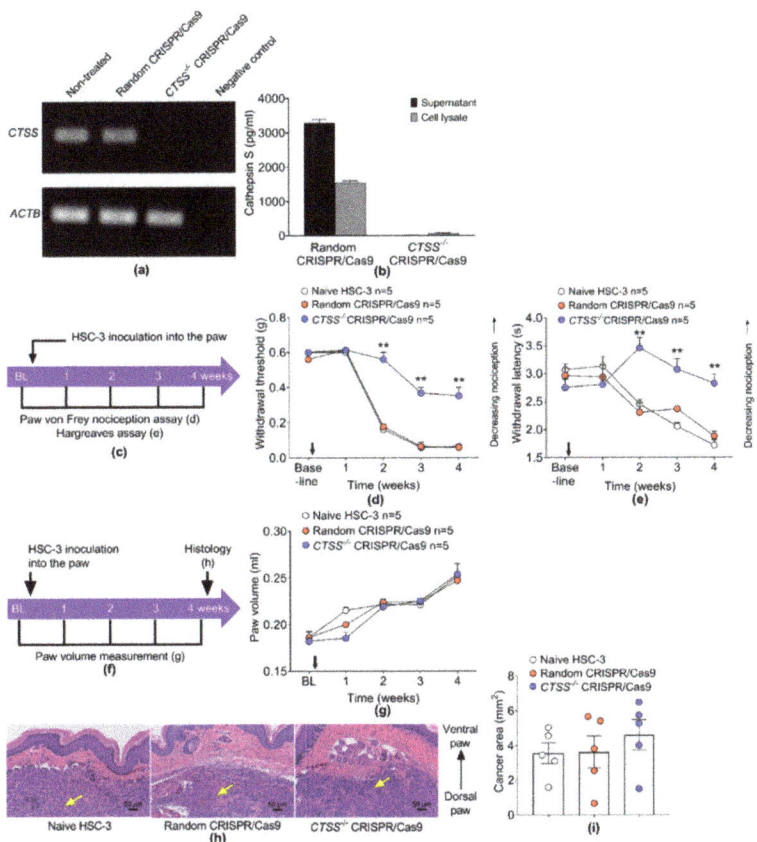

Figure 9. Deletion of *CTSS* with CRISPR/Cas9 in HSC-3 attenuates nociception, but not tumor volume or cancer area, in the mouse oral cancer xenograft model. (**a**) RT-PCR semi-quantitative analysis of *CTSS* expression in non-treated HSC-3 and HSC-3 treated with random CRISPR/Cas9 or $CTSS^{-/-}$ CRISPR/Cas9. No *CTSS* mRNA signal was detected in the HSC-3 $CTSS^{-/-}$ cells. Beta actin (*ACTB*) was used as a control. (**b**) $CTSS^{-/-}$ CRISPR/Cas9 reduced cathepsin S protein in supernatant and whole-cell lysate from HSC-3. (**c**) The experiment timeline for the inoculation of HSC-3 or HSC-3 $CTSS^{-/-}$ into the left hind paw of $NU/J\ Foxn1^{nu}$ mice. The mice were tested with (**d**) paw von Frey nociception assay and (**e**) Hargreaves thermal assay. Cancer mice generated with HSC-3 $CTSS^{-/-}$ exhibited (**d**) a withdrawal threshold and (**e**) a withdrawal latency higher than cancer mice generated with HSC-3 treated with random CRISPR/Cas9. ** $p < 0.01$ HSC-3 $CTSS^{-/-}$ mice versus HSC-3 random CRISPR/Cas9 mice, two-way ANOVA. (**f**) In vivo experiment timeline of inoculation of HSC-3 $CTSS^{-/-}$ into the paw of $NU/J\ Foxn1^{nu}$ mice for the measurement of tumor volume and cancer area. We measured the volume of the cancer paw before inoculation (BL), and every week until 4 weeks after inoculation. The cancer paws were collected for histological H&E staining at 4 weeks after inoculation. (**g**) HSC-3 $CTSS^{-/-}$ did not increase cancer paw volume in mice compared to cancer mice inoculated with HSC-3 treated with random CRISPR/Cas9. (**h**) Representative histological H&E images of the cancer (yellow arrow) in the paw inoculated with naive HSC-3 (left image), HSC-3 treated with random CRISPR/Cas9 (middle image), or HSC-3 $CTSS^{-/-}$ (right image). (**i**) Quantification of cancer area in each mouse.

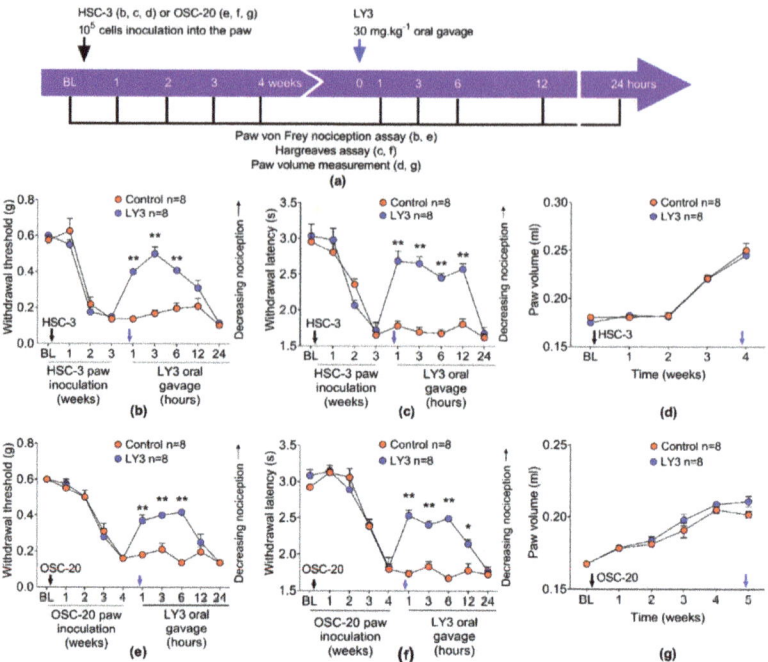

Figure 10. The cathepsin S inhibitor, LY3000328, attenuates nociception in paw xenograft models generated with HSC-3 or OSC-20. (**a**) Experiment timeline for the inoculation of HSC-3 or OSC-20 into the left hind paw of the NU/J *Foxn1nu* mice, subsequent treatment with the cathepsin S inhibitor, LY3000328, and simultaneous nociceptive behavioral testing. The mice were evaluated with (**b,e**) the paw von Frey nociception assay, (**c,f**) Hargreaves thermal assay, and (**d,g**) cancer paw volume before (BL or Baseline) and at 1, 2, 3, and 4 weeks after inoculation to monitor cancer nociception and cancer paw volume. When the mice developed cancer nociception in two consecutive weeks (i.e., week 2, 3 in HSC-3 paw cancer mice or week 3, 4 in OSC-20 paw cancer mice), the mice were administered LY3000328 (blue arrow). The (**b,e**) paw von Frey nociception assay and the (**c,f**) Hargreaves thermal assay were conducted at 1, 3, 6, 12, and 24 h after LY3000328 treatment. LY3000328 increased (**b,e**) withdrawal threshold and (**c,f**) withdrawal latency relative to LY3000328 vehicle control (i.e., 30% DMSO in normal saline without LY3000328). (**d,g**) LY3000328 did not increase paw cancer volume relative to the control at 24 h after oral gavage of LY3000328. * $p < 0.05$; ** $p < 0.01$ LY3000328 versus control, two-way ANOVA.

4. Discussion

The primary question addressed by the present study was whether cathepsin S produces cancer pain. We also sought to determine whether the putative nociceptive mechanism involves PAR$_2$ on neurons; a role for PAR$_2$ is likely as we previously demonstrated that PAR$_2$ plays a central role regulating cancer pain [35–37]. Specifically, mice completely lacking PAR$_2$ exhibit reduced cancer-associated allodynia and orofacial dysfunction [35,36]. Mice lacking PAR$_2$ specifically in nociceptive neurons (Par$_2$Na$_v$1.8 mice) also exhibit attenuated nociception, indicating a central role for neuronal PAR$_2$ in cancer pain [27]. Furthermore, we also demonstrated that PAR$_2$-activating proteases (e.g., TMPRSS2 and legumain) contribute to cancer pain in a PAR$_2$-dependent manner [27,37].

We first characterized cathepsin S expression and activity in human oral squamous cell carcinoma tissues and patient-matched normal oral mucosa using cathepsin S-specific antibodies and BMV157, an activity-based probe that enables the assessment of the proteolytically active fraction of cathepsin S. Total and active cathepsin S were increased in cancer tissues compared to normal tissues. In breast, prostate, colorectal and metastatic brain cancers, cathepsin S is supplied by the tumor cells and associated stromal cells, predominantly macrophages [9,38,39]. In accordance with other cancers, we observed cathepsin S production by both keratin$^+$ tumor cells and CD68$^+$ macrophages of oral cancer specimens collected from four patients. Cathepsin S expression in adjacent normal tissue was minimal. We also demonstrated that cathepsin S activity is upregulated in immortalized human oral cancer cell lines compared to dysplastic oral keratinocytes. We demonstrated that cathepsin S is secreted by oral cancer cells, and that it cleaves human PAR$_2$. The orthotopic xenografts of human oral cancer cells also exhibited increased cathepsin S activity compared to naïve mouse tongue tissue.

Furthermore, purified cathepsin S was able to invoke facial nociception in vivo, also in an activity-dependent and PAR$_2$-dependent manner, suggesting that cathepsin S would be capable of provoking oral cancer pain.

We next investigated the ability of tumor-supplied cathepsin S to provoke oral cancer pain. The deletion of cathepsin S specifically from HSC-3 tumor cells resulted in a reduction of mechanical allodynia and thermal hyperalgesia (58.7% and 87.0%, respectively) produced by paw xenografts. In the future, complementary studies involving the inoculation of HSC-3 cells into wild-type and cathepsin S-deficient nude mice would shed light on the contribution of stromal (macrophage)-supplied cathepsin S to cancer pain. Ultimately, we showed that the administration of a single dose of a cathepsin S-selective inhibitor LY3000328, which targets both tumor and stromal-supplied cathepsin S, was able to attenuate cancer pain for at least 12 h in two independent xenograft models [16].

The treatment of oral cancer pain is challenging because cancers are heterogeneous and because oral cancers produce and secrete several nociceptive mediators. Nociceptive mediators produced and secreted by oral cancer include, but are not limited to, nerve growth factor, ATP, endothelin-1 and other proteases [30,40,41]. The cathepsin S/PAR$_2$ axis is a strategic target for cancer pain. Cathepsin S is active in the extracellular environment of the cancer and associated neurons. Accordingly, it could be antagonized without cellular uptake, as opposed to other cathepsins, which are active in lysosomes. Furthermore, PAR$_2$ activates several types of TRP channels, including TRPV4 [42], TRPV1 [43,44] and TRPA1 [45], which amplify the action of cathepsin S. As a result, nociceptors responsive to several algesic mediator types are sensitized and induce hyperexcitability and sustained nociception. In addition, PAR$_2$ transactivates the epidermal growth factor receptor (EGFR), which also mediates nociception [46–48]. Thus, if we could prevent the activation of PAR$_2$ by cathepsin S, we could potentially abrogate the sensitization of the receptors that mediate the nociceptive action of myriad mediators produced and secreted by cancers. A potential concern with the inhibition of cathepsin S is that antigen processing, which is critical to the immune response to cancers, might be affected. This argument is countered by the finding that cathepsin S is upregulated by several cancers. Moreover, to the degree that evolutionary mechanisms underlie tumor progression, the natural selection of tumor cells may be less likely to favor the overexpression of cathepsin S if proliferation were reduced. In fact, the inhibition or deletion of the gene for cathepsin S reverses several hallmarks of cancer [13]. Because of the previous studies reporting that cathepsin S mediates carcinogenesis, we measured the proliferation and tumor volume following the genetic deletion and pharmacologic antagonism of cathepsin S. The antinociceptive effect that we demonstrated could reflect reduced proliferation and decreased tumor burden. We found that neither the deletion of *CTSS* nor a single dose of the cathepsin S inhibitor, LY3000328, affected the tumor volume; therefore, the mechanism of preventing the expression or inhibiting cathepsin S is antinociceptive. The nociceptive mechanisms that we demonstrated in oral cancer (a notoriously painful malignancy) likely overlap with other cancer pain mechanisms, including bone cancer pain. Nociceptive mediators/mechanisms common to oral cancer and bone cancer include, but are not limited to, endothelin, NGF, and PAR$_2$ [30,40,41,49,50]. Cathepsin S also might contribute to visceral pain associated with gastrointestinal cancers including pancreatic cancer. Cathepsins, including cathepsin

S, also mediate pancreatitis [51]. Because cathepsin S inhibitors have been clinically used and show good safety profiles, we are considering a trial to test their efficacy for the management of cancer pain [6].

5. Conclusions

Cathepsin S, a lysosomal cysteine protease, is present and active in the oral cancer microenvironment. The protease cleaves protease-activated receptor-2 (PAR_2) on neurons to contribute to the severe pain that is associated with oral cancer. In humans, cathepsin S activity correlates with reported pain. Genetic deletion of the gene for cathepsin S in a human oral cancer cell line reverses nociception in a mouse cancer model generated with the cancer cell line. We conclude that cathepsin S is responsible for oral cancer pain through PAR_2 on neurons.

Supplementary Materials: The following are available online at https://www.mdpi.com/article/10.3390/cancers13184697/s1, Figure S1: Uncropped western blot figures of Figure 1a, Figure S2: Uncropped western blot figures of Figure 5a, Figure S3: Uncropped western blot figures of Figure 6a.

Author Contributions: Conceptualization, N.W.B., L.E.E.-M. and B.L.S.; methodology, N.H.T., K.I., R.L., N.W.B., L.E.E.-M. and B.L.S.; formal analysis, N.H.T.; K.I., E.C. and M.N.J.; investigation, N.H.T.; K.I., E.C., B.M.A., C.M.S., N.N.S., H.D.T., D.H.K., R.G.A., L.Y., R.L., J.C.D., C.Z.L., D.D.J.; writing—original draft preparation, B.L.S.; writing—review and editing, N.H.T., J.C.D., N.W.B. and L.E.E.-M.; funding acquisition, N.W.B., L.E.E.-M. and B.L.S. All authors have read and agreed to the published version of the manuscript.

Funding: Supported by grants from the National Institutes of Health (NS102722, DE026806, DK118971, DE029951, N.W.B., B.L.S.) and Department of Defense (W81XWH1810431, N.W.B., B.L.S.). L.E.M. was supported by a Priority-Driven Collaborative Cancer Research grant (co-funded by Cancer Australia and Cure Cancer, GNT1157171), a Grimwade Fellowship from the Russell and Mab Grimwade Miegunyah Fund at The University of Melbourne, and a DECRA Fellowship from the Australian Research Council (ARC, DE180100418).

Institutional Review Board Statement: This study was conducted according to the guidelines of the Declaration of Helsinki, and approved by the Institutional Review Board of New York University (IRB# 10-01261 and date of approval 09/15/2020).

Informed Consent Statement: Informed consent was obtained from all subjects involved in the study.

Data Availability Statement: The data are presented in the article.

Acknowledgments: We thank members of the Experimental Pathology Research Laboratory, which is partially supported by the Cancer Center Support Grant P30CA016087 at NYU Langone's Laura and Isaac Perlmutter Cancer Center. The Akoya/PerkinElmer Vectra Polaris® multispectral imaging system was acquired through a Shared Instrumentation Grant S10 OD021747. The images of the cancer cell and neuron in the graphical abstract are from TogoTV (©2016 DBCLS TogoTV).

Conflicts of Interest: N.W.B. is a founding scientist of Endosome Therapeutics Inc. Research in NWB's laboratory is partly supported by Takeda Pharmaceuticals International. J.C.D. fabricates dolognawmeter™ assay devices through Gnatheon Scientific LLC.

References

1. Riese, R.J.; Mitchell, R.N.; Villadangos, J.A.; Shi, G.P.; Palmer, J.T.; Karp, E.R.; De Sanctis, G.T.; Ploegh, H.L.; Chapman, H.A. Cathepsin S activity regulates antigen presentation and immunity. *J. Clin. Investig.* **1998**, *101*, 2351–2363. [CrossRef] [PubMed]
2. Chapman, H.A.; Riese, R.J.; Shi, G.P. Emerging roles for cysteine proteases in human biology. *Annu. Rev. Physiol.* **1997**, *59*, 63–88. [CrossRef] [PubMed]
3. Overall, C.M.; Lopez-Otin, C. Strategies for MMP inhibition in cancer: Innovations for the post-trial era. *Nat. Rev. Cancer* **2002**, *2*, 657–672. [CrossRef] [PubMed]
4. Maciewicz, R.A.; Etherington, D.J. A comparison of four cathepsins (B, L, N and S) with collagenolytic activity from rabbit spleen. *Biochem. J.* **1988**, *256*, 433–440. [CrossRef] [PubMed]
5. Morton, P.A.; Zacheis, M.L.; Giacoletto, K.S.; Manning, J.A.; Schwartz, B.D. Delivery of nascent MHC class II-invariant chain complexes to lysosomal compartments and proteolysis of invariant chain by cysteine proteases precedes peptide binding in B-lymphoblastoid cells. *J. Immunol.* **1995**, *154*, 137–150.

6. Brown, R.; Nath, S.; Lora, A.; Samaha, G.; Elgamal, Z.; Kaiser, R.; Taggart, C.; Weldon, S.; Geraghty, P. Cathepsin S: Investigating an old player in lung disease pathogenesis, comorbidities, and potential therapeutics. *Respir. Res.* **2020**, *21*, 111. [CrossRef]
7. Burden, R.E.; Gormley, J.A.; Jaquin, T.J.; Small, D.M.; Quinn, D.J.; Hegarty, S.M.; Ward, C.; Walker, B.; Johnston, J.A.; Olwill, S.A.; et al. Antibody-mediated inhibition of cathepsin S blocks colorectal tumor invasion and angiogenesis. *Clin. Cancer Res* **2009**, *15*, 6042–6051. [CrossRef]
8. Flannery, T.; Gibson, D.; Mirakhur, M.; McQuaid, S.; Greenan, C.; Trimble, A.; Walker, B.; McCormick, D.; Johnston, P.G. The clinical significance of cathepsin S expression in human astrocytomas. *Am. J. Pathol.* **2003**, *163*, 175–182. [CrossRef]
9. Kos, J.; Sekirnik, A.; Kopitar, G.; Cimerman, N.; Kayser, K.; Stremmer, A.; Fiehn, W.; Werle, B. Cathepsin S in tumours, regional lymph nodes and sera of patients with lung cancer: Relation to prognosis. *Br. J. Cancer* **2001**, *85*, 1193–1200. [CrossRef]
10. Flannery, T.; McConnell, R.S.; McQuaid, S.; McGregor, G.; Mirakhur, M.; Martin, L.; Scott, C.; Burden, R.; Walker, B.; McGoohan, C.; et al. Detection of cathepsin S cysteine protease in human brain tumour microdialysates in vivo. *Br. J. Neurosurg.* **2007**, *21*, 204–209. [CrossRef]
11. Gocheva, V.; Wang, H.W.; Gadea, B.B.; Shree, T.; Hunter, K.E.; Garfall, A.L.; Berman, T.; Joyce, J.A. IL-4 induces cathepsin protease activity in tumor-associated macrophages to promote cancer growth and invasion. *Genes Dev.* **2010**, *24*, 241–255. [CrossRef]
12. Joyce, J.A.; Baruch, A.; Chehade, K.; Meyer-Morse, N.; Giraudo, E.; Tsai, F.Y.; Greenbaum, D.C.; Hager, J.H.; Bogyo, M.; Hanahan, D. Cathepsin cysteine proteases are effectors of invasive growth and angiogenesis during multistage tumorigenesis. *Cancer Cell* **2004**, *5*, 443–453. [CrossRef]
13. Wang, X.; Xiong, L.; Yu, G.; Li, D.; Peng, T.; Luo, D.; Xu, J. Cathepsin S silencing induces apoptosis of human hepatocellular carcinoma cells. *Am. J. Transl. Res.* **2015**, *7*, 100–110. [PubMed]
14. Gocheva, V.; Zeng, W.; Ke, D.; Klimstra, D.; Reinheckel, T.; Peters, C.; Hanahan, D.; Joyce, J.A. Distinct roles for cysteine cathepsin genes in multistage tumorigenesis. *Genes Dev.* **2006**, *20*, 543–556. [CrossRef]
15. Wang, B.; Sun, J.; Kitamoto, S.; Yang, M.; Grubb, A.; Chapman, H.A.; Kalluri, R.; Shi, G.P. Cathepsin S controls angiogenesis and tumor growth via matrix-derived angiogenic factors. *J. Biol. Chem.* **2006**, *281*, 6020–6029. [CrossRef] [PubMed]
16. Sevenich, L.; Bowman, R.L.; Mason, S.D.; Quail, D.F.; Rapaport, F.; Elie, B.T.; Brogi, E.; Brastianos, P.K.; Hahn, W.C.; Holsinger, L.J.; et al. Analysis of tumour- and stroma-supplied proteolytic networks reveals a brain-metastasis-promoting role for cathepsin S. *Nat. Cell Biol.* **2014**, *16*, 876–888. [CrossRef]
17. Hsieh, M.-J.; Lin, C.-W.; Chen, M.-K.; Chien, S.-Y.; Lo, Y.-S.; Chuang, Y.-C.; Hsi, Y.-T.; Lin, C.-C.; Chen, J.-C.; Yang, S.-F. Inhibition of cathepsin S confers sensitivity to methyl protodioscin in oral cancer cells via activation of p38 MAPK/JNK signaling pathways. *Sci. Rep.* **2017**, *7*, 45039. [CrossRef] [PubMed]
18. Vergnolle, N.; Wallace, J.L.; Bunnett, N.W.; Hollenberg, M.D. Protease-activated receptors in inflammation, neuronal signaling and pain. *Trends Pharmacol. Sci.* **2001**, *22*, 146–152. [CrossRef]
19. Clark, A.K.; Yip, P.K.; Grist, J.; Gentry, C.; Staniland, A.A.; Marchand, F.; Dehvari, M.; Wotherspoon, G.; Winter, J.; Ullah, J.; et al. Inhibition of spinal microglial cathepsin S for the reversal of neuropathic pain. *Proc. Natl. Acad. Sci. USA* **2007**, *104*, 10655–10660. [CrossRef] [PubMed]
20. Connelly, S.T.; Schmidt, B.L. Evaluation of pain in patients with oral squamous cell carcinoma. *J. Pain* **2004**, *5*, 505–510. [CrossRef] [PubMed]
21. Kolokythas, A.; Connelly, S.T.; Schmidt, B.L. Validation of the University of California San Francisco Oral Cancer Pain Questionnaire. *J. Pain* **2007**, *8*, 950–953. [CrossRef]
22. Jimenez-Vargas, N.N.; Pattison, L.A.; Zhao, P.; Lieu, T.; Latorre, R.; Jensen, D.D.; Castro, J.; Aurelio, L.; Le, G.T.; Flynn, B.; et al. Protease-activated receptor-2 in endosomes signals persistent pain of irritable bowel syndrome. *Proc. Natl. Acad. Sci. USA* **2018**, *115*, E7438–E7447. [CrossRef]
23. Stirling, L.C.; Forlani, G.; Baker, M.D.; Wood, J.N.; Matthews, E.A.; Dickenson, A.H.; Nassar, M.A. Nociceptor-specific gene deletion using heterozygous NaV1.8-Cre recombinase mice. *Pain* **2005**, *113*, 27–36. [CrossRef] [PubMed]
24. Oresic Bender, K.; Ofori, L.; van der Linden, W.A.; Mock, E.D.; Datta, G.K.; Chowdhury, S.; Li, H.; Segal, E.; Sanchez Lopez, M.; Ellman, J.A.; et al. Design of a highly selective quenched activity-based probe and its application in dual color imaging studies of cathepsin S activity localization. *J. Am. Chem. Soc.* **2015**, *137*, 4771–4777. [CrossRef] [PubMed]
25. Verdoes, M.; Oresic Bender, K.; Segal, E.; van der Linden, W.A.; Syed, S.; Withana, N.P.; Sanman, L.E.; Bogyo, M. Improved quenched fluorescent probe for imaging of cysteine cathepsin activity. *J. Am. Chem. Soc.* **2013**, *135*, 14726–14730. [CrossRef] [PubMed]
26. Edgington-Mitchell, L.E.; Bogyo, M.; Verdoes, M. Live Cell Imaging and Profiling of Cysteine Cathepsin Activity Using a Quenched Activity-Based Probe. *Methods Mol. Biol.* **2017**, *1491*, 145–159. [CrossRef] [PubMed]
27. Tu, N.H.; Jensen, D.D.; Anderson, B.M.; Chen, E.; Jimenez-Vargas, N.N.; Scheff, N.N.; Inoue, K.; Tran, H.D.; Dolan, J.C.; Meek, T.A.; et al. Legumain Induces Oral Cancer Pain by Biased Agonism of Protease-Activated Receptor-2. *J. Neurosci.* **2021**, *41*, 193–210. [CrossRef] [PubMed]
28. Deseure, K.; Koek, W.; Adriaensen, H.; Colpaert, F.C. Continuous administration of the 5-hydroxytryptamine1A agonist (3-Chloro-4-fluoro-phenyl)-[4-fluoro-4-[[(5-methyl-pyridin-2-ylmethyl) -amino]-methyl]piperidin-1-yl]-methadone (F 13640) attenuates allodynia-like behavior in a rat model of trigeminal neuropathic pain. *J. Pharmacol. Exp. Ther.* **2003**, *306*, 505–514. [CrossRef]
29. Ye, Y.; Bae, S.S.; Viet, C.T.; Troob, S.; Bernabe, D.; Schmidt, B.L. IB4(+) and TRPV1(+) sensory neurons mediate pain but not proliferation in a mouse model of squamous cell carcinoma. *Behav. Brain Funct.* **2014**, *10*, 5. [CrossRef]

30. Ye, Y.; Dang, D.; Zhang, J.; Viet, C.T.; Lam, D.K.; Dolan, J.C.; Gibbs, J.L.; Schmidt, B.L. Nerve growth factor links oral cancer progression, pain, and cachexia. *Mol. Cancer Ther.* **2011**, *10*, 1667–1676. [CrossRef]
31. Chaplan, S.R.; Bach, F.W.; Pogrel, J.W.; Chung, J.M.; Yaksh, T.L. Quantitative assessment of tactile allodynia in the rat paw. *J. Neurosci. Methods* **1994**, *53*, 55–63. [CrossRef]
32. Pickering, V.; Gupta, J.R.; Quang, P.; Jordan, R.C.; Schmidt, B.L. Effect of peripheral endothelin-1 concentration on carcinoma-induced pain in mice. *Eur. J. Pain* **2007**, *12*, 293–300. [CrossRef]
33. Yamano, S.; Viet, C.T.; Dang, D.; Dai, J.; Hanatani, S.; Takayama, T.; Kasai, H.; Imamura, K.; Campbell, R.; Ye, Y.; et al. Ex vivo nonviral gene delivery of mu-opioid receptor to attenuate cancer-induced pain. *Pain* **2017**, *158*, 240–251. [CrossRef] [PubMed]
34. Zhao, P.; Lieu, T.; Barlow, N.; Metcalf, M.; Veldhuis, N.A.; Jensen, D.D.; Kocan, M.; Sostegni, S.; Haerteis, S.; Baraznenok, V.; et al. Cathepsin S causes inflammatory pain via biased agonism of PAR2 and TRPV4. *J. Biol. Chem.* **2014**, *289*, 27215–27234. [CrossRef]
35. Lam, D.K.; Schmidt, B.L. Serine proteases and protease-activated receptor 2-dependent allodynia: A novel cancer pain pathway. *Pain* **2010**, *149*, 263–272. [CrossRef]
36. Lam, D.K.; Dang, D.; Zhang, J.; Dolan, J.C.; Schmidt, B.L. Novel animal models of acute and chronic cancer pain: A pivotal role for PAR2. *J. Neurosci.* **2012**, *32*, 14178–14183. [CrossRef]
37. Lam, D.K.; Dang, D.; Flynn, A.N.; Hardt, M.; Schmidt, B.L. TMPRSS2, a novel membrane-anchored mediator in cancer pain. *Pain* **2015**, *156*, 923–930. [CrossRef]
38. Lindahl, C.; Simonsson, M.; Bergh, A.; Thysell, E.; Antti, H.; Sund, M.; Wikström, P. Increased levels of macrophage-secreted cathepsin S during prostate cancer progression in TRAMP mice and patients. *Cancer Genom. Proteom.* **2009**, *6*, 149–159.
39. Small, D.M.; Burden, R.E.; Jaworski, J.; Hegarty, S.M.; Spence, S.; Burrows, J.F.; McFarlane, C.; Kissenpfennig, A.; McCarthy, H.O.; Johnston, J.A.; et al. Cathepsin S from both tumor and tumor-associated cells promote cancer growth and neovascularization. *Int. J. Cancer* **2013**, *133*, 2102–2112. [CrossRef] [PubMed]
40. Ye, Y.; Dolan, J.; Schmidt, B. ATP correlates with pain in cancer patients and produces nociception in an oral cancer mouse model. In Proceedings of the The International Association for the Study of Pain: The 14th World Congress on Pain, Milan, Italy, 27–31 August 2012.
41. Schmidt, B.L.; Pickering, V.; Liu, S.; Quang, P.; Dolan, J.; Connelly, S.T.; Jordan, R.C. Peripheral endothelin A receptor antagonism attenuates carcinoma-induced pain. *Eur. J. Pain* **2007**, *11*, 406–414. [CrossRef] [PubMed]
42. Zhao, P.; Lieu, T.; Barlow, N.; Sostegni, S.; Haerteis, S.; Korbmacher, C.; Liedtke, W.; Jimenez-Vargas, N.N.; Vanner, S.J.; Bunnett, N.W. Neutrophil Elastase Activates Protease-activated Receptor-2 (PAR2) and Transient Receptor Potential Vanilloid 4 (TRPV4) to Cause Inflammation and Pain. *J. Biol. Chem.* **2015**, *290*, 13875–13887. [CrossRef] [PubMed]
43. Amadesi, S.; Cottrell, G.S.; Divino, L.; Chapman, K.; Grady, E.F.; Bautista, F.; Karanjia, R.; Barajas-Lopez, C.; Vanner, S.; Vergnolle, N.; et al. Protease-activated receptor 2 sensitizes TRPV1 by protein kinase Cepsilon- and A-dependent mechanisms in rats and mice. *J. Physiol.* **2006**, *575*, 555–571. [CrossRef] [PubMed]
44. Sostegni, S.; Diakov, A.; McIntyre, P.; Bunnett, N.; Korbmacher, C.; Haerteis, S. Sensitisation of TRPV4 by PAR2 is independent of intracellular calcium signalling and can be mediated by the biased agonist neutrophil elastase. *Pflug. Arch.* **2015**, *467*, 687–701. [CrossRef]
45. Lieu, T.; Jayaweera, G.; Zhao, P.; Poole, D.P.; Jensen, D.; Grace, M.; McIntyre, P.; Bron, R.; Wilson, Y.M.; Krappitz, M.; et al. The bile acid receptor TGR5 activates the TRPA1 channel to induce itch in mice. *Gastroenterology* **2014**, *147*, 1417–1428. [CrossRef]
46. Verma, V.; Khoury, S.; Parisien, M.; Cho, C.; Maixner, W.; Martin, L.J.; Diatchenko, L. The dichotomous role of epiregulin in pain. *Pain* **2020**, *161*, 1052–1064. [CrossRef]
47. Martin, L.J.; Smith, S.B.; Khoutorsky, A.; Magnussen, C.A.; Samoshkin, A.; Sorge, R.E.; Cho, C.; Yosefpour, N.; Sivaselvachandran, S.; Tohyama, S.; et al. Epiregulin and EGFR interactions are involved in pain processing. *J. Clin. Investig.* **2017**, *127*, 3353–3366. [CrossRef] [PubMed]
48. Caruso, R.; Pallone, F.; Fina, D.; Gioia, V.; Peluso, I.; Caprioli, F.; Stolfi, C.; Perfetti, A.; Spagnoli, L.G.; Palmieri, G.; et al. Protease-activated receptor-2 activation in gastric cancer cells promotes epidermal growth factor receptor trans-activation and proliferation. *Am. J. Pathol.* **2006**, *169*, 268–278. [CrossRef]
49. Halvorson, K.G.; Kubota, K.; Sevcik, M.A.; Lindsay, T.H.; Sotillo, J.E.; Ghilardi, J.R.; Rosol, T.J.; Boustany, L.; Shelton, D.L.; Mantyh, P.W. A blocking antibody to nerve growth factor attenuates skeletal pain induced by prostate tumor cells growing in bone. *Cancer Res.* **2005**, *65*, 9426–9435. [CrossRef] [PubMed]
50. Peters, C.M.; Lindsay, T.H.; Pomonis, J.D.; Luger, N.M.; Ghilardi, J.R.; Sevcik, M.A.; Mantyh, P.W. Endothelin and the tumorigenic component of bone cancer pain. *Neuroscience* **2004**, *126*, 1043–1052. [CrossRef] [PubMed]
51. Lyo, V.; Cattaruzza, F.; Kim, T.N.; Walker, A.W.; Paulick, M.; Cox, D.; Cloyd, J.; Buxbaum, J.; Ostroff, J.; Bogyo, M.; et al. Active cathepsins B, L, and S in murine and human pancreatitis. *Am. J. Physiol. Gastrointest. Liver Physiol.* **2012**, *303*, G894–G903. [CrossRef] [PubMed]

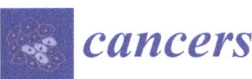

Review

De-Escalation of Therapy for Patients with Early-Stage Squamous Cell Carcinoma of the Anus

Eric Miller and Jose Bazan *

Department of Radiation Oncology at the Arthur G. James Cancer Hospital and Richard J. Solove Research Institute, The Ohio State University Comprehensive Cancer Center, Columbus, OH 43210, USA; eric.miller@osumc.edu
* Correspondence: jose.bazan2@osumc.edu; Tel.: +1-614-688-7371

Simple Summary: Management of early-stage squamous cell carcinoma of the anus (SCCA) remains controversial. The current standard of care treatment of chemotherapy combined with radiation therapy can result in both acute and late toxicity. Alternative therapies, including radiation therapy alone or local excision, may be less toxic, but the role of these therapies in early-stage SCCA remains unclear. Additional options for reducing the intensity of therapy for early-stage SCCA include reduction of radiation dose, altering treatment volumes, modifying chemotherapy type and dosage, and using intensity-modulated radiation therapy to reduce the radiation dose to adjacent normal tissues. Multiple prospective studies are actively investigating the role of de-escalation of therapy in patients with early-stage SCCA.

Abstract: The incidence of squamous cell carcinoma of the anus (SCCA) is increasing, particularly in the elderly, with increased mortality in this age group. While the current standard of care for localized SCCA remains chemoradiation (CRT), completion of this treatment can be challenging with risks for severe acute and late toxicity. It remains unclear if full course CRT is required for the management of early-stage SCCA or if de-escalation of treatment is possible without compromising patient outcomes. Alternative therapies include radiation therapy alone or local excision for appropriate patients. Modifying standard CRT may also reduce toxicity including the routine use of intensity-modulated radiation therapy for treatment delivery, modification of treatment volumes, and selection and dosing of concurrent systemic therapy agents. Finally, we provide an overview of currently accruing prospective trials focused on defining the role of de-escalation of therapy in patients with early-stage SCCA.

Keywords: anal cancer; radiation therapy; chemoradiation; de-escalation of therapy

1. Introduction

Squamous cell carcinoma of the anus (SCCA) remains a relatively rare malignancy, representing less than 1% of all cancer cases in the United States [1]. However, the incidence of SCCA is increasing, particularly in the elderly, with an almost 5% increase in mortality due to this malignancy in the most vulnerable [2]. While the current standard of care treatment for localized SCCA is radiation therapy (RT) with concurrent multiagent chemotherapy, questions remain if this potentially toxic and morbid treatment is appropriate for those with early-stage disease (e.g., T1–2 N0) [3–6]. In other HPV-related malignancies, such as head and neck cancer, there has been a recent emphasis placed on careful de-escalation of therapy to potentially mitigate against acute and late treatment-related toxicity while not adversely impacting patient outcomes [7]. Similarly, in SCCA, any adjustments to the currently accepted standard of care treatment that may potentially improve tolerability and reduce the risk of toxicity while delivering the same level of cancer control are welcome. This is of particular importance in early-stage SCCA, where rates of overall survival (OS) and disease-free survival (DFS) at 5 years are anticipated to be 86% and 80%, respectively, following treatment for patients with T2 N0 disease based on the results of RTOG-9811 [8]. Further, progress in imaging, resulting in better detection of metastatic or locally advanced disease [9,10], adds an additional layer of complexity in interpreting the results of earlier studies and evaluating treatment of patients considered to have early-stage disease. In this review, we will summarize the available literature focused on de-escalation of therapy for early-stage SCCA, including modifications in treatment modality as well as alterations in the currently accepted standard of care. We will also discuss modifications to standard chemoradiation (CRT) to decrease toxicity and ongoing prospective clinical trials that seek to finally define the role of de-escalation of therapy for early-stage SCCA.

2. Chemoradiation versus Radiation Therapy Alone

Organ preservation therapy for SCCA was borne out of the pioneering work of Norman Nigro, who first used preoperative chemotherapy and radiation therapy (RT) to convert unresectable patients to resectable and incidentally found high response rates at the time of surgery, prompting him to ultimately forego resection [11,12]. Initial reports showed favorable outcomes with both RT alone as well as CRT. However, CRT was secured as the standard of care treatment for localized SCCA following two key trials, namely the United Kingdom Coordinating Committee on Cancer Research (UKCCCR) Anal Cancer Trial (ACT I) and the European Organization for Research and Treatment of Cancer (EORTC) trial [13–15]. In ACT I, patients treated with CRT had a reduced risk of local failure and death from anal cancer compared to the RT alone arm [13]. On long-term follow-up, CRT remained associated with a reduction in the risk of locoregional relapse, improved relapse-free and colostomy-free survival (CFS), and a reduction in the risk of dying from SCCA [15]. The outcomes of the EORTC trial were similar, with CRT resulting in improved locoregional recurrence (LRR) rates and colostomy-free interval compared to RT alone [14]. In ACT I, more acute toxicity was observed in the CRT group, with similar rates of late toxicity between the two arms [13]. While nearly 40% of patients randomized on ACT I had T1–2 N0 disease [16], patients with similar early-stage disease were excluded from the EORTC trial [14] making decisive treatment decisions challenging for this patient population. It is important to highlight that patients included in ACT I underwent essentially clinical staging alone, potentially limiting any conclusions about treatment of early-stage patients included in this trial compared to contemporary treatment that incorporates modern imaging.

Given the limited number of patients with early-stage disease included in the randomized trials that defined CRT as the standard of care for localized SCCA, questions remain as to whether RT alone is sufficient treatment for the smaller proportion of patients with early-stage disease. A summary of select studies reporting on RT alone for early-stage SCCA is shown in Table 1. In a subset analysis of patients with T1–2 N0 disease included on ACT I, a clear advantage in treatment of these patients with CRT compared to RT alone was observed for local failure (RR = 0.49, 95% CI 0.29–0.71, p = 0.0005) [16]. However, multiple retrospective series have shown favorable results using RT alone, particularly in those with early-stage disease [17–19]. A small series of 69 patients from 17 French institutions evaluated outcomes of patients with either Tis or T1 SCCA with tumor size $\leq$1 cm found on clinical exam or endosonography treated with RT or local excision (LE) alone [20]. Of the 69 patients included in the study, three patients with Tis underwent LE alone, while the remaining 66 were treated with RT, with 26 of those patients undergoing LE before RT. Of the 66 patients who received RT, eight underwent brachytherapy alone. The 5-year OS, CFS, and DFS rates were 94%, 85%, and 89%, respectively.

Table 1. Select studies evaluating radiation therapy (RT) alone or comparing chemoradiation (CRT) to RT in early-stage anal cancer.

Author	Inclusion	Key Results
Ortholan et al. [20]	69 patients: 12 patients with Tis, 57 patients with T1, all ≤1 cm; 66 received RT, 3 Tis treated with local excision alone	91% local control in RT group; 5-year OS 94%, CFS 85%, and DFS 89%
Fallai et al. [21]	62 patients: 9 stage I, with 8 patients treated with CRT	5-year OS and LRC both 100% for stage I patients
Zilli et al. [22]	146 patients: 29 patients with T1, 117 with T2 disease; RT alone in 71 and CRT in 75	5-year LRC of 75.5% for RT vs. 86.8% for CRT, $p = 0.155$; 5-year CSS of 88.5% for RT vs. 94.9% for CRT, $p = 0.161$
De Bari et al. [23]	122 patients: 24 patients with T1, 98 patients with T2; RT alone in 52 and CRT in 70	CRT improved LC on multivariate analysis (RR = 0.34, 95% CI 0.16–0.75, $p = 0.007$)
Miller et al. [4]	3839 stage I patients: RT alone in 287 and CRT in 3552	CRT associated with a 31% reduction in the risk of death compared to RT alone (HR = 0.69, 95% CI 0.50–0.95, $p = 0.023$)
Buckstein et al. [3]	299 stage I patients: RT alone in 99 and CRT in 200	After propensity score matching, no difference in OS, CSS, CFS, or DFS between the groups.

Several smaller retrospective studies have also reported on outcomes of CRT vs. RT in patients with early-stage SCCA. Fallai et al. reported on 62 elderly (age ≥70 years) patients treated with RT or CRT for clinically staged SCCA [21]. Only 15% of patients included in the study were stage I, while 47% were stage II and 39% had stage III disease. Eight of the nine patients with stage I disease were treated with CRT with 5-year OS and locoregional control (LRC) rates of 100%. Overall, use of CRT was associated with improved 3-year outcomes, including DFS (85% vs. 46%, $p = 0.013$), local control (LC) (80% vs. 60%, $p = 0.032$), and LRC (81% vs. 61%, $p = 0.037$), but not OS (85% vs. 67%, $p = 0.3$). A review of 146 patients with T1–2 N0 SCCA treated at Geneva University Hospital in Switzerland was conducted to study the impact of concurrent chemotherapy on LRC and cancer-specific survival (CSS) [22]. Staging was completed per the treatment period, with physical examination, abdominal ultrasound, and chest radiography used initially and incorporation of abdominopelvic computed tomography (CT), transrectal echoendoscopy, pelvic magnetic resonance imaging (MRI), and fluorodeoxyglucose positron emission tomography (PET) scans for patients treated more recently. Of the patients included in the study, 80% were T2 N0 and 48% were treated with RT alone, with 91% receiving split course treatment and over half of patients receiving a brachytherapy boost to the primary tumor. The mean ± SD tumor size in the RT and CRT groups was 2.9 ± 1.2 cm and 3.2 ± 0.9 cm, respectively, $p = 0.168$. The 5-year rate of LRC for RT alone was 75.5% compared to 86.8% for patients treated with CRT, $p = 0.155$. On multivariate analysis, treatment with CRT showed a trend toward significance for LRC (HR = 2.23, 95% CI 0.95–5.23, $p = 0.065$). De Bari et al. reported on 122 patients with T1–2 N0 SCCA treated with CRT (70 patients) or RT alone (52 patients) [23]. Similar to Zilli et al., imaging for staging was dependent on the treatment time period, with only 16% of patients undergoing staging pelvic MRI. Of note, only 29% of patients treated received prophylactic inguinal irradiation, and a brachytherapy boost to the primary tumor was delivered in 68% of patients. Delivery of CRT statistically improved LC (RR = 0.34, 95% CI 0.16–0.75, $p = 0.007$).

The questionable benefit of CRT over RT alone for early-stage SCCA has also been investigated using large database studies. Buckstein et al. performed a cohort analysis comparing CRT to RT in elderly patients with stage I SCCA using the Surveillance, Epidemiology, and End Results (SEER) registry linked to Medicare [3]. The final study population consisted of 99 patients treated with RT alone and 200 patients treated with CRT. Unadjusted analysis showed that patients treated with RT alone had inferior OS at

5 years compared to those receiving CRT (61% vs. 73%, $p = 0.002$), but no difference in cause-specific survival, DFS, or rate of abdominoperineal resection was observed. Following propensity score matching, there was no significant difference in OS ($p = 0.08$) and no significant difference in the other oncologic outcomes assessed. In the matched population, CRT was associated with a higher frequency of acute toxicity but no difference in late toxicity. We sought to determine if RT alone was sufficient for treatment of patients with stage I SCCA using the National Cancer Database (NCDB) [4]. We identified 3552 stage I SCCA patients treated with CRT and 287 treated with RT alone. Patients treated with CRT were more likely to be ≥70 years old (33.1% vs. 19.7%, $p < 0.001$) and less likely to be female (63.1% vs. 71.0%, $p < 0.001$). Following propensity score matching, treatment with CRT compared to RT alone was associated with a 31% reduction in the risk of death (HR = 0.69, 95% CI 0.50–0.95, $p = 0.023$).

Talwar et al. performed a systematic review and meta-analysis comparing RT to CRT for stage I SCCA patients [5]. The authors included five retrospective studies with 3784 patients treated with CRT and 415 patients treated with RT. The 5-year OS was significantly higher for patients treated with CRT compared to RT alone (RR = 1.18, 95% CI 1.10–1.26, $p < 0.00001$). No difference in DFS between the groups was observed, although that endpoint was not reported in all of the studies included in the meta-analysis. Finally, of the studies able to report on toxicity, higher rates of both acute and late toxicity were reported in patients who received CRT.

3. Local Excision versus Chemoradiation

While the standard of care for localized SCCA is CRT, there has been some debate as to whether CRT is the optimal approach for patients with early-stage SCCA, particularly T1 N0 disease. This is because patients with T1 N0 disease represented a very small proportion of patients treated on the major randomized studies of SCCA [13,14,24–26]. The number of series that report LC results of local excision alone are few, all with a small number of patients, some including T1 and T2 tumors, and all demonstrating local recurrence rates ranging 0–60% [27–31]. In a recent retrospective study of 57 patients with T1 N0 SCCA, 13 received local excision alone and 44 received CRT [32]. Local recurrences occurred in two of the 13 patients treated with LE (15% rate, both salvaged with surgery) and one of the 44 patients with CRT. There was no difference in 5-year progression-free survival (PFS) between the two cohorts (91% vs. 83%, $p = 0.57$). A large retrospective study of patients with T1 N0 SCCA identified from the NCDB compared OS amongst 503 patients treated with local excision alone compared to 1740 patients treated with CRT from 2004 to 2012 [33]. The authors found that the use of local excision alone increased steadily during the study period from a rate of 17.3% in 2004 to 30.8% in 2012. The 5-year OS rate was similar in patients treated with local excision alone compared to CRT (85.3% vs. 86.8%, $p = 0.93$). Interestingly, a comprehensive NCDB analysis of treatment outcomes in patients with stage I SCCA from 2004 to 2015 found slightly worse OS in patients treated with excision alone compared to CRT in a propensity-score-matched cohort (4-year OS 82.8% vs. 85.6%, $p = 0.045$) [4]. While these OS data from the NCDB studies are somewhat conflicting in a statistical manner, the OS rates of 83–85% for excision alone compared to 86–87% are numerically similar and likely not clinically significant differences. Therefore, excision alone can be considered for select patients with T1 N0 disease, which is supported by the NCCN guidelines [34].

4. Modifications to Systemic Therapy

Radiation therapy with concurrent 5-FU and mitomycin C (MMC) remains the current standard of care for localized SCCA based on the results of multiple large randomized trials. The addition of MMC to 5-FU and RT was investigated in RTOG 87-04/ECOG 1289 [25]. Adding MMC improved the 4-year local failure rate (34% vs. 16%, $p = 0.0008$), DFS (51% vs. 73%, $p = 0.0003$), and CFS (59% vs. 71%, $p = 0.014$) with no significant difference in OS (67% vs. 76%, $p = 0.31$) but at the cost of increased grade 4–5 toxicity (8%

vs. 26%, $p < 0.001$). In an attempt to replace MMC, several studies compared replacing MMC for cisplatin with concurrent 5-FU and RT [24,26,35]. RTOG 98-11 was a phase III randomized trial comparing 5-FU plus cisplatin induction chemotherapy followed by RT with concurrent 5-FU plus cisplatin to RT with concurrent 5-FU plus MMC [24]. The initial results showed an improvement in colostomy rate with the use of MMC (10% with MMC vs. 19% with cisplatin, $p = 0.02$), but no difference in 5-year LR, DFS, or OS despite higher rates of severe acute grade 3–4 hematologic toxicity with MMC (61% with MMC vs. 42% with cisplatin, $p < 0.001$). At longer follow-up, DFS (67.8% vs. 57.8%, $p = 0.006$) and OS (78.3% vs. 70.7%, $p = 0.026$) at 5 years were statistically better for RT with concurrent 5-FU plus MMC compared to 5-FU plus cisplatin [35]. In addition, a trend for improved CFS (71.9% vs. 65.0%, $p = 0.05$), locoregional failure (20.0% vs. 26.4%, $p = 0.087$), and colostomy failure (11.9% vs. 17.3%, $p = 0.074$) with the addition of MMC was also reported. ACT II was a 2 × 2 factorial trial that investigated if replacing MMC with cisplatin improves response and if maintenance chemotherapy following CRT improves PFS [26]. Patients were randomized to receive either MMC or cisplatin with concurrent 5-FU and RT with or without two additional courses of 5-FU and cisplatin. No difference in 3-year PFS was observed between the MMC and cisplatin groups (HR = 0.95, 95% CI 0.75–1.19, $p = 0.63$) or in those patients receiving maintenance chemotherapy. Of note, similar toxicity was observed in the MMC and cisplatin groups.

Modifications to this standard regimen have resulted in similar rates of efficacy with potential improvements in toxicity. The replacement of 5-FU by capecitabine has been investigated in multiple smaller phase II trials and retrospective reports. A multicenter phase II pilot study was performed in the United Kingdom that investigated the use of capecitabine delivered at a dose of 825 mg/m^2 twice daily during RT instead of 5-FU using the ACT II radiation regimen (50.4 Gy with concurrent MMC 12 mg/m^2 delivered on day 1) [36]. The LC rate based on exam, imaging, or both at 6 months following completion of treatment was 90%. When evaluating compliance with treatment, 58% of patients completed both chemotherapy and RT as planned. Grade 3–4 acute toxicity was observed in 45% of patients. Oliveira et al. conducted a phase II trial consisting of 43 patient with either T2–4 N0 M0 or Tany N1–3 M0 SCCA treated with capecitabine 825 mg/m^2 twice daily during RT with a single dose of MMC 15 mg/m^2 on day 1 [37]. The primary endpoint of the study was LC at 6 months determined by clinical exam and imaging with either pelvic CT or MRI. The rate of LRC at 6 months was 86%. The main grade 3–4 toxicities were grade 3 radiation dermatitis (23.2%), grade 3 lymphopenia (11.6%), and grade 3 neutropenia (6.9%). Treatment interruption of capecitabine was required in 55.8% of patients for a mean duration of 11.2 ± 11.0 days due to primarily grade 3 radiation dermatitis and grade 2–3 hematologic toxicity.

Treatment in a larger cohort of patients receiving more modern treatment was conducted by Jones et al., who reviewed SCCA patients treated with intensity-modulated radiation therapy (IMRT) with concurrent MMC (single-dose on day 1) and either 5-FU or capecitabine from 50 centers in the United Kingdom [38]. Data from 40 centers with 147 patients were included in the study, 35.4% of whom were treated with concurrent capecitabine/MMC and 64.6% treated with concurrent 5-FU/MMC. Although limited by available data, the 1-year relapse-free rates were not significantly different between the two groups (76.2% in the capecitabine/MMC vs. 79.3% in the 5-FU/MMC, $p = 0.80$), nor were the 1-year CFS rates (77.5% in the capecitabine/MMC vs. 90.7% in the 5-FU/MMC, $p = 0.09$). While no difference was observed in overall rates of grade 3 or 4 toxicity (45% for capecitabine/MMC vs. 55% for 5-FU/MMC), less grade 3–4 hematologic toxicity was observed in the capecitabine/MMC cohort (4% vs. 27%, $p < 0.001$). A single institution series by Goodman et al. compared 107 patients with SCCA treated with IMRT and concurrent MMC (day 1 and 29 at 10 mg/m^2) with 5-FU (63 patients) or capecitabine (44 patients) [39]. The 2-year oncologic outcomes between the groups were similar, including OS (87% for 5-FU vs. 98% for capecitabine, $p = 0.12$), LRR (6.5% for 5-FU vs. 8.2% for capecitabine, $p = 0.78$), distant metastasis (14.7% for 5-FU vs. 7.6% for capecitabine,

$p = 0.26$), and colostomy rate (5% for 5-FU vs. 9% for capecitabine, $p = 0.65$). More grade 3 to 4 neutropenia was observed in the 5-FU group compared to the capecitabine group (52% vs. 20%, $p = 0.001$). Treatment breaks due to toxicity were more likely in the 5-FU group compared to the capecitabine group (41% vs. 14%, $p = 0.006$) with a median treatment duration significantly longer for patients receiving 5-FU (39 days, range 32–52 days vs. 37 days, range 32–44 days, $p < 0.001$). Finally, dose reductions were more likely in the 5-FU group (52% vs. 16%, $p < 0.001$). A meta-analysis of five trials reported pooled outcomes, including a complete response rate of 88% (83–94%) at 6 months post-treatment with an overall complete response rate evaluated at different time intervals of 91% (87–95%), with 93.5–100% of patients completing the planned RT dose [40]. This result further highlights that capecitabine is an effective and convenient alternative to 5-FU for treatment of SCCA.

Dosing of MMC has varied between North American and European trials. While in North American trials, MMC has been dosed as 10 mg/m^2 delivered in two doses, European trials typically deliver 12–15 mg/m^2 on day 1 of RT [13,14,24–26]. Reducing the dose of MMC conceivably would reduce toxicity. White et al. performed a single-institution retrospective review of 217 patients receiving definitive CRT for localized SCCA, comparing treatment outcomes and toxicity in patients who received one (154 patients) vs. two (63 patients) cycles of concurrent MMC [41]. At 2-years, no significant differences in oncologic outcomes were observed between the two groups (one vs. two cycles), including PFS (78% vs. 85%, $p = 0.39$), CSS (88% vs. 94%, $p = 0.11$), CFS (87% vs. 92%, $p = 0.51$), and OS (84% vs. 91%, $p = 0.16$). Rates of grade ≥ 2 acute toxicity were higher in the two cycle group, including overall hematologic (89% vs. 73%, $p = 0.01$), skin (97% vs. 84%, $p = 0.006$), genitourinary (19% vs. 8%, $p = 0.04$), and treatment-related death (5% vs. 0%, $p = 0.02$). While limited, the results of this study indicate that a single dose of MMC is efficacious and may result in less acute treatment-related toxicity than two cycles. Of course, this result needs to be confirmed in prospective trials.

5. Advancements in Radiation Therapy

5.1. Intensity-Modulated Radiation Therapy (IMRT)

While CRT is the standard of care for management of localized SCCA, acute toxicities of this therapy represent a major challenge for patients. Until the early 2000s, most patients were treated with conventional RT, which refers to the use of either two-dimensional (2D) or three-dimensional (3D) conformal radiation therapy (3DCRT) techniques. The field design for 2D/3DCRT generally included an anterior–posterior (AP) field and a posterior–anterior (PA) field, where the whole pelvis (superior border at L5/S1) was treated to 30.6 Gy. At that point, the superior border of the AP/PA fields was then reduced to the bottom of the sacroiliac joints to a total dose of 45 Gy. The fields would be reduced again, and the primary tumor would then receive an additional boost dose of radiation. The inguinal nodes were generally either included in the AP field by widening the field size (wide AP/narrow PA; "thunderbird technique"), or the inguinal nodes were supplemented using electrons [42,43]. While RT is intended to target the primary tumor and regional lymphatics, the conventional 2D/3DCRT techniques described above result in the irradiation of many other organs and normal tissues (small bowel, large bowel, bladder, bone marrow, genitalia, and external skin). The acute toxicities that subsequently develop from irradiation of these nontarget structures may result in radiation treatment interruptions, thereby prolonging the overall treatment time. Rates of grade 3 or higher nonhematologic toxicities are as high as 61% [13,14,35,44]. These severe acute toxicities include dermatitis, diarrhea, dysuria, and proctitis. Furthermore, grade 3 or higher hematologic toxicity rates are as high as 60% in studies that have incorporated MMC [25,35,45]. In addition to these severe acute effects of concurrent chemoradiation, long-term toxicities, such as anal stenosis, sphincter dysfunction, sexual dysfunction, and fibrosis, are common long-term effects of CRT for anal cancer. In a systematic review of the literature, Pan et al. found that the overall incidence of late gastrointestinal toxicity in over 130 studies of anal cancer ranged from 7% to 64.5%, with grade 3 and higher toxicities reported in up to 33.3% of patients [46]. The most common late toxicities were fecal incontinence (up to 44%), diarrhea (up to 27%), and ulceration (up to 23%) [46]. These severe and common acute and long-term effects of CRT for patients with SCCA underscores the need for improved radiation techniques as well as the need for de-escalation of radiation dose in appropriate situations.

Approximately 15 years ago, the first reports of IMRT for the treatment of SCCA began to emerge [47,48]. IMRT uses an inverse-planning algorithm that varies beam intensities from multiple different angles to allow the prescription dose to conform tightly around the target volumes while decreasing radiation dose to surrounding normal tissues. IMRT can be delivered with static, fixed fields or with rotational therapy (i.e., volumetric modulated arc therapy, VMAT). Early proof of principle studies demonstrated that IMRT can reduce radiation dose to surrounding structures, such as the bladder, bowel, and perineal skin, with resulting acceptable toxicity and clinical outcome profile [47,48]. There have been no randomized studies of IMRT compared to conventional radiation therapy techniques, but several retrospective studies have compared the clinical outcomes and toxicities in patients with SCCA treated with IMRT versus 2D/3DCRT [42,49,50]. The first study to compare these approaches demonstrated that, compared to patients treated with 2D/3DCRT ($N = 17$), patients treated with IMRT ($N = 29$) had less acute grade >2 nonhematologic toxicities (65% 2D/3DCRT vs. 21% IMRT, $p = 0.003$), reduced need for treatment breaks (88% 2D/3DCRT vs. 34.5% IMRT, $p = 0.001$), and shorter treatment duration (57 days 2D/3DCRT vs. 40 days IMRT, $p < 0.0001$) [42]. One of the early concerns with IMRT was that the more conformal dose to the target volumes and steep dose gradient might actually result in an increased risk of LRR. However, early results of patients treated with IMRT in these retrospective studies showed 2–3 year local–regional control rates of 87–91% compared to 57–87% with 2D/3DCRT [42,49]. Finally, in a large, retrospective study ($N = 376$ IMRT; $N = 403$ 2D/3DCRT) utilizing the Veterans Affairs database, Bryant et al. demonstrated that patients treated with IMRT had significantly lower rates of treatment breaks ≥ 5 days, increased rates of receiving both doses of MMC, and decreased risk of colostomy related to tumor recurrence or progression [50]. These authors found no difference in CSS in patients treated with IMRT vs. 2D/3DCRT.

Prospective evaluation of IMRT for SCCA has been conducted in the RTOG 0529 clinical trial [45]. In this study, dose-painted IMRT (DP-IMRT) was used to treat elective nodal volumes to a lower dose (42 Gy in 28 fractions for T2 N0 disease and 45 Gy in 30 fractions for T3–4 N0–3 disease) while simultaneously treating the gross disease to a higher dose (50.4 Gy in 28 fractions to the primary tumor for T2 N0 disease, 54 Gy in 30 fractions to the primary tumor for T3–4 N0–3 disease, 50.4 Gy in 30 fractions for gross nodal disease ≤ 3 cm, and 54 Gy in 30 fractions for gross nodal disease >3 cm). Compared to the control arm from the RTOG 98-11 study (5-FU/MMC/RT), there was a significant reduction in acute grade 2+ hematologic toxicity (73% vs. 85%, $p = 0.03$), grade 3+ gastrointestinal toxicity (21% vs. 36%, $p = 0.0082$), and grade 3+ dermatologic toxicity (23% vs. 49%, $p < 0.0001$) with DP-IMRT [45]. Long-term cancer control outcomes from this study have not yet been published.

With respect to acute hematologic toxicities, there have been a series of studies over the past 10–15 years investigating the association of radiation dose to the pelvic bone marrow (PBM) and the subsequent development of acute hematologic toxicities. These early studies demonstrated that low dose to the pelvic bone marrow (5–20 Gy) is associated with endpoints such as grade ≥ 2 hematologic toxicities [51–53]. Subsequent studies have used advanced imaging modalities now used in the staging of SCCA, including PET/CT, to identify the active portions of the bone marrow to help further facilitate bone marrow sparing [54–56]. There are now prospective data to support the use of IMRT for bone marrow sparing in an effort to reduce acute severe hematologic toxicities [57].

Recently, a couple of retrospective studies reported long-term results of treating patients with SCCA with IMRT. Investigators from the Mayo Clinic reported results of 127 patients with SCCA treated from 2003 to 2019 with IMRT with a median follow-up of 4 years [58]. The 4-year LRR was 9%. Acute grade 3+ toxicity rates were 31% hematologic,

17% gastrointestinal, and 16% dermatologic, comparing favorably with the RTOG 0529 study. Grade 3+ long-term effects were uncommon and included 3% gastrointestinal toxicity, 2% genitourinary toxicity, and 1% pain. With a median follow-up of nearly 6 years, de Meric de Bellefon et al. reported long-term results of 193 patients with SCCA treated with IMRT [59]. In a heterogeneous cohort that included 63% of patients with stage III disease, the long-term LC was excellent at 89%. With longer follow-up, these authors did find that there was a 24% rate of grade 3 late toxicities (the most common included vaginal stricture/pain with intercourse/discharge or rectovaginal fistula in 27 patients, proctitis or rectal ulcer in 14 patients, and diarrhea in 12 patients) and one patient with late grade 4 hematuria.

Taken together, these data suggest that radiation therapy with IMRT should be a standard of care for patients with localized SCCA. There is substantial evidence that has accumulated to demonstrate that acute toxicities and treatment breaks/delays are significantly lower in patients treated with IMRT compared to conventional radiation therapy techniques. In addition, more evidence has accumulated that IMRT results in at least the same cancer control outcomes compared with conventional techniques.

5.2. Adjusting Radiation Therapy Volumes

IMRT represents an avenue of radiation de-escalation by reducing the dose to surrounding critical structures. Another avenue of interest in radiation de-escalation has been omission of RT to the inguinal nodal basins in patients that present with uninvolved inguinal nodes. Irradiation of the inguinal nodes increases the risk of acute dermatologic toxicity and may also be associated with long-term complications, such as lower extremity lymphedema. However, inguinal nodal irradiation has been a component of early randomized clinical trials [24–26], though it was systematically omitted in one study [14] and left to the physicians' choice in another [60]. In order to help answer the question regarding necessity of elective inguinal irradiation, Ortholan et al. conducted a retrospective, multicenter study involving four cancer centers in south France that treated SCCA between 2000 and 2004 [61]. Patients were staged by clinical exam, ultrasound, endorectal ultrasonography, and CT without use of PET. Amongst 181 patients with uninvolved inguinal nodes, the decision to treat the inguinal lymph nodes was per the discretion of the physician: 75 received elective inguinal irradiation (45 Gy in 25 fractions) and 106 did not. The groups were well balanced with the exception that those that received inguinal irradiation tended to have larger tumors and be of younger age. The cumulative rate of inguinal recurrence was 2% in those that received irradiation vs. 16% in those that did not. When analyzed by T stage, those that did not receive inguinal irradiation had >10% risk of inguinal nodal recurrence (12% for T1–2 tumors and 30% for T3–T4 tumors).

There are some contrasting data to the Ortholan et al. study. Crowley et al. reported results of 30 patients with SCCA, none of whom had inguinal nodal or pelvic nodal involvement based on clinical exam and cross-sectional imaging, treated with CRT at a single center from 1998 to 2004 [62]. The radiation fields did not include the inguinal nodes in any cases, and all patients had T1–3 N0 disease. At a median follow-up of 41 months, there was only one patient with an inguinal nodal relapse, suggesting that omission of inguinal nodal RT may be safe. Similarly, in a study from the Samsung Medical Center in Korea, Kim et al. retrospectively reviewed 33 patients treated with CRT for SCCA between 1994 and 2013, all of whom had no inguinal nodal involvement at diagnosis based on clinical exam and CT scans in the majority of patients and pelvic MRI (42.4%) and PET (21.2%) in the minority [63]. None of these patients received elective inguinal nodal irradiation. At a median follow-up of 50 months, the authors found no cases of inguinal nodal recurrence.

While the data from these two small studies are compelling, the data from Ortholan et al. strongly suggest that all patients with T3–4 disease should receive inguinal irradiation. At this time, there is insufficient data to suggest that omission of inguinal nodal irradiation is safe even for T1–2 tumors, especially in light of the 12% risk of inguinal nodal relapse seen in these patients in the Ortholan et al. study. However, in the modern era with excellent staging techniques, including use of PET/CT, prospective evaluation of omission of inguinal nodal RT or lower doses of inguinal nodal RT is worthy of study in low-risk patients (T1–2 N0).

5.3. Adjusting Radiation Therapy Dose

Finally, another method of radiation de-escalation is to lower the total RT dose to some or all of the target volumes. In the original Nigro protocol [12], the RT dose described was 3000 cGy in 15 fractions to the full pelvis along with 5-FU/MMC and was intended to be given as preoperative therapy prior to APR. In all three of the patients initially described, the tumor had a complete clinical response. Subsequent updates in larger patient numbers continued this approach of 3000 cGy in 15 fractions with 5-FU/MMC and showed excellent LC rates [11,64]. The approach of lowering the total dose may be adequate for smaller tumors. For instance, Smith et al. reported results of 42 consecutive patients treated with 30 Gy/15 fractions along with 5-FU/MMC [65]. The LC was 90% for patients with T1–2 tumors but only 38% for patients with T3–4 disease. In a separate series of 21 patients with T1 N0 disease based on clinical exam and CT treated with 30 Gy/15 fractions + 5-FU/MMC, Hatfield et al. found that only one patient experienced a local relapse at a median follow-up of 42 months [66]. In addition to treating these patients with reduced-dose RT, 18 of the 21 patients also had treatment fields that were of smaller volume encompassing the gross tumor with a 3 cm margin in all directions as opposed to larger fields that encompassed the whole pelvis. The approach of reduced-dose RT has also been examined by Charnley et al. in a group of elderly patients (>75 years old) with poor performance status precluding the use of standard-dose CRT [67]. In this retrospective study, 16 patients (10 T2 N0 and 6 T3–4 N0–3; 81% completed CT scans for staging) received 30 Gy in 15 fractions to fields encompassing the gross tumor + 3 cm in all directions along with 5-FU (no MMC). Median follow-up was 16 months, and the LC rate was 73%.

In summary, there are some data for reduced-dose RT. Reducing RT dose appears to be a promising treatment strategy for patients with small, node-negative tumors (e.g., T1–2 N0) and is now the subject of at least two prospective trials. The optimal treatment approach for elderly patients and/or those with poor PS that may preclude standard-dose RT and chemotherapy regimens also remains an area worthy of future investigation.

6. Current Prospective Trials

De-escalation of therapy for early-stage SCCA is currently being investigated in multiple prospective clinical trials as summarized in Table 2. DECREASE is a clinical trial evaluating lower-dose CRT in early-stage SCCA (T1–2 (with tumor size ≤ 4 cm) N0 M0) currently accruing through the Eastern Cooperative Oncology Group (NCT04166318). Patients complete staging studies with specific criteria to assess risk of cancer involvement based on imaging modality and are then randomized to standard-dose CRT or deintensified CRT. In standard-dose CRT, the primary tumor receives 50.4 Gy, and the elective nodal regions, including the full pelvis and inguinal nodes, receive a dose of 42 Gy in 28 fractions with concurrent MMC (single dose of 12 mg/m^2) and two cycles of 5-FU or concurrent capecitabine. With deintensified CRT, the primary tumor and pelvis/inguinals receive a dose of 36 and 32 Gy in 20 fractions, respectively, for T1 N0 disease and 41.4 and 34.5 Gy in 23 fractions, respectively, for T2 N0 disease with concurrent MMC (single dose of 10 mg/m^2) and one cycle of 5-FU or capecitabine. The coprimary endpoint of the study is to determine if deintensified CRT can maintain 2-year disease control of 85% or higher while improving anorectal health-related quality of life compared to standard-dose CRT.

Table 2. Summary of current de-escalation studies for early-stage squamous cell carcinoma of the anus.

Study	Key Inclusion Criteria	Study Design/Treatment	Primary Endpoint
DECREASE (NCT04166318)	T1–2 (with tumor size ≤4 cm) N0 anal canal or anal margin squamous cell carcinoma; specific radiographic criteria for lymph node evaluation.	Randomized phase II in 1:2 fashion to standard-dose CRT vs. deintensified CRT. Doses of RT based on T stage.	To determine if deintensified CRT results in 2-year disease control ≥85% while improving health-related quality of life compared to standard CRT.
ACT 3 (ISRCTN88455282)	T1 N0 anal margin squamous cell carcinoma treated with local excision.	Nonrandomized phase II: patients with tumor margins >1 mm will undergo observation, while those with margins ≤1 mm will receive adjuvant CRT.	To assess the 3-year locoregional failure rate.
ACT 4 (ISRCTN88455282)	T1–2 (with tumor size ≤4 cm) N0 anal canal or T2 (with tumor size ≤4 cm) N0 anal margin squamous cell carcinoma.	Randomized phase II in 1:2 fashion to standard-dose CRT vs. deintensified CRT.	To assess the 3-year locoregional failure rate.

The PLATO (PersonaLising Anal cancer radioTherapy dOse) umbrella trial (ISRCTN88455282) is being conducted by Cancer Research UK and includes clinical trials ACT 3 and 4. ACT 3 is a nonrandomized phase II study evaluating local excision with selective postoperative CRT for patients with T1 N0 anal margin tumors. Patients with surgical margins >1 mm will receive no additional treatment, while those with margins ≤1 mm receive additional CRT with reduced doses (41.4 Gy in 23 fractions with single dose MMC and concurrent capecitabine) [68]. ACT 4 is a randomized phase II trial comparing reduced-dose (41.4 Gy in 23 fractions) to standard-dose (50.4 Gy in 28 fractions) CRT for patients with T1–2 (<4 cm) N0 SCCA with the goal of decreasing toxicity while maintaining high rates of LRC [69].

The dosimetric advantages of proton therapy may also be a useful method to reduce toxicity and spare adjacent organs at risk in the management of SCCA. Use of proton therapy to treat localized SCCA while sparing the pelvic kidney in transplant recipients has been reported in a small case series [70]. In a multi-institutional single-arm pilot study, patients with localized SCCA were treated with pencil beam scanning proton beam RT with concurrent 5-FU and MMC [71]. Of the 25 patients enrolled in the protocol, 23 completed treatment per protocol. The primary endpoint was feasibility of combination treatment with a grade 3+ dermatologic toxicity rate less than 48% (from RTOG 98–11). The grade 3+ radiation dermatitis rate was 24% with an overall clinical complete response rate of 88%. There are two ongoing trials investigating the use of proton beam therapy for SCCA. One study is a pilot study in patients with locally advanced disease evaluating the feasibility of intensity-modulated proton beam therapy with concurrent 5-FU and MMC to reduce toxicity in SCCA, being conducted at the University of Cincinnati (NCT03018418). The primary endpoint of the study is to evaluate rates of grade 3+ acute hematologic, gastrointestinal, genitourinary, and dermatologic toxicity. The second study is a phase II feasibility trial at MD Anderson Cancer Center (NCT03690921) investigating the use of linear energy transfer-optimized intensity-modulated proton therapy for definitive chemoradiation (concurrent cisplatin and 5-FU) of stages I–III SCCA. The primary endpoint is physician-reported grade 3+ gastrointestinal, genitourinary, and hematologic toxicity. If the results of such studies are promising, proton beam therapy may be another method to further reduce toxicity in the treatment of patients with early-stage SCCA.

7. Conclusions

Determining appropriate de-escalation of therapy for early-stage SCCA is of utmost importance given the aging population at risk of this malignancy and is an active area of clinical investigation, with multiple currently enrolling critical clinical trials. While the results of these trials will start to shed light on the appropriate use of reducing intensity of treatment in the general population of early-stage patients, additional questions remain regarding the optimal treatment of the elderly or those with a less favorable performance status. Perhaps future studies will take advantage of advances in radiation delivery, such as proton beam therapy and novel biomarkers, to further customize therapy and in turn reduce toxicity in these favorable prognosis early-stage SCCA patients.

Author Contributions: Conceptualization, E.M. and J.B.; writing—original draft preparation, E.M. and J.B.; writing—review and editing, E.M. and J.B. Both authors have read and agreed to the published version of the manuscript.

Funding: This publication was supported in part by the National Institutes of Health, [Grant Number P30 CA16058].

Data Availability Statement: The data presented in this study are available in this article.

Conflicts of Interest: J.B. declares no conflict of interest. E.M. is the Alliance Champion for ECOG-ACRIN EA2182, the DECREASE study.

References

1. Siegel, R.L.; Miller, K.D.; Jemal, A. Cancer statistics, 2020. *CA Cancer J. Clin.* **2020**, *70*, 7–30. [CrossRef]
2. Deshmukh, A.; Suk, R.; Shiels, M.S.; Sonawane, K.; Nyitray, A.G.; Liu, Y.; Gaisa, M.M.; Palefsky, J.M.; Sigel, K. Recent Trends in Squamous Cell Carcinoma of the Anus Incidence and Mortality in the United States, 2001–2015. *J. Natl. Cancer Inst.* **2020**, *112*, 829–838. [CrossRef]
3. Buckstein, M.; Arens, Y.; Wisnivesky, J.; Gaisa, M.; Goldstone, S.; Sigel, K. A Population-Based Cohort Analysis of Chemoradiation Versus Radiation Alone for Definitive Treatment of Stage I Anal Cancer in Older Patients. *Dis. Colon Rectum* **2018**, *61*, 787–794. [CrossRef]
4. Miller, E.; Nalin, A.; Pardo, D.D.; Arnett, A.; Abushahin, L.; Husain, S.; Jin, N.; Williams, T.; Bazan, J. Stage I Squamous Cell Carcinoma of the Anus: Is Radiation Therapy Alone Sufficient Treatment? *Cancers* **2020**, *12*, 3248. [CrossRef]
5. Talwar, G.; Daniel, R.; McKechnie, T.; Levine, O.; Eskicioglu, C. Radiotherapy alone versus chemoradiotherapy for stage I anal squamous cell carcinoma: A systematic review and meta-analysis. *Int. J. Color. Dis.* **2021**, 1–12. [CrossRef]
6. Youssef, I.; Osborn, V.; Lee, A.; Katsoulakis, E.; Kavi, A.; Choi, K.; Safdieh, J.; Schreiber, D. Survival benefits and predictors of use of chemoradiation compared with radiation alone for early stage (T1-T2N0) anal squamous cell carcinoma. *J. Gastrointest. Oncol.* **2019**, *10*, 616–622. [CrossRef] [PubMed]
7. Mehanna, H.; Rischin, D.; Wong, S.J.; Gregoire, V.; Ferris, R.; Waldron, J.; Le, Q.-T.; Forster, M.; Gillison, M.; Laskar, S.; et al. De-Escalation After DE-ESCALATE and RTOG 1016: A Head and Neck Cancer InterGroup Framework for Future De-Escalation Studies. *J. Clin. Oncol.* **2020**, *38*, 2552–2557. [CrossRef]
8. Gunderson, L.L.; Moughan, J.; Ajani, J.A.; Pedersen, J.E.; Winter, K.A.; Benson, A.B.; Thomas, C.R.; Mayer, R.J.; Haddock, M.G.; Rich, T.A.; et al. Anal Carcinoma: Impact of TN Category of Disease on Survival, Disease Relapse, and Colostomy Failure in US Gastrointestinal Intergroup RTOG 98-11 Phase 3 Trial. *Int. J. Radiat. Oncol.* **2013**, *87*, 638–645. [CrossRef] [PubMed]
9. Cotter, S.E.; Grigsby, P.W.; Siegel, B.A.; Dehdashti, F.; Malyapa, R.S.; Fleshman, J.W.; Birnbaum, E.H.; Wang, X.; Abbey, E.; Tan, B.; et al. FDG-PET/CT in the evaluation of anal carcinoma. *Int. J. Radiat. Oncol.* **2006**, *65*, 720–725. [CrossRef]
10. Roach, S.; Hulse, P.; Moulding, F.; Wilson, R.; Carrington, B. Magnetic resonance imaging of anal cancer. *Clin. Radiol.* **2005**, *60*, 1111–1119. [CrossRef]
11. Leichman, L.; Nigro, N.; Vaitkevicius, V.K.; Considine, B.; Buroker, T.; Bradley, G.; Seydel, H.G.; Olchowski, S.; Cummings, G.; Leichman, C.; et al. Cancer of the anal canal. Model for preoperative adjuvant combined modality therapy. *Am. J. Med.* **1985**, *78*, 211–215. [CrossRef]
12. Nigro, N.D.; Vaitkevicius, V.K.; Considine, B. Combined therapy for cancer of the anal canal. *Dis. Colon Rectum* **1974**, *17*, 354–356. [CrossRef] [PubMed]
13. Epidermoid anal cancer: Results from the UKCCCR randomised trial of radiotherapy alone versus radiotherapy, 5-fluorouracil, and mitomycin. UKCCCR Anal Cancer Trial Working Party. UK Co-ordinating Committee on Cancer Research. *Lancet* **1996**, *348*, 1049–1054. [CrossRef]

14. Bartelink, H.; Roelofsen, F.; Eschwege, F.; Rougier, P.; Bosset, J.F.; Gonzalez, D.G.; Peiffert, D.; Van Glabbeke, M.; Pierart, M. Concomitant radiotherapy and chemotherapy is superior to radiotherapy alone in the treatment of locally advanced anal cancer: Results of a phase III randomized trial of the European Organization for Research and Treatment of Cancer Radiotherapy and Gastrointestinal Cooperative Groups. *J. Clin. Oncol.* **1997**, *15*, 2040–2049. [CrossRef] [PubMed]
15. Northover, J.; Glynne-Jones, R.; Sebag-Montefiore, D.; James, R.; Meadows, H.; Wan, S.; Jitlal, M.; Ledermann, J. Chemoradiation for the treatment of epidermoid anal cancer: 13-year follow-up of the first randomised UKCCCR Anal Cancer Trial (ACT I). *Br. J. Cancer* **2010**, *102*, 1123–1128. [CrossRef]
16. Northover, J.; Meadows, H.; Ryan, C.; Gray, R. Combined radiotherapy and chemotherapy for anal cancer. *Lancet* **1997**, *349*, 205–206. [CrossRef]
17. Deniaud-Alexandre, E.; Touboul, E.; Tiret, E.; Sezeur, A.; Houry, S.; Gallot, D.; Parc, R.; Huang, R.; Qu, S.-H.; Huart, J.; et al. Results of definitive irradiation in a series of 305 epidermoid carcinomas of the anal canal. *Int. J. Radiat. Oncol.* **2003**, *56*, 1259–1273. [CrossRef]
18. James, R.D.; Pointon, R.S.; Martin, S. Local radiotherapy in the management of squamous carcinoma of the anus. *BJS* **1985**, *72*, 282–285. [CrossRef]
19. Newman, G.; Calverley, D.; Acker, B.; Manji, M.; Haya, J.; Flores, A. The management of carcinoma of the anal canal by external beam radiotherapy, experience in Vancouver 1971–1988. *Radiother. Oncol.* **1992**, *25*, 196–202. [CrossRef]
20. Ortholan, C.; Ramaioli, A.; Peiffert, D.; Lusinchi, A.; Romestaing, P.; Chauveinc, L.; Touboul, E.; Peignaux, K.; Bruna, A.; De La Roche, G.; et al. Anal canal carcinoma: Early-stage tumors ≤10 mm (T1 or Tis): Therapeutic options and original pattern of local failure after radiotherapy. *Int. J. Radiat. Oncol.* **2005**, *62*, 479–485. [CrossRef]
21. Fallai, C.; Cerrotta, A.; Valvo, F.; Badii, D.; Olmi, P. Anal carcinoma of the elderly treated with radiotherapy alone or with concomitant radio-chemotherapy. *Crit. Rev. Oncol.* **2007**, *61*, 261–268. [CrossRef]
22. Zilli, T.; Schick, U.; Ozsahin, M.; Gervaz, P.; Roth, A.D.; Allal, A.S. Node-negative T1–T2 anal cancer: Radiotherapy alone or concomitant chemoradiotherapy? *Radiother. Oncol.* **2012**, *102*, 62–67. [CrossRef]
23. De Bari, B.; Lestrade, L.; Pommier, P.; Maddalo, M.; Buglione, M.; Magrini, S.M.; Carrie, C. Could Concomitant Radio-Chemotherapy Improve the Outcomes of Early-Stage Node Negative Anal Canal Cancer Patients? A Retrospective Analysis of 122 Patients. *Cancer Investig.* **2015**, *33*, 114–120. [CrossRef]
24. Ajani, J.A.; Winter, K.A.; Gunderson, L.L.; Pedersen, J.; Benson, A.B.; Thomas, C.R.; Mayer, R.J.; Haddock, M.G.; Rich, T.A.; Willett, C. Fluorouracil, Mitomycin, and Radiotherapy vs Fluorouracil, Cisplatin, and Radiotherapy for Carcinoma of the Anal Canal. *JAMA* **2008**, *299*, 1914–1921. [CrossRef]
25. Flam, M.; John, M.; Pajak, T.F.; Petrelli, N.; Myerson, R.; Doggett, S.; Quivey, J.; Rotman, M.; Kerman, H.; Coia, L.; et al. Role of mitomycin in combination with fluorouracil and radiotherapy, and of salvage chemoradiation in the definitive nonsurgical treatment of epidermoid carcinoma of the anal canal: Results of a phase III randomized intergroup study. *J. Clin. Oncol.* **1996**, *14*, 2527–2539. [CrossRef]
26. James, R.D.; Glynne-Jones, R.; Meadows, H.M.; Cunningham, D.; Myint, A.S.; Saunders, M.P.; Maughan, T.; McDonald, A.; Essapen, S.; Leslie, M.; et al. Mitomycin or cisplatin chemoradiation with or without maintenance chemotherapy for treatment of squamous-cell carcinoma of the anus (ACT II): A randomised, phase 3, open-label, 2×2 factorial trial. *Lancet Oncol.* **2013**, *14*, 516–524. [CrossRef]
27. Alfa-Wali, M.; Pria, A.D.; Nelson, M.; Tekkis, P.; Bower, M. Surgical excision alone for stage T1 anal verge cancers in people living with HIV. *Eur. J. Surg. Oncol. (EJSO)* **2016**, *42*, 813–816. [CrossRef] [PubMed]
28. Boman, B.M.; Moertel, C.G.; O'Connell, M.J.; Scott, M.; Weiland, L.H.; Beart, R.W.; Gunderson, L.L.; Spencer, R.J. Carcinoma of the anal canal, a clinical and pathologic study of 188 cases. *Cancer* **1984**, *54*, 114–125. [CrossRef]
29. Faynsod, M.; Vargas, H.I.; Tolmos, J.; Udani, V.M.; Dave, S.; Arnell, T.; Stabile, B.E.; Stamos, M.J. Patterns of recurrence in anal canal carcinoma. *Arch. Surg.* **2000**, *135*, 1090–1095. [CrossRef]
30. Frost, D.B.; Richards, P.C.; Montague, E.D.; Giacco, G.G.; Martin, R.G. Epidermoid cancer of the anorectum. *Cancer* **1984**, *53*, 1285–1293. [CrossRef]
31. Klas, J.V.; Rothenberger, D.A.; Wong, W.D.; Madoff, R.D. Malignant tumors of the anal canal: The spectrum of disease, treatment, and outcomes. *Cancer* **1999**, *85*, 1686–1693. [CrossRef]
32. Chakrabarti, S.; Jin, Z.; Huffman, B.M.; Yadav, S.; Graham, R.P.; Lam-Himlin, R.M.; Lightner, A.L.; Hallemeier, C.L.; Mahipal, A. Local excision for patients with stage I anal canal squamous cell carcinoma can be curative. *J. Gastrointest. Oncol.* **2019**, *10*, 171–178. [CrossRef]
33. Chai, C.Y.; Cao, H.S.T.; Awad, S.; Massarweh, N.N. Management of Stage I Squamous Cell Carcinoma of the Anal Canal. *JAMA Surg.* **2018**, *153*, 209–215. [CrossRef]
34. NCCN Clinical Practice Guidelines in Oncology: Anal Carcinoma. Version 1.2021. Available online: www.nccn.org/professionals/physician_gls/pdf/anal.pdf (accessed on 8 April 2021).
35. Gunderson, L.L.; Winter, K.A.; Ajani, J.A.; Pedersen, J.E.; Moughan, J.; Benson, A.B., Jr, C.R.T.; Mayer, R.J.; Haddock, M.G.; Rich, T.A.; et al. Long-Term Update of US GI Intergroup RTOG 98-11 Phase III Trial for Anal Carcinoma: Survival, Relapse, and Colostomy Failure With Concurrent Chemoradiation Involving Fluorouracil/Mitomycin Versus Fluorouracil/Cisplatin. *J. Clin. Oncol.* **2012**, *30*, 4344–4351. [CrossRef]

36. Glynne-Jones, R.; Meadows, H.; Wan, S.; Gollins, S.; Leslie, M.; Levine, E.; McDonald, A.C.; Myint, S.; Samuel, L.; Sebag-Montefiore, D. EXTRA—A Multicenter Phase II Study of Chemoradiation Using a 5 Day per Week Oral Regimen of Capecitabine and Intravenous Mitomycin C in Anal Cancer. *Int. J. Radiat. Oncol.* **2008**, *72*, 119–126. [CrossRef] [PubMed]
37. Oliveira, S.C.R.; Moniz, C.M.V.; Riechelmann, R.P.; Alex, A.K.; Braghirolli, M.I.; Bariani, G.; Nahas, C.S.R.; Hoff, P.M.G. Phase II Study of Capecitabine in Substitution of 5-FU in the Chemoradiotherapy Regimen for Patients with Localized Squamous Cell Carcinoma of the Anal Canal. *J. Gastrointest. Cancer* **2016**, *47*, 75–81. [CrossRef] [PubMed]
38. Jones, C.M.; Adams, R.; Downing, A.; Glynne-Jones, R.; Harrison, M.; Hawkins, M.; Sebag-Montefiore, D.; Gilbert, D.C.; Muirhead, R. Toxicity, Tolerability, and Compliance of Concurrent Capecitabine or 5-Fluorouracil in Radical Management of Anal Cancer With Single-dose Mitomycin-C and Intensity Modulated Radiation Therapy: Evaluation of a National Cohort. *Int. J. Radiat. Oncol.* **2018**, *101*, 1202–1211. [CrossRef] [PubMed]
39. Goodman, K.A.; Julie, D.; Cercek, A.; Cambridge, L.; Woo, K.M.; Zhang, Z.; Wu, A.J.; Reidy, D.L.; Segal, N.H.; Stadler, Z.K.; et al. Capecitabine With Mitomycin Reduces Acute Hematologic Toxicity and Treatment Delays in Patients Undergoing Definitive Chemoradiation Using Intensity Modulated Radiation Therapy for Anal Cancer. *Int. J. Radiat. Oncol.* **2017**, *98*, 1087–1095. [CrossRef]
40. Souza, K.T.; Pereira, A.; Araujo, R.L.; Oliveira, S.C.R.; Hoff, P.M.; Riechelmann, R.P. Replacing 5-fluorouracil by capecitabine in localised squamous cell carcinoma of the anal canal: Systematic review and meta-analysis. *Ecancermedicalscience* **2016**, *10*, 699. [CrossRef]
41. White, E.C.; Goldman, K.; Aleshin, A.; Lien, W.W.; Rao, A.R. Chemoradiotherapy for squamous cell carcinoma of the anal canal: Comparison of one versus two cycles mitomycin-C. *Radiother. Oncol.* **2015**, *117*, 240–245. [CrossRef] [PubMed]
42. Bazan, J.G.; Hara, W.; Hsu, A.; Kunz, P.A.; Ford, J.; Fisher, G.A.; Welton, M.L.; Shelton, A.; Kapp, D.S.; Koong, A.C.; et al. Intensity-modulated radiation therapy versus conventional radiation therapy for squamous cell carcinoma of the anal canal. *Cancer* **2011**, *117*, 3342–3351. [CrossRef]
43. Lee, N.Y.; Lu, J.J. *Target Volume Delineation and Field Setup: A Practical Guide for Conformal and Intensity-Modulated Radiation Therapy*; Springer-Verlag Berlin Heidelberg: Heidelberg, Germany, 2013.
44. Brooks, C.; Lee, Y.; Aitken, K.; Hansen, V.; Tait, D.; Hawkins, M. Organ-sparing Intensity-modulated Radiotherapy for Anal Cancer using the ACTII Schedule: A Comparison of Conventional and Intensity-modulated Radiotherapy Plans. *Clin. Oncol.* **2013**, *25*, 155–161. [CrossRef] [PubMed]
45. Kachnic, L.A.; Winter, K.; Myerson, R.J.; Goodyear, M.D.; Willins, J.; Esthappan, J.; Haddock, M.G.; Rotman, M.; Parikh, P.J.; Safran, H.; et al. RTOG 0529: A Phase 2 Evaluation of Dose-Painted Intensity Modulated Radiation Therapy in Combination With 5-Fluorouracil and Mitomycin-C for the Reduction of Acute Morbidity in Carcinoma of the Anal Canal. *Int. J. Radiat. Oncol.* **2013**, *86*, 27–33. [CrossRef]
46. Bin Pan, Y.; Maeda, Y.; Wilson, A.; Glynne-Jones, R.; Vaizey, C.J. Late gastrointestinal toxicity after radiotherapy for anal cancer: A systematic literature review. *Acta Oncol.* **2018**, *57*, 1427–1437. [CrossRef] [PubMed]
47. Milano, M.T.; Jani, A.B.; Farrey, K.J.; Rash, C.; Heimann, R.; Chmura, S.J. Intensity-modulated radiation therapy (IMRT) in the treatment of anal cancer: Toxicity and clinical outcome. *Int. J. Radiat. Oncol.* **2005**, *63*, 354–361. [CrossRef] [PubMed]
48. Salama, J.K.; Mell, L.K.; Schomas, D.A.; Miller, R.C.; Devisetty, K.; Jani, A.B.; Mundt, A.J.; Roeske, J.C.; Liauw, S.L.; Chmura, S.J. Concurrent Chemotherapy and Intensity-Modulated Radiation Therapy for Anal Canal Cancer Patients: A Multicenter Experience. *J. Clin. Oncol.* **2007**, *25*, 4581–4586. [CrossRef] [PubMed]
49. Dasgupta, T.; Rothenstein, D.; Chou, J.F.; Zhang, Z.; Wright, J.L.; Saltz, L.B.; Temple, L.K.; Paty, P.B.; Weiser, M.R.; Guillem, J.G.; et al. Intensity-modulated radiotherapy vs. conventional radiotherapy in the treatment of anal squamous cell carcinoma: A propensity score analysis. *Radiother. Oncol.* **2013**, *107*, 189–194. [CrossRef] [PubMed]
50. Bryant, A.K.; Huynh-Le, M.-P.; Simpson, D.R.; Mell, L.K.; Gupta, S.; Murphy, J.D. Intensity Modulated Radiation Therapy Versus Conventional Radiation for Anal Cancer in the Veterans Affairs System. *Int. J. Radiat. Oncol.* **2018**, *102*, 109–115. [CrossRef] [PubMed]
51. Bazan, J.G.; Luxton, G.; Mok, E.C.; Koong, A.C.; Chang, D.T. Normal Tissue Complication Probability Modeling of Acute Hematologic Toxicity in Patients Treated With Intensity-Modulated Radiation Therapy for Squamous Cell Carcinoma of the Anal Canal. *Int. J. Radiat. Oncol.* **2012**, *84*, 700–706. [CrossRef]
52. Julie, D.A.R.; Oh, J.H.; Apte, A.P.; Deasy, J.O.; Tom, A.; Wu, A.J.; Goodman, K.A. Predictors of acute toxicities during definitive chemoradiation using intensity-modulated radiotherapy for anal squamous cell carcinoma. *Acta Oncol.* **2016**, *55*, 208–216. [CrossRef]
53. Mell, L.K.; Schomas, D.A.; Salama, J.K.; Devisetty, K.; Aydogan, B.; Miller, R.C.; Jani, A.B.; Kindler, H.L.; Mundt, A.J.; Roeske, J.C.; et al. Association Between Bone Marrow Dosimetric Parameters and Acute Hematologic Toxicity in Anal Cancer Patients Treated With Concurrent Chemotherapy and Intensity-Modulated Radiotherapy. *Int. J. Radiat. Oncol.* **2008**, *70*, 1431–1437. [CrossRef]
54. Lesca, A.; Arcadipane, F.; Ragona, R.; Lesca, A.; Gallio, E.; Mistrangelo, M.; Cassoni, P.; Arena, V.; Bustreo, S.; Faletti, R.; et al. Dose to specific subregions of pelvic bone marrow defined with FDG-PET as a predictor of hematologic nadirs during concomitant chemoradiation in anal cancer patients. *Med Oncol.* **2016**, *33*, 72. [CrossRef]

55. Liang, Y.; Bydder, M.; Yashar, C.M.; Rose, B.S.; Cornell, M.; Hoh, C.K.; Lawson, J.D.; Einck, J.; Saenz, C.; Fanta, P.; et al. Prospective Study of Functional Bone Marrow-Sparing Intensity Modulated Radiation Therapy With Concurrent Chemotherapy for Pelvic Malignancies. *Int. J. Radiat. Oncol.* **2013**, *85*, 406–414. [CrossRef] [PubMed]
56. Rose, B.S.; Jee, K.-W.; Niemierko, A.; Murphy, J.E.; Blaszkowsky, L.S.; Allen, J.N.; Lee, L.K.; Wang, Y.; Drapek, L.C.; Hong, T.S.; et al. Irradiation of FDG-PET–Defined Active Bone Marrow Subregions and Acute Hematologic Toxicity in Anal Cancer Patients Undergoing Chemoradiation. *Int. J. Radiat. Oncol.* **2016**, *94*, 747–754. [CrossRef]
57. Arcadipane, F.; Silvetti, P.; Olivero, F.; Gastino, A.; De Luca, V.; Mistrangelo, M.; Cassoni, P.; Racca, P.; Gallio, E.; Lesca, A.; et al. Bone Marrow-Sparing IMRT in Anal Cancer Patients Undergoing Concurrent Chemo-Radiation: Results of the First Phase of a Prospective Phase II Trial. *Cancers* **2020**, *12*, 3306. [CrossRef]
58. Jethwa, K.R.; Day, C.N.; Sandhyavenu, H.; Gonuguntla, K.; Harmsen, W.S.; Breen, W.G.; Routman, D.M.; Garda, A.E.; Hubbard, J.M.; Halfdanarson, T.R.; et al. Intensity modulated radiotherapy for anal canal squamous cell carcinoma: A 16-year single institution experience. *Clin. Transl. Radiat. Oncol.* **2021**, *28*, 17–23. [CrossRef]
59. Bellefon, M.D.M.D.; Lemanski, C.; Castan, F.; Samalin, E.; Mazard, T.; Lenglet, A.; Demontoy, S.; Riou, O.; Llacer-Moscardo, C.; Fenoglietto, P.; et al. Long-term follow-up experience in anal canal cancer treated with Intensity-Modulated Radiation Therapy: Clinical outcomes, patterns of relapse and predictors of failure. *Radiother. Oncol.* **2020**, *144*, 141–147. [CrossRef] [PubMed]
60. Peiffert, D.; Tournier-Rangeard, L.; Gérard, J.-P.; Lemanski, C.; François, E.; Giovannini, M.; Cvitkovic, F.; Mirabel, X.; Bouché, O.; Luporsi, E.; et al. Induction Chemotherapy and Dose Intensification of the Radiation Boost in Locally Advanced Anal Canal Carcinoma: Final Analysis of the Randomized UNICANCER ACCORD 03 Trial. *J. Clin. Oncol.* **2012**, *30*, 1941–1948. [CrossRef] [PubMed]
61. Ortholan, C.; Resbeut, M.; Hannoun-Levi, J.-M.; Teissier, E.; Gerard, J.-P.; Ronchin, P.; Zaccariotto, A.; Minsat, M.; Benezery, K.; François, E.; et al. Anal Canal Cancer: Management of Inguinal Nodes and Benefit of Prophylactic Inguinal Irradiation (CORS-03 Study). *Int. J. Radiat. Oncol.* **2012**, *82*, 1988–1995. [CrossRef]
62. Crowley, C.; Winship, A.; Hawkins, M.; Morris, S.; Leslie, M. Size Does Matter: Can we Reduce the Radiotherapy Field Size for Selected Cases of Anal Cancer Undergoing Chemoradiation? *Clin. Oncol.* **2009**, *21*, 376–379. [CrossRef] [PubMed]
63. Kim, H.; Park, H.C.; Yu, J.I.; Choi, O.H.; Ahn, Y.C.; Kim, S.T.; Park, J.O.; Park, Y.S.; Kim, H.C. Can we omit prophylactic inguinal nodal irradiation in anal cancer patients? *Radiat. Oncol. J.* **2015**, *33*, 83–88. [CrossRef]
64. Nigro, N.D.; Seydel, H.G.; Considine, B.; Vaitkevicius, V.K.; Leichman, L.; Kinzie, J.J. Combined preoperative radiation and chemotherapy for squamous cell carcinoma of the anal canal. *Cancer* **1983**, *51*, 1826–1829. [CrossRef]
65. E Smith, D.; Shah, K.H.; Rao, A.R.; Frost, D.B.; Latino, F.; Anderson, P.J.; Peddada, A.V.; Kagan, A.R. Cancer of the anal canal: Treatment with chemotherapy and low-dose radiation therapy. *Radiology* **1994**, *191*, 569–572. [CrossRef]
66. Hatfield, P.; Cooper, R.; Sebag-Montefiore, D. Involved-Field, Low-Dose Chemoradiotherapy for Early-Stage Anal Carcinoma. *Int. J. Radiat. Oncol.* **2008**, *70*, 419–424. [CrossRef]
67. Charnley, N.; Choudhury, A.; Chesser, P.; A Cooper, R.; Sebag-Montefiore, D. Effective treatment of anal cancer in the elderly with low-dose chemoradiotherapy. *Br. J. Cancer* **2005**, *92*, 1221–1225. [CrossRef] [PubMed]
68. Renehan, A.G.; Berkman, L.; McParland, L.; Sebag-Montefiore, D.; Muirhead, R.; Adams, R.; Harrison, M.; Hawkins, M.; Glynne-Jones, R.; Gilbert, D.; et al. Early stage anal margin cancer: Towards evidence-based management. *Color. Dis.* **2019**, *21*, 387–391. [CrossRef] [PubMed]
69. Sebag-Montefiore, D.; Adams, R.; Bell, S.; Berkman, L.; Gilbert, D.; Glynne-Jones, R.; Goh, V.; Gregory, W.; Harrison, M.; Kachnic, L.; et al. The Development of an Umbrella Trial (PLATO) to Address Radiation Therapy Dose Questions in the Locoregional Management of Squamous Cell Carcinoma of the Anus. *Int. J. Radiat. Oncol.* **2016**, *96*, E164–E165. [CrossRef]
70. Buchberger, D.; Kreinbrink, P.; Kharofa, J. Proton Therapy in the Treatment of Anal Cancer in Pelvic Kidney Transplant Recipients: A Case Series. *Int. J. Part. Ther.* **2019**, *6*, 28–34. [CrossRef]
71. Wo, J.Y.; Plastaras, J.P.; Metz, J.M.; Jiang, W.; Yeap, B.Y.; Drapek, L.C.; Adams, J.; Baglini, C.; Ryan, D.P.; Murphy, J.E.; et al. Pencil Beam Scanning Proton Beam Chemoradiation Therapy With 5-Fluorouracil and Mitomycin-C for Definitive Treatment of Carcinoma of the Anal Canal: A Multi-institutional Pilot Feasibility Study. *Int. J. Radiat. Oncol.* **2019**, *105*, 90–95. [CrossRef] [PubMed]

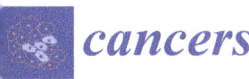

Article

Genomic Signature of Oral Squamous Cell Carcinomas from Non-Smoking Non-Drinking Patients

Kendrick Koo [1,2,3,4], Dmitri Mouradov [1,2], Christopher M. Angel [5], Tim A. Iseli [3], David Wiesenfeld [3,4], Michael J. McCullough [4], Antony W. Burgess [1,2,3] and Oliver M. Sieber [1,2,3,6,*]

1. Personalised Oncology Division, The Walter and Eliza Hall Institute of Medial Research, Parkville, VIC 3052, Australia; kendrick.koo@unimelb.edu.au (K.K.); mouradov.d@wehi.edu.au (D.M.); tburgess@wehi.edu.au (A.W.B.)
2. Department of Medical Biology, The University of Melbourne, Parkville, VIC 3052, Australia
3. Department of Surgery, The Royal Melbourne Hospital, The University of Melbourne, Parkville, VIC 3050, Australia; iselient@hotmail.com (T.A.I.); david.wiesenfeld@mh.org.au (D.W.)
4. Melbourne Dental School, The University of Melbourne, Carlton, VIC 3053, Australia; m.mccullough@unimelb.edu.au
5. Peter MacCallum Cancer Centre, Parkville, VIC 3000, Australia; christopher.angel@petermac.org
6. Department of Biochemistry and Molecular Biology, Monash University, Clayton, VIC 3800, Australia
* Correspondence: sieber.o@wehi.edu.au

Citation: Koo, K.; Mouradov, D.; Angel, C.M.; Iseli, T.A.; Wiesenfeld, D.; McCullough, M.J.; Burgess, A.W.; Sieber, O.M. Genomic Signature of Oral Squamous Cell Carcinomas from Non-Smoking Non-Drinking Patients. *Cancers* **2021**, *13*, 1029. https://doi.org/10.3390/cancers13051029

Academic Editor: Amanda Psyrri

Received: 1 February 2021
Accepted: 22 February 2021
Published: 1 March 2021

Publisher's Note: MDPI stays neutral with regard to jurisdictional claims in published maps and institutional affiliations.

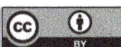

Copyright: © 2021 by the authors. Licensee MDPI, Basel, Switzerland. This article is an open access article distributed under the terms and conditions of the Creative Commons Attribution (CC BY) license (https://creativecommons.org/licenses/by/4.0/).

Simple Summary: A clinically distinct cohort of non-smoking non-drinking patients who develop oral cavity squamous cell carcinomas has been identified, with previous work suggesting that these patients tend to be older, female, and have poor outcomes. Our study characterised tumour molecular alterations in these patients, identifying differences in genomic profiles as compared to patients who smoke and/or drink. Associations between molecular alterations and other clinical and pathological characteristics were also explored.

Abstract: Molecular alterations in 176 patients with oral squamous cell carcinomas (OSCC) were evaluated to delineate differences in non-smoking non-drinking (NSND) patients. Somatic mutations and DNA copy number variations (CNVs) in a 68-gene panel and human papilloma virus (HPV) status were interrogated using targeted next-generation sequencing. In the entire cohort, *TP53* (60%) and *CDKN2A* (24%) were most frequently mutated, and the most common CNVs were *EGFR* amplifications (9%) and deletions of *BRCA2* (5%) and *CDKN2A* (4%). Significant associations were found for *TP53* mutation and nodal disease, lymphovascular invasion and extracapsular spread, *CDKN2A* mutation or deletion with advanced tumour stage, and *EGFR* amplification with perineural invasion and extracapsular spread. *PIK3CA* mutation, *CDKN2A* deletion, and *EGFR* amplification were associated with worse survival in univariate analyses ($p < 0.05$ for all comparisons). There were 59 NSND patients who tended to be female and older than patients who smoke and/or drink, and showed enrichment of *CDKN2A* mutations, *EGFR* amplifications, and *BRCA2* deletions ($p < 0.05$ for all comparisons), with a younger subset showing higher mutation burden. HPV was detected in three OSCC patients and not associated with smoking and drinking habits. NSND OSCC exhibits distinct genomic profiles and further exploration to elucidate the molecular aetiology in these patients is warranted.

Keywords: oral cancer; tobacco; alcohol; human papilloma virus; targeted sequencing; DNA copy number; *TP53*; *CDKN2A*; *EGFR*; *PIK3CA*

1. Introduction

Squamous cell carcinomas of the head and neck (HNSCC) are a heterogeneous group of cancers arising in the upper aerodigestive tract, with oral cavity cancers being the most common. HNSCC is traditionally viewed as a disease of smokers [1] and drinkers [2], but non-smoking non-drinking patients (NSND) also develop HNSCC. Chronic exposures to heavy metals from sources other than tobacco, such as contaminated food and soil, may also constitute a risk factor [3]. The human papilloma virus (HPV) is more common in oropharyngeal patients with no tobacco risk factors [4] and has a clear role in the development of oropharyngeal SCCs, but its role in oral cavity SCC (OSCC) patients without tobacco or alcohol risk factors remains poorly defined [5].

Retrospective audits of OSCC patients at our centre have revealed a larger than expected group of non-smoking (40%) and NSND (24%) patients who are predominantly female, have a bimodal age distribution, and a predilection for disease on the oral tongue. Furthermore, NSND patients with OSCC appear to have worse disease-specific mortality than smoking or drinking (SD) patients [6,7]. Other retrospective studies have also explored this NSND group, and whilst they concur that the group is more likely to be female and have oral cavity tumours, no consensus pattern in age distribution or survival outcomes has emerged [8–15]. One previous study reported poorer survival in the NSND group, but this was confined to young NSND patients [12], whilst another found a non-significant trend towards improved survival in the NSND group as a whole [11].

NSND patients are unlikely to be a homogenous group, and the suggested bimodal age distribution and adverse clinical outcomes of NSND patients highlight these patients as an important group requiring further study. Delineation of molecular alterations in NSND patients may provide insights into the aetiology of OSCC in these patients.

Recent high-throughput sequencing studies have defined the broad mutation landscape and key genomic drivers of HNSCC [16–30]. A few papers have specifically examined oral cavity tumours [20,22–24,27,29,30] but many combine HNSCC from all anatomical sites, and only a few publications separate out HPV-positive and HPV-negative tumours [16,17,19,21,28]. None of these previous papers have reported on mutations characteristic of NSND patients. A summary of principal molecular findings from previous studies of HNSCC cohorts is provided in Figure 1 [16–30]. Overall, these data highlight the central role of p53 inactivation in HNSCC development, with 60% of tumours (1187/1969, 60%) across studies harbouring *TP53* mutations. *CDKN2A* (315/1969, 16%), *PIK3CA* (302/1969, 15%), *NOTCH1* (230/1969, 12%) and *FAT1* (180/1969, 9%) constitute the next four most frequently mutated genes. HPV-positive tumours show distinct molecular profiles as compared to HPV-negative tumours, with less frequent mutations in *TP53* (4%, 10/236 vs. 68%, 1177/1733, $p < 0.001$), *HRAS* (2%, 4/236 vs. 7%, 110/1683, $p < 0.01$), *CASP8* (1%, 1/134 vs. 14%, 117/838, $p < 0.001$) and *CDKN2A* (0%, 0/236 vs. 20%, 315/1585, $p < 0.001$), and an enrichment of *PIK3CA* mutations (29%, 68/236 vs. 14%, 234/1673, $p < 0.001$). Comparing studies specific for OSCC to those including all head and neck sites, there is an enrichment for *CASP8* (28%, 82/288 vs. 5%, 36/684, $p < 0.001$) and *FAT1* mutations (30%, 87/288 vs. 14%, 93/652, $p < 0.001$).

The impact of risk factors on somatic mutation load may also contribute to the clinical course of NSND patients: Tobacco use has been associated with a distinct somatic mutation signature in HNSCC with an enrichment of C > A transversions, although this signature appears much more pronounced in laryngeal cancers than OSCC [31]. Furthermore, a mutation signature related to APOBEC cytidine deaminase editing has been identified in HPV-positive HNSCC [32]. Notably, alcohol consumption has been associated with T > C transitions in oesophageal [33] and hepatocellular [34] carcinomas, although this has not been reported for HNSCC.

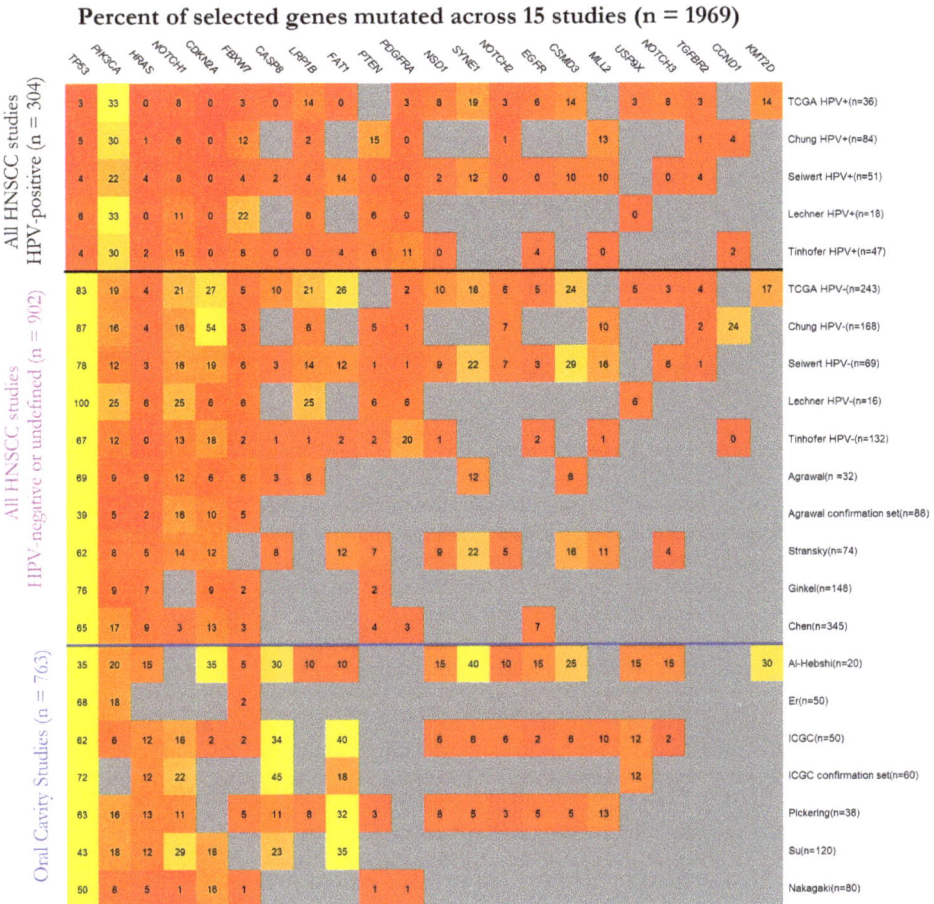

Figure 1. Summary of Squamous cell carcinomas of the head and neck (HNSCC) gene mutations reported in 15 previous studies [16–30], stratified by human papilloma virus (HPV) status as available. Studies dedicated to oral squamous cell carcinomas (OSCC) are shown separately. Percentage of patients with a gene mutation are shown; red indicates low percentages and yellow indicates high percentages. Grey boxes indicate that no data were available for that gene for a particular publication.

Apart from somatic mutations, HNSCCs exhibit significant genomic instability. Many HNSCCs show abundant DNA copy number variations (CNV), with prominent amplifications of chromosome 3q26/28 (the locus containing the *PIK3CA* oncogene), deletions of chromosome 9p21.3 (containing the *CDKN2A* tumour suppressor) as well as focal amplifications of *EGFR* and *CCND1*, and deletions of *FAT1* and *NOTCH1* [28]. There is one report on CNVs in a small cohort of non-smokers with oral tongue cancers that found no genomic differences as compared to smokers [35], but CNVs in the NSND group of HNSCC patients has not been addressed previously.

To refine our understanding of gene mutation profiles and somatic CNVs in OSCC and to elucidate potential genomic associations with tobacco and alcohol consumption, we performed targeted sequencing of 176 OSCCs from a community-based patient cohort for a panel of 68 frequently mutated HNSCC genes. To examine the involvement of HPV in OSCC from NSND and SD patients, our amplicon panel also included the genomes of the four most prevalent HPV risk subtypes (HPV subtypes 16, 18, 33, and 35). Mutation data were interrogated for associations with patient reported smoking and drinking habits, HPV status, clinicopathologic data, and survival outcomes.

2. Materials and Methods

Patients. A total of 176 patients with newly diagnosed OSCC presenting to the Royal Melbourne Hospital, Parkville, Australia, were examined. This study was approved by the relevant Human Research Ethics committees (RMH HREC 2013.087, RMH HREC 2012.071). For 103 patients diagnosed between January 2007 and August 2010, archival tumour blocks were retrieved from pathology archives. Regions of tumour with >50% neoplastic cell content were marked out by a specialist head and neck pathologist (C.M.A.) based on hematoxylin and eosin (H&E) stained sections, and macrodissected from 10 μm unstained serial sections. For 73 patients diagnosed between January 2014 and July 2016, fresh tumour and blood samples were obtained at surgery. Fresh-frozen tumour tissue was embedded in OCT medium and assessed for adequate (>50%) neoplastic cell content based on H&E-stained sections.

Disease stage at presentation was classified according to the AJCC 7th edition [36]. Patient smoking and drinking habits were recorded. Individuals who had smoked less than 100 cigarettes in their lifetime were classified as non-smokers, with all patients who were current or former smokers classified as smokers. Individuals without regular alcohol consumption (<1 standard drink per week) were classified as non-drinkers. All patients were treated by radical intent surgery and referred for adjuvant radiotherapy (with or without chemotherapy) as clinically appropriate. Clinical, treatment, and follow-up details were collected in a dedicated database, with a census date set at 1/1/2020 (minimum patient follow-up time of 3.5 years). Follow up was performed in line with current clinical guidelines, with disease-free patients discharged after 5 years.

Targeted gene panel sequencing. HNSCC somatic mutation and RNASeq data for 313 patients with oral cavity SCC were retrieved from the TCGA data portal and analysed to select genes for the curation of a dedicated 500 kb custom Agilent SureSelect XT2 amplicon panel for next-generation sequencing. Gene selection was based on mutation prevalence, RNA expression, and likelihood of contributing to oncogenesis as assessed by two previously described algorithms, OncodriveClust [37] and MutSigCV [38]. The finalised panel included 68 candidate genes, achieving a mean coverage of 95% (range 86–100%, Supplementary Table S1). To enable tumour typing for HPV status, HPV genomes for the four main high-risk subtypes (HPV subtypes 16, 18, 33, and 35) were included. DNA was extracted using the DNeasy Blood & Tissue, AllPrep DNA/RNA Mini and GeneRead FFPE extraction kits (Qiagen), according to manufacturer's instructions. Libraries were prepared using the Agilent SureSelect XT2 system and single-end sequencing performed on an Illumina Next-Seq platform.

Mutation detection. Raw data were processed and mutation calling performed using GATK software [39,40]. Local realignment and base recalibration steps were performed prior to variant calling. Identified SNPs and indels were filtered and annotated with SnpEff [41]. Mutations identified exclusively on forward or reverse reads were found to be enriched in the FFPE samples as compared to the fresh-frozen samples, a known FFPE sequencing artefact [42]. Accordingly, a strand bias filter removing any mutation calls based solely on forward or reverse reads was applied across all samples to remove such sequencing artifacts.

For fresh-frozen tumour samples, somatic mutations were identified based on the sequencing data from the matched blood samples. Matched normal samples were not available for FFPE tumour samples, and putative somatic mutations were identified by filtering against germline variants identified in the 1000 Genomes Project, the normal samples from our prospective cohort and a previously curated database created for identification of somatic mutations in colorectal cancer cell lines [43]. Pathogenicity prediction was performed using the previously published PolyPhen-2 algorithm, with scores above 0.85 considered to be likely pathogenic [44].

HPV detection. Read counts mapping to viral sequences were normalised against library size. Samples with post-normalisation read counts for any single HPV subtype of greater than 1000 were considered to be HPV-positive.

DNA copy number analysis. DNA copy number analysis was conducted using ExomeDepth [45], which has been demonstrated to be a robust technique for determination of CNVs from targeted capture sequencing data [46]. A variant of the standard ExomeDepth pipeline was used [47], whereby low mappability regions as computed for 36-mers were removed from the SureSelect probe set prior to read mapping [48], with blood samples used as a reference set.

Statistical Analysis. All statistical analyses were performed using the R software for statistical computing [49]. Differences between groups were assessed using Fisher's exact test for categorical variables and the Kruskal Wallis test for continuous variables. Mutation counts were compared between groups of interest using a generalised linear model [50]. Each gene mutated in at least 5% of patients (mutations in >10 cases) and with at least 50% of mutations assigned as likely pathogenic were correlated to clinicopathologic variables. Between-group survival differences by mutation status were assessed using Kaplan–Meier analysis and Cox-proportional hazard models adjusting for clinicopathologic variables. Overall survival was defined as time from diagnosis to death, with censoring done where patients were alive at last contact. Two-sided p-values < 0.05 were considered statistically significant.

3. Results

3.1. Patient Clinical Characteristics and HPV Status

Clinical details of 176 OSCC patients examined in this study are summarised in Table 1. A total of 82 patients had early stage (stage I/II) disease and 94 patients had local or regionally advanced disease (stage III/IV). All patients were treated with radical intent surgery and were referred for radiotherapy and/or chemotherapy following discussion at a multidisciplinary team meeting. Sixty-three percent (110/176) of patients received adjuvant radiotherapy and 22% (39/176) were treated with chemotherapy.

Clinicopathologic details and treatment delivery were similar between retrospective patients (n = 103) diagnosed between January 2007 and August 2010 and prospectively recruited patients (n = 73) diagnosed between January 2014 and July 2016. However, the proportions of non-drinkers and NSND patients were higher in the prospective cohort, consistent with the reported trend of reduced alcohol consumption among Australians over this time period [51] (Supplementary Table S2).

Presence of HPV was identified through our targeted sequencing approach in 3 out of 176 (1.7%) OSCCs (Figure 2); one case was positive for HPV-16 and two cases for HPV-33. This HPV detection rate is consistent with a previous study from our centre, which used orthogonal methods (PCR-ELISA and RNA in situ hybridization) to identify HPV [52] and all of the overlapping patients between the two studies had concordant HPV detection results (39/39 patients, 2/39 HPV-positive), supporting accuracy of targeted next generation sequencing for virus detection. As a further control, a small set of prospectively collected oropharyngeal tumours, which are known to have high prevalence of HPV infection [5], were also sequenced with 57% (4 out of 7) tumours found to be positive for HPV-16, consistent with the prevalence reported by a previous systematic review [53]. A single OSCC NSND patient (1.7%, 1/59) was HPV-positive, similar to the HPV-positive rate in SD patients (1.7%, 2/117, p = 1). There were no significant associations between HPV status and clinicopathologic variables in OSCC patients (Supplementary Table S3).

Table 1. Clinical characteristics of 176 OSCC patients in this study. Percentages for groups are shown in brackets. NSND = non-smoker and non-drinker.

Characteristic		All Patients (n = 176)
Gender	Female	76 (43.2)
	Male	100 (56.8)
Age	Median (range)	66 (33–98)
	Non-smoker	86 (48.9)
	Non-drinker	79 (44.9)
	NSND	59 (33.5)
T stage	1	39 (22.2)
	2	66 (37.5)
	3	14 (8.0)
	4	57 (32.4)
N stage	N0	115 (65.3)
	N+	61 (34.7)
AJCC stage	I	32 (18.2)
	II	50 (28.4)
	III	37 (21.0)
	IV	57 (32.4)
Perineural invasion	Present	32 (18.2)
	Absent	144 (81.8)
Lymphovascular invasion	Present	18 (10.2)
	Absent	158 (89.8)
Extracapsular spread	Present	20 (11.4)
	Absent	156 (88.6)
HPV status	Positive	3 (1.7)
	Negative	173 (98.3)
Radiotherapy	Yes	110 (62.5)
	No	66 (37.5)
Chemotherapy	Yes	39 (22.2)
	No	137 (77.8)

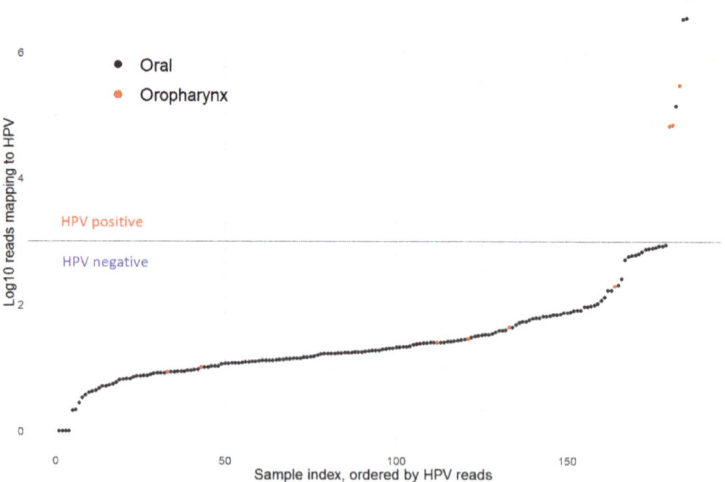

Figure 2. HPV prevalence in 176 OSCC patients for high-risk HPV subtypes 16, 18, 33, and 35 based on genomic sequencing. Tumour samples with normalised HPV read counts >1000 were considered HPV-positive. Seven oropharyngeal tumours, which are known to have a high prevalence of HPV infection, were included as control.

NSND patients were significantly older than SD patients (mean age of 70 years vs. 64 years, $p = 0.004$). However, there was evidence for a bimodal age distribution (Figure 3), consistent with our previously reported findings that included a subset of the current cohort [6]. As anticipated, a significantly higher proportion of NSND patients (73%, 43/59) were female as compared to SD patients (28%, 28/117; $p < 0.001$), while other clinical features were similar (Supplementary Table S4). NSND patients showed poorer five-year overall survival as compared to SD patients in univariate analysis (HR 1.7, 95% CI 1.0–2.8, $p = 0.05$, Supplementary Figure S1), although this was not maintained in multivariate analysis adjusting for clinicopathologic features (Supplementary Table S5).

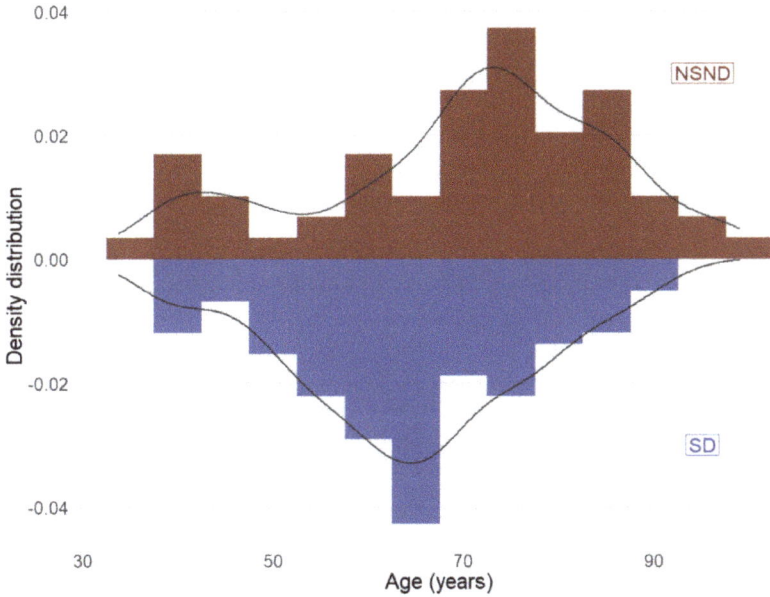

Figure 3. Age of diagnosis distribution for 176 OSCC patients by drinking and smoking status. NSND = non-smoker and non-drinker; SD = smokers and/or drinker.

3.2. Genomic Alterations and Clinical Associations for OSCC Patients

Non-synonymous somatic mutations in 68 cancer genes were identified in 93% (164/176) of OSCC patients (Supplementary Data) with similar mutation frequencies in tumours from prospective and retrospective patients ($p = 0.25$ by Kruskal-Wallis).

Seven genes had mutations in greater than 10% of samples, including *TP53* (60%, 106/176), *CDKN2A* (24%, 42/176), *FLG* (22%, 39/176), *NOTCH1* (17%, 30/176), *FAT1* (15%, 26/176), *NBPF1* (12%, 21/176), and *PIK3CA* (11%, 21/176) (Figure 4). Frequently mutated sites in key driver genes *TP53*, *CDKN2A*, and *PIK3CA* corresponded to hotspots identified by the Catalogue of Somatic Mutations in Cancer (COSMIC) database (Supplementary Figures S2–S4).

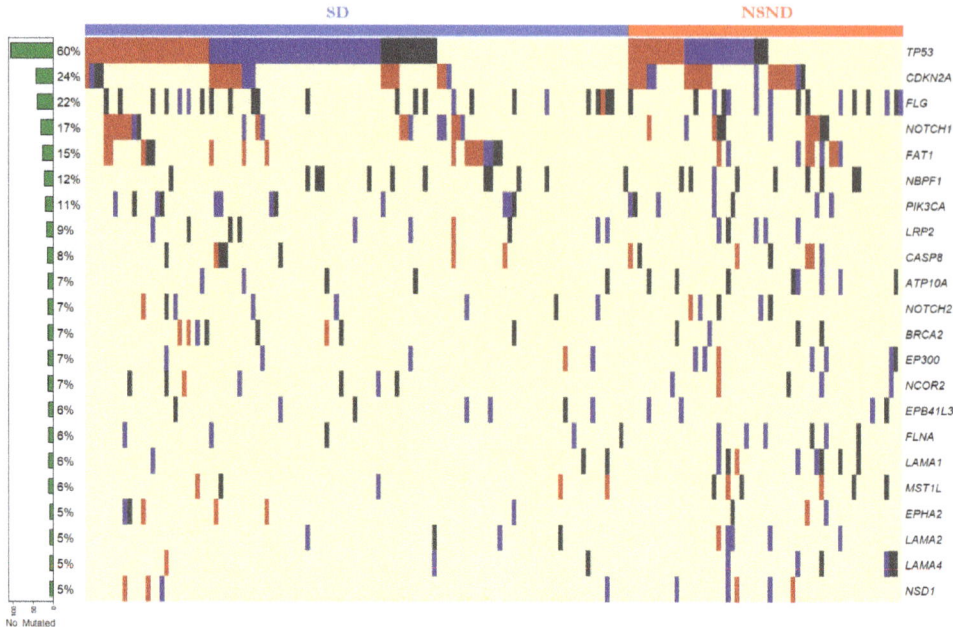

Figure 4. Mutation map for 23 candidate genes mutated in at least 5% (9/176) of tumours from OSCC patients. Nonsense and indel mutations are indicated by red bars, missense mutations with a PolyPhen-2 score > 0.85 are indicated by purple bars, missense mutations with a PolyPhen-2 score < 0.85 indicated by grey bars. The row at the bottom indicates patients with no detected mutations in the targeted sequencing panel. The colour bar at the top denotes smokers and/or drinkers (SD, blue) and non-smokers and non-drinkers (NSND, red).

Based on the predicted pathogenicity score from the PolyPhen-2 algorithm or nonsense/indel mutation status, the majority of mutations in *TP53* (85%, 91/106), *CDKN2A* (93%, 39/42), *NOTCH1* (83%, 25/30), *FAT1* (85%, 22/26), *PIK3CA* (62%, 13/21) were likely pathogenic. In contrast, smaller proportions of mutations were assigned as likely pathogenic for *FLG* (31%, 12/39) and *NBPF1* (5%, 1/21). Additionally, likely pathogenicity was assigned for the majority of mutations in 12 out of 16 genes that exhibited mutation frequencies between 5% and 10%. These genes included *CASP8* (57%, 8/14), *NOTCH2* (69%, 9/13), *EP300* (92%, 11/12), *NCOR2* (58%, 7/12), *EPHA2* (78%, 7/9), and *LAMA2* (78%, 7/9) (Supplementary Table S6). Low levels (<5%) of mutations were found in 45 genes with no mutations detected in 4 of our candidate genes.

DNA copy-number aberrations of one or more candidate genes were identified in 64% (113/176) of tumours (Supplementary Data), with fewer CNVs detected for patients in the retrospective cohort (mean 1.0, range 0–5) as compared to the prospective cohort (mean 2.0, range 0–7, $p < 0.01$), potentially related to differential algorithm sensitivity in archival versus fresh-frozen specimens. Out of CNVs identified at similar frequencies in both groups of patients, the most frequent amplifications were detected in *EGFR* (9%, 16/176), *MMP12* (6%, 10/176) and *PRKDC* (5%, 8/176), while the most frequent deletions were in *BRCA2* (5%, 9/176 patients) and *CDKN2A* (4%, 7/176) (Supplementary Table S7). Read ratios for representative samples with *EGFR* amplification and *CDKN2A* deletion are shown in Supplementary Figures S5 and S6. No deletions characteristic of EGFRvIII were identified.

A total of 17 genes were mutated in at least 5% of patients and had at least 50% of mutations assigned likely pathogenic. Associations with clinicopathologic variables were examined for these genes as well as the five genes with recurrent CNVs (Table 2).

Table 2. Univariate analysis for selected gene mutations and copy number alterations against clinicopathologic variables. "Group 1" indicates the referent variable, whilst "Group 2" indicates the comparison variable. Only comparisons where $p < 0.05$ are shown. NSND = non-smoker and non-drinker; SD = smokers and/or drinker; LN = lymph node; LVI = lymphovascular invasion; PNI = perineural invasion; ECS = extracapsular spread; OR = odds ratio, CI = confidence interval; * $p < 0.05$.

Group 1 vs. Group 2	Gene	Group 1 n (%)	Group 2 n (%)	OR (95% CI)	p
Male vs. Female	TP53 mut	67/100 (67.0)	39/76 (51.3)	1.9 (1.0–3.7)	0.043 *
	CASP8 mut	3/100 (3.0)	11/76 (14.5)	0.2 (0.0–0.7)	0.009 *
Smokers vs. Non-smokers	CDKN2A mut	15/90 (16.7)	27/86 (31.4)	0.4 (0.2–0.9)	0.033 *
Drinkers vs. Non-drinkers	CASP8 mut	4/97 (4.1)	10/79 (12.7)	0.3 (0.1–1.1)	0.050 *
	LAMA4 mut	1/97 (1.0)	8/79 (10.1)	0.1 (0.0–0.7)	0.012 *
NSND vs. SD	CDKN2A mut	21/59 (35.6)	21/117 (17.9)	2.5 (1.2–5.5)	0.014 *
	EGFR amp	10/59 (16.9)	6/117 (5.1)	3.7 (1.2–13.3)	0.023 *
	BRCA2 del	7/59 (11.9)	2/117 (1.7)	7.6 (1.4–77.8)	0.007 *
T3/4 tumours vs. T1/2 tumours	CDKN2A mut	26/71 (36.6)	16/105 (15.2)	3.2 (1.5–7.1)	0.002 *
	CDKN2A del	7/71 (9.9)	0/105 (0)	Inf (2.3–Inf)	0.001 *
	BRCA2 del	8/71 (11.3)	1/105 (1.0)	13 (1.7–590.0)	0.003 *
LN+ vs. LN−	TP53 mut	48/61 (78.7)	58/115 (50.4)	3.6 (1.7–8.1)	<0.001 *
	BRCA2 del	7/61 (11.5)	2/115 (1.7)	7.2 (1.3–73.5)	0.009 *
LVI+ vs. LVI−	TP53 mut	15/18 (83.3)	91/158 (57.6)	3.7 (1.0–20.0)	0.042 *
	NCOR2 mut	4/18 (22.2)	8/156 (5.1)	5.3 (1.0–22.9)	0.023 *
PNI+ vs. PNI−	EGFR amp	7/32 (21.9)	9/144 (6.2)	4.2 (1.2–13.9)	0.012 *
ECS+ vs. ECS−	CDKN2A mut	9/20 (45.0)	33/156 (21.2)	3 (1.0–8.8)	0.026 *
	TP53 mut	19/20 (95.0)	87/156 (55.8)	15 (2.3–633.0)	<0.001 *
	EGFR amp	5/20 (25.0)	11/156 (7.1)	4.3 (1.0–16.0)	0.022 *
	BRCA2 del	4/20 (20.0)	5/156 (3.2)	7.4 (1.3–38.4)	0.011 *

TP53 mutations were significantly associated with male gender (Male: 67/100 vs. Female: 39/76, $p = 0.043$), nodal disease (N+: 48/61 vs. N0: 58/115, $p < 0.001$), lymphovascular invasion (LVI+: 15/18 vs. LVI-: 91/158, $p = 0.042$) and extracapsular spread (ECS+: 19/20 vs. ECS-: 87/156, $p < 0.001$). CDKN2A mutations were more frequent in non-smokers (Non-smokers: 27/86 vs. Smokers: 15/90, $p = 0.033$) and NSND patients (NSND: 21/59 vs. SD: 21/117, $p = 0.014$) and associated with advanced tumour stage (T3/4: 26/71 vs. T1/2: 16/105, $p = 0.002$) and extracapsular spread (ECS+: 9/20 vs. ECS-: 33/156, $p = 0.026$). CASP8 mutations were associated with female gender (Male: 3/100 vs. Female: 11/76, $p = 0.009$) and non-drinking status (Non-drinkers: 10/79 vs. Drinkers: 4/97, $p = 0.0497$). No associations with gender, drinking status, smoking status, tumour stage, nodal involvement, LVI, ECS and HPV status were observed for FAT1 or PIK3CA mutated tumours. No HPV-positive patient (0/3) had a TP53 mutation, but this did not reach statistical significance. EGFR amplification was associated with NSND status (NSND: 10/59 vs. SD: 6/117, $p = 0.023$), perineural invasion (PNI+: 7/32 vs. PNI-: 9/144, $p = 0.012$) and extracapsular spread (ECS+: 5/20 vs. ECS-: 11/156, $p = 0.022$). Copy number loss of CDKN2A was associated with advanced tumour stage (T3/4: 7/71 vs. T1/2: 0/105, $p = 0.001$) and loss of BRCA2 was associated with advanced tumour stage (T3/4: 8/71 vs. T1/2: 1/105, $p = 0.003$), nodal disease (N+: 7/61 vs. N0: 2/115, $p = 0.009$), extracapsular spread (ECS+: 4/20 vs. ECS-: 5/156, $p = 0.011$) and NSND status (NSND: 7/59 vs. SD: 2/117, $p = 0.007$).

Univariate analysis for five-year overall survival was not significant for TP53 (Figure 5), CDKN2A, and FAT1 (Supplementary Figure S7) mutations ($p > 0.05$). Significantly poorer outcomes were observed for patients with PIK3CA mutated tumours as compared to patients with PIK3CA wild-type tumours (HR 2.0, 95% CI 1.0–3.9, $p = 0.045$) (Figure 5) although this did not remain significant in a multivariate analysis adjusting for clinicopathologic variables (Table 3). No other gene mutation was associated with a statistically significant survival difference (Supplementary Table S8). *EGFR* amplification was significantly associated with poorer survival (HR 2.7, CI 1.4–5.4, $p = 0.004$) as was *CDKN2A* deletion (HR 2.8, CI 1.1–7.1, $p = 0.026$) in univariate analyses (Figure 5), but this was not maintained when adjusting for other variables (Table 3).

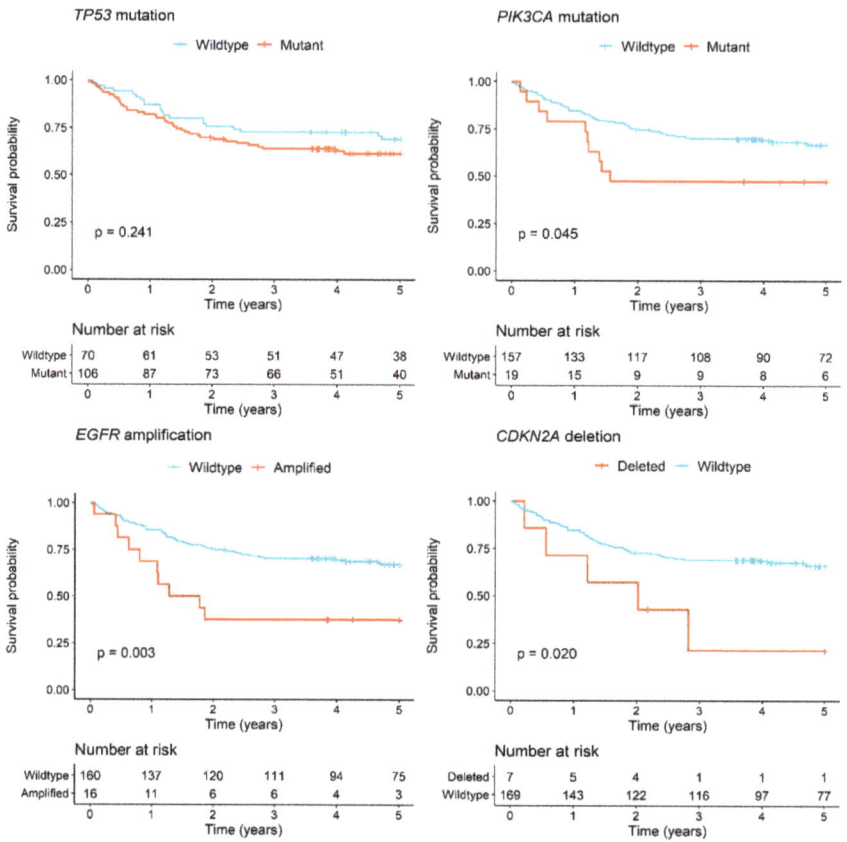

Figure 5. Kaplan–Meier survival curves for OSCC patients by *TP53* mutation, *PIK3CA* mutation, *EGFR* amplification, or *CDKN2A* deletion status. p values are for the log rank test.

3.3. Mutation Differences between NSND and SD Patients

We observed more mutated genes in non-drinkers (mean 4.3 vs. 3.4 in drinkers, $p = 0.001$), non-smokers (mean 4.2 vs. 3.4 in smokers, $p = 0.008$), and the NSND patients (mean 4.7 vs. mean 3.3 in SD patients, $p < 0.001$). The mutation spectrum comparing NSND to SD patients is visualised in Supplementary Figure S8. Examination of mutation counts identified five patients among the NSND group who had higher numbers of mutations (>12) as compared to the SD group (Figure 6).

Table 3. Univariate and multivariate Cox proportional hazards analysis assessing *PIK3CA* mutation, *EGFR* amplification or *CDKN2A* mutation and clinicopathologic variables in OSCC patients. NSND = non-smoker and non-drinker; SD = smokers and/or drinker; LN = lymph node; PNI = perineural invasion; LVI = lymphovascular invasion; HR = hazard ratio, AHR = adjusted hazard ratio, CI = confidence interval; * $p < 0.05$.

	Univariate Analysis			Multivariate Analysis		
	HR	95% CI	p	AHR	95% CI	p
***PIK3CA* Mutation**	2.0	1.0–3.9	0.050 *	1.4	0.7–2.9	0.303
Male vs. female	0.8	0.5–1.3	0.406	1.1	0.6–1.9	0.808
Age (in decades)	1.7	1.2–1.8	<0.001 *	1.6	1.3–2.0	<0.001 *
NSND vs. SD	1.7	1.0–2.8	0.050 *	1.2	0.6–2.1	0.630
T3/4 vs. T1/2	2.9	1.7–5.0	<0.001 *	2.6	1.5–4.4	0.001 *
LN+ vs. LN-	2.3	1.4–3.8	0.001 *	2.0	1.1–3.6	0.019 *
PNI+ vs. PNI-	1.7	1.0–3.1	0.064	1.5	0.8–2.7	0.211
LVI+ vs. LVI-	2.0	1.0–4.0	0.064	1.4	0.6–3.1	0.443
***EGFR* Amplification**	2.7	1.4–5.4	0.004 *	1.8	0.9–3.6	0.118
Male vs. female	0.8	0.5–1.3	0.406	1.1	0.6–1.9	0.861
Age (in decades)	1.7	1.2–1.8	<0.001 *	1.6	1.3–2.1	<0.001 *
NSND vs. SD	1.7	1.0–2.8	0.050 *	1.1	0.6–2.0	0.829
T3/4 vs. T1/2	2.9	1.7–5.0	<0.001 *	2.4	1.4–4.2	0.001 *
LN+ vs. LN-	2.3	1.4–3.8	0.001 *	2.0	1.1–3.7	0.016 *
PNI+ vs. PNI-	1.7	1.0–3.1	0.064	1.4	0.7–2.6	0.301
LVI+ vs. LVI-	2.0	1.0–4.0	0.064	1.5	0.6–3.3	0.360
***CDKN2A* Deletion**	2.8	1.1–7.1	0.026 *	1.8	0.6–5.0	0.261
Male vs. female	0.8	0.5–1.3	0.406	1.0	0.6–1.9	0.932
Age (in decades)	1.7	1.2–1.8	<0.001 *	1.6	1.3–2.0	<0.001 *
NSND vs. SD	1.7	1.0–2.8	0.050 *	1.2	0.6–2.3	0.556
T3/4 vs. T1/2	2.9	1.7–5.0	<0.001 *	2.3	1.3–4.1	0.004 *
LN+ vs. LN-	2.3	1.4–3.8	0.001 *	2.2	1.2–4.1	0.009 *
PNI+ vs. PNI-	1.7	1.0–3.1	0.064	1.5	0.8–2.8	0.172
LVI+ vs. LVI-	2.0	1.0–4.0	0.064	1.2	0.5–2.8	0.654

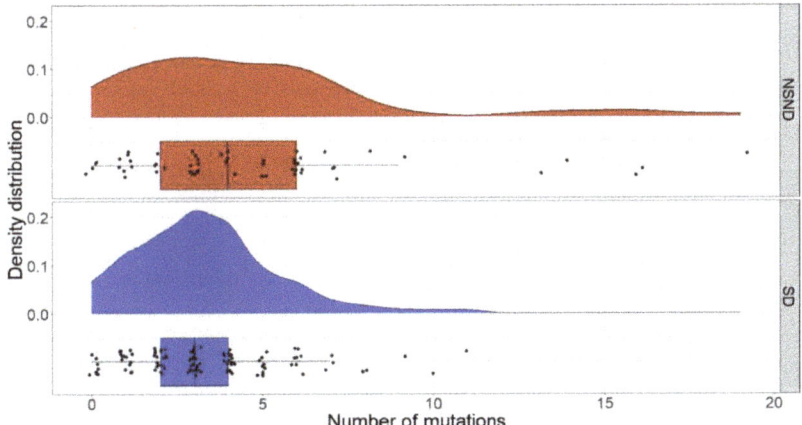

Figure 6. Distribution of mutation counts, comparing the NSND and the SD groups. NSND = non-smoker and non-drinker; SD = smokers and/or drinker.

These five patients were younger than the remainder of the NSND group (mean 53 years vs. 71 years, $p = 0.013$). The distribution of mutation types (transitions, transversions, and indels) in these five patients were compared to the distribution in other NSND patients as well as the SD group (Table 4). There was no significant difference between this high mutation group and the remainder of the NSND group ($p = 0.297$). However, compared to the SD group, there was a decrease in proportion of insertions/deletions, and an enrichment of T > C transitions ($p = 0.019$ for the NSND high mutation group, $p = 0.067$ for the NSND group as a whole). There was no evidence of enrichment of tobacco-associated enrichment of C > A transversions or alcohol-associated enrichment of T > C transitions among SD patients.

Table 4. Distribution of mutational alterations, comparing the SD group with the entire NSND group or subset of with low or high mutation load. NSND = non-smoker and non-drinker; SD = smokers and/or drinker. * $p < 0.05$.

Alteration	SD (n = 117, 434 Mutations)	NSND, All (n = 59, 366 Mutations)	NSND, Low Mutation Group (n = 54, 233 Mutations)	NSND, High Mutation Group (n = 5, 133 Mutations)
C > A	60 (13.8)	39 (10.7)	27 (11.6)	12 (9.6)
C > G	44 (10.1)	42 (11.5)	27 (11.6)	15 (12.0)
C > T	178 (41.0)	164 (44.8)	107 (45.9)	57 (45.6)
T > A	33 (7.6)	12 (3.3)	6 (2.6)	6 (4.8)
T > C	47 (10.8)	61 (16.7)	35 (15.0)	26 (20.8)
T > G	18 (4.1)	16 (4.4)	7 (3.0)	9 (7.2)
Indel	54 (12.4)	32 (8.7)	24 (10.3)	8 (6.0)
Compared to SD		$p = 0.010$ *	$p = 0.067$	$p = 0.019$ *
Compared to NSND				$p = 0.297$

4. Discussion

This study surveyed the molecular profiles of 176 OSCC patients, 34% of which were NSND patients, providing insights into the aetiology of this subgroup. HPV was excluded as a major contributor to carcinogenesis in oral cavity cancers in the NSND group, with a similar low prevalence in both this subgroup (1.7%) and SD patients (1.7%). Nonetheless, none of the HPV-positive OSCCs in this study harboured a *TP53* mutations, consistent with the well-established role of HPV E6 protein as an inhibitor of *TP53* [54].

In the context of the targeted gene panel, a subset of our NSND OSCC patients had a higher mutation burden than SD patients. This was an unexpected finding as the *a priori* expectation was that smokers/drinkers would accumulate more mutations over time as a result of carcinogen exposure. The increase in mutation burden, particularly of T > C transitions, in the NSND group could imply an underlying mutational process, but with our limited targeted sequencing, mutational signatures could not be explored in depth. An alternate hypothesis is that the oncogenes and tumour suppressor genes targeted by our sequencing panel may play a more dominant role in NSND patients. Sequencing of the entire exome or genome and replication in an independent cohort would be required to differentiate between these possibilities.

In NSND patients, the well described tumour suppressor *CDKN2A* was found to be mutated at almost twice the frequency of SD patients (35.6% vs. 17.9%), and this was also evident when comparing smokers to non-smokers. However, the frequency of *CDKN2A* deletions was not significantly different between groups (NSND: 1/59, 1.7%; SD 6/117, 5.1%). Notably, *CDKN2A* promoter methylation is another mechanism of *CDKN2A* inactivation, which is known to be common in HNSCC as a whole (20% of cases in TCGA data [28]) but could not be evaluated in our cohort. Whilst an association between smoking and *CDKN2A* inactivation has not previously been identified in OSCC, a meta-analysis in non-small cell lung carcinoma (NSCLC) has reported a positive association between p16 promoter methylation and smoking [55].

Amplification of *EGFR* was more common in the NSND group than the SD group (16.9% vs. 5.1%). Overexpression of EGFR has been found to be correlated with smoking and poorer overall survival in oropharyngeal SCC [56], and in NSCLC, *EGFR* mutations are more common in non-smokers than smokers and is clinically helpful in guiding the use of targeted therapy [57]. In a similar vein, exploration of *EGFR* as a biomarker for EGFR-directed therapy in NSND OSCC patients may be warranted. *BRCA2* deletions were more frequently identified in the NSND group than the SD group (11.9% vs. 1.7%) although the significance of these deletions is uncertain.

Our study also highlighted a number of more general molecular associations in OSCC. *TP53* mutation was associated with nodal disease, lymphovascular invasion, and extracapsular spread, consistent with previous reports in the OSCC literature [58]. Mutations and deletions of *CDKN2A* were independently associated with advanced tumour stage in our cohort and some investigators have associated *CDKN2A* copy number loss with poor prognosis in HNSCC [59], which was also observed in univariate analysis in our patients. Finally, *EGFR* amplification was associated with poor overall survival in univariate analysis and was associated with perineural invasion and extracapsular spread. Extracapsular spread has previously been associated with *EGFR* amplification [60] or high expression levels of EGFR [61,62], as has perineural invasion [63]. Whilst overexpression of EGFR has been associated with worse survival in oropharyngeal cancers [56], previous work has not identified an association between *EGFR* amplification and survival [64]. Finally, *PIK3CA* mutations were found to be associated with poor prognosis in OSCC patients in univariate analysis, which has previously been reported in a cohort of HPV-positive oropharyngeal SCCs [65].

Caveats of our study are that tobacco and alcohol histories were self-reported and exposure to second-hand tobacco is difficult to quantify, which may lead to some erroneous classifications of NSND status. The cohort size in our study was limited although molecular findings were broadly consistent with the OSCC literature. Our survey of molecular alterations was limited to a panel of genes, precluding more detailed examination of mutation signatures or larger-scale DNA copy-number or structural alterations that may drive oncogenesis in the NSND group. In addition, transcriptomic and epigenomic alterations may contribute to OSCC in NSND patients. Examination of independent cohorts will be required to validate our findings. As the proportion of NSND HNSCC patients is relatively small, this will likely require aggregation of clinically annotated HNSCC sequencing datasets across multiple institutions.

5. Conclusions

In summary, we have excluded HPV as a primary driver underlying oral carcinogenesis in NSND patients and have identified significant molecular differences between the NSND and SD groups in OSCC including cancer gene alterations and mutation burden based on our targeted gene panel. Further studies are warranted to elucidate the molecular aetiology of OSCC in NSND patients.

Supplementary Materials: The following are available online at https://www.mdpi.com/2072-6694/13/5/1029/s1: Supplementary Table S1. Coverage statistics for the Agilent®SureSelect XT2 amplicon panel for 68 selected candidate HNSCC genes, Supplementary Table S2. Clinical characteristics of 73 prospective and 103 retrospective OSCC patients, Supplementary Table S3. Clinical characteristics of HPV-negative OSCC patients compared against HPV-positive patients, Supplementary Table S4. Clinical characteristics of OSCC patients in the NSND group compared to the SD group, Supplementary Table S5. Univariate and multivariate and Cox proportional hazards analyses assessing smoking/drinking status and clinicopathologic variables in 176 OSCC patients, Supplementary Table S6. Pathogenicity predictions by the PolyPhen-2 algorithm for missense mutations detected in tumours from 176 OSCC patients, Supplementary Table S7. Gene amplifications and deletions in 176 OSCC patients as determined by ExomeDepth, Supplementary Table S8. Univariate and multivariate and Cox proportional hazards analyses assessing genes mutated in at least 5% of OSCC patients, Supplementary Figure S1. Kaplan-Meier survival curves for 176 OSCC patients by smoking/drinking status, Supplementary Figure S2. Amino acid positions for TP53 mutations detected in our OSCC cohort against mutations reported for aerodigestive tumours in the COSMIC database, Supplementary Figure S3. Amino acid positions for CDKN2A mutations detected in our OSCC cohort against mutations reported for aerodigestive tumours in the COSMIC database, Supplementary Figure S4. Amino acid positions for PIK3CA mutations detected in our OSCC cohort against mutations reported for aerodigestive tumours in the COSMIC database, Supplementary Figure S5. ExomeDepth CNV plot for a representative OSCC sample with a detected EGFR amplification, Supplementary Figure S6. ExomeDepth CNV plot for a representative OSCC sample with a detected CDKN2A deletion, Supplementary Figure S7. Kaplan-Meier survival curves for 176 OSCC patients by CDKN2A, FAT1, NOTCH1 or CASP8 mutation status, Supplementary Figure S8. Spectrum of missense mutations in OSCC tumours from NSND patients as compared to SD patients: Supplementary_Figures_Tables.docx. Supplementary Data. Somatic mutations and DNA copy number variants detected in 176 OSCC patients: Supplementary_Data.xlsx.

Author Contributions: Conceptualization, K.K., D.W., T.A.I., M.J.M., O.M.S. and A.W.B.; methodology, K.K., D.M., O.M.S. and A.W.B.; software, K.K. and D.M.; formal analysis, K.K. and D.M.; investigation, K.K., D.M. and C.M.A., resources, D.W., C.M.A., T.A.I., O.M.S. and A.W.B.; data curation, K.K. and D.M.; writing—original draft preparation, K.K.; writing—review and editing, O.M.S., A.W.B., M.J.M., D.W., T.A.I. and D.M.; supervision, A.W.B., O.M.S. and M.J.M.; funding acquisition, A.W.B. and D.W. All authors have read and agreed to the published version of the manuscript.

Funding: This study was supported by the Jack Tindall Bequest, the Price Family Foundation, an Australian and New Zealand Head and Neck Cancer Society Grant, an Independent Research Institutes Infrastructure Support Scheme Grant and a Victorian State Government Operational Infrastructure Support Grant. K.K. was supported by a PhD scholarship from the Garnett Passe and Rodney Williams Memorial Foundation. O.M.S. is a National Health and Medical Research Council (NHMRC) Senior Research Fellows (APP1136119).

Institutional Review Board Statement: This study was approved by the Royal Melbourne Hospital Human Research Ethics committees (RMH HREC 2013.087, RMH HREC 2012.071).

Informed Consent Statement: Informed consent was obtained from prospective subjects involved in the study (HREC 2013.087). A waiver of informed consent for retrospectively recruited patients was granted by the relevant Ethics committee (HREC 2012.071).

Data Availability Statement: The molecular data presented in this study are available in the Supplementary Data. Associated clinical data cannot be provided to maintain patient confidentiality.

Acknowledgments: The author would like to acknowledge Stephen Wilcox for his assistance with DNA sequencing and Chris Love for collection of patient survival data.

Conflicts of Interest: The authors declare no conflict of interest.

References

1. Centers for Disease Control (CDC). Smoking and cancer. *MMWR Morb. Mortal. Wkly Rep.* **1982**, *31*, 77–80.
2. Tuyns, A.J. Epidemiology of alcohol and cancer. *Cancer Res.* **1979**, *39 Pt 2*, 2840–2843.
3. Chen, F.; Wang, J.; Chen, J.; Yan, L.; Hu, Z.; Wu, J.; Bao, X.; Lin, L.; Wang, R.; Cai, L.; et al. Serum copper and zinc levels and the risk of oral cancer: A new insight based on large-scale case-control study. *Oral Dis.* **2019**, *25*, 80–86. [CrossRef]
4. Ang, K.K.; Harris, J.; Wheeler, R.; Weber, R.; Rosenthal, D.I.; Nguyen-Tan, P.F.; Westra, W.H.; Chung, C.H.; Jordan, R.C.; Lu, C.; et al. Human papillomavirus and survival of patients with oropharyngeal cancer. *N. Engl. J. Med.* **2010**, *363*, 24–35. [CrossRef] [PubMed]
5. *IARC Monographs on the Evaluation of Carcinogenic Risks to Humans*; Human Papillomaviruses: Lyon, France, 2007; Volume 90.
6. Koo, K.; Barrowman, R.; McCullough, M.; Iseli, T.; Wiesenfeld, D. Non-smoking non-drinking elderly females: A clinically distinct subgroup of oral squamous cell carcinoma patients. *Int. J. Oral. Maxillofac. Surg.* **2013**, *42*, 929–933. [CrossRef]
7. DeAngelis, A.; Breik, O.; Koo, K.; Iseli, T.; Nastri, A.; Fua, T.; Rischin, D.; McCullough, M.; Wiesenfeld, D. Non-smoking, non-drinking elderly females, a 5year follow-up of a clinically distinct cohort of oral squamous cell carcinoma patients. *Oral Oncol.* **2018**, *86*, 113–120. [CrossRef]
8. Wiseman, S.M.; Swede, H.; Stoler, D.L.; Anderson, G.R.; Rigual, N.R.; Hicks, W.L., Jr.; Douglas, W.G.; Tan, D.; Loree, T.R. Squamous cell carcinoma of the head and neck in nonsmokers and nondrinkers: An analysis of clinicopathologic characteristics and treatment outcomes. *Ann. Surg. Oncol.* **2003**, *10*, 551–557. [CrossRef]
9. Farshadpour, F.; Hordijk, G.J.; Koole, R.; Slootweg, P.J. Non-smoking and non-drinking patients with head and neck squamous cell carcinoma: A distinct population. *Oral Dis.* **2007**, *13*, 239–243. [CrossRef]
10. Dahlstrom, K.R.; Little, J.A.; Zafereo, M.E.; Lung, M.; Wei, Q.; Sturgis, E.M. Squamous cell carcinoma of the head and neck in never smoker-never drinkers: A descriptive epidemiologic study. *Head Neck* **2008**, *30*, 75–84. [CrossRef]

11. Harris, S.L.; Kimple, R.J.; Hayes, D.N.; Couch, M.E.; Rosenman, J.G. Never-smokers, never-drinkers: Unique clinical subgroup of young patients with head and neck squamous cell cancers. *Head Neck* **2010**, *32*, 499–503. [CrossRef] [PubMed]
12. Bachar, G.; Hod, R.; Goldstein, D.P.; Irish, J.C.; Gullane, P.J.; Brown, D.; Gilbert, R.W.; Hadar, T.; Feinmesser, R.; Shpitzer, T. Outcome of oral tongue squamous cell carcinoma in patients with and without known risk factors. *Oral Oncol.* **2011**, *47*, 45–50. [CrossRef] [PubMed]
13. Albuquerque, R.; Lopez-Lopez, J.; Mari-Roig, A.; Jane-Salas, E.; Rosello-Llabres, X.; Santos, J.R. Oral tongue squamous cell carcinoma (OTSCC): Alcohol and tobacco consumption versus non-consumption. A study in a Portuguese population. *Braz. Dent. J.* **2011**, *22*, 517–521. [CrossRef]
14. Kruse, A.L.; Bredell, M.; Luebbers, H.T.; Gratz, K.W. Head and neck cancer in the elderly: A retrospective study over 10 years (1999–2008). *Head Neck Oncol.* **2010**, *2*, 25. [CrossRef]
15. Laco, J.; Vosmikova, H.; Novakova, V.; Celakovsky, P.; Dolezalova, H.; Tucek, L.; Nekvindova, J.; Vosmik, M.; Cermakova, E.; Ryska, A. The role of high-risk human papillomavirus infection in oral and oropharyngeal squamous cell carcinoma in non-smoking and non-drinking patients: A clinicopathological and molecular study of 46 cases. *Virchows Arch.* **2011**, *458*, 179–187. [CrossRef] [PubMed]
16. Lechner, M.; Frampton, G.M.; Fenton, T.; Feber, A.; Palmer, G.; Jay, A.; Pillay, N.; Forster, M.; Cronin, M.T.; Lipson, D.; et al. Targeted next-generation sequencing of head and neck squamous cell carcinoma identifies novel genetic alterations in HPV+ and HPV-tumors. *Genome Med.* **2013**, *5*, 49. [CrossRef]
17. Seiwert, T.Y.; Zuo, Z.; Keck, M.K.; Khattri, A.; Pedamallu, C.S.; Stricker, T.; Brown, C.; Pugh, T.J.; Stojanov, P.; Cho, J.; et al. Integrative and comparative genomic analysis of HPV-positive and HPV-negative head and neck squamous cell carcinomas. *Clin. Cancer Res.* **2015**, *21*, 632–641. [CrossRef]
18. van Ginkel, J.H.; de Leng, W.W.; de Bree, R.; van Es, R.J.; Willems, S.M. Targeted sequencing reveals TP53 as a potential diagnostic biomarker in the post-treatment surveillance of head and neck cancer. *Oncotarget* **2016**, *7*, 61575–61586. [CrossRef]
19. Chung, C.H.; Guthrie, V.B.; Masica, D.L.; Tokheim, C.; Kang, H.; Richmon, J.; Agrawal, N.; Fakhry, C.; Quon, H.; Subramaniam, R.M.; et al. Genomic alterations in head and neck squamous cell carcinoma determined by cancer gene-targeted sequencing. *Ann. Oncol.* **2015**, *26*, 1216–1223. [CrossRef]
20. Chen, S.J.; Liu, H.; Liao, C.T.; Huang, P.J.; Huang, Y.; Hsu, A.; Tang, P.; Chang, Y.S.; Chen, H.C.; Yen, T.C. Ultra-deep targeted sequencing of advanced oral squamous cell carcinoma identifies a mutation-based prognostic gene signature. *Oncotarget* **2015**, *6*, 18066–18080. [CrossRef]
21. Tinhofer, I.; Budach, V.; Saki, M.; Konschak, R.; Niehr, F.; Johrens, K.; Weichert, W.; Linge, A.; Lohaus, F.; Krause, M.; et al. Targeted next-generation sequencing of locally advanced squamous cell carcinomas of the head and neck reveals druggable targets for improving adjuvant chemoradiation. *Eur. J. Cancer* **2016**, *57*, 78–86. [CrossRef]
22. Er, T.K.; Wang, Y.Y.; Chen, C.C.; Herreros-Villanueva, M.; Liu, T.C.; Yuan, S.S. Molecular characterization of oral squamous cell carcinoma using targeted next-generation sequencing. *Oral Dis.* **2015**, *21*, 872–878. [CrossRef]
23. Al-Hebshi, N.N.; Li, S.; Nasher, A.T.; El-Setouhy, M.; Alsanosi, R.; Blancato, J.; Loffredo, C. Exome sequencing of oral squamous cell carcinoma in users of Arabian snuff reveals novel candidates for driver genes. *Int. J. Cancer* **2016**, *139*, 363–372. [CrossRef]
24. Pickering, C.R.; Zhang, J.; Yoo, S.Y.; Bengtsson, L.; Moorthy, S.; Neskey, D.M.; Zhao, M.; Ortega Alves, M.V.; Chang, K.; Drummond, J.; et al. Integrative genomic characterization of oral squamous cell carcinoma identifies frequent somatic drivers. *Cancer Discov.* **2013**, *3*, 770–781. [CrossRef]
25. Stransky, N.; Egloff, A.M.; Tward, A.D.; Kostic, A.D.; Cibulskis, K.; Sivachenko, A.; Kryukov, G.V.; Lawrence, M.S.; Sougnez, C.; McKenna, A.; et al. The mutational landscape of head and neck squamous cell carcinoma. *Science* **2011**, *333*, 1157–1160. [CrossRef] [PubMed]
26. Agrawal, N.; Frederick, M.J.; Pickering, C.R.; Bettegowda, C.; Chang, K.; Li, R.J.; Fakhry, C.; Xie, T.X.; Zhang, J.; Wang, J.; et al. Exome sequencing of head and neck squamous cell carcinoma reveals inactivating mutations in NOTCH1. *Science* **2011**, *333*, 1154–1157. [CrossRef]
27. India Project Team of the International Cancer Genome Consortium. Mutational landscape of gingivo-buccal oral squamous cell carcinoma reveals new recurrently-mutated genes and molecular subgroups. *Nat. Commun.* **2013**, *4*, 2873. [CrossRef]
28. The Cancer Genome Atlas Network. Comprehensive genomic characterization of head and neck squamous cell carcinomas. *Nature* **2015**, *517*, 576–582. [CrossRef] [PubMed]
29. Nakagaki, T.; Tamura, M.; Kobashi, K.; Omori, A.; Koyama, R.; Idogawa, M.; Ogi, K.; Hiratsuka, H.; Tokino, T.; Sasaki, Y. Targeted next-generation sequencing of 50 cancer-related genes in Japanese patients with oral squamous cell carcinoma. *Tumour. Biol.* **2018**, *40*. [CrossRef] [PubMed]
30. Su, S.C.; Lin, C.W.; Liu, Y.F.; Fan, W.L.; Chen, M.K.; Yu, C.P.; Yang, W.E.; Su, C.W.; Chuang, C.Y.; Li, W.H.; et al. Exome Sequencing of Oral Squamous Cell Carcinoma Reveals Molecular Subgroups and Novel Therapeutic Opportunities. *Theranostics* **2017**, *7*, 1088–1099. [CrossRef] [PubMed]
31. Alexandrov, L.B.; Ju, Y.S.; Haase, K.; Van Loo, P.; Martincorena, I.; Nik-Zainal, S.; Totoki, Y.; Fujimoto, A.; Nakagawa, H.; Shibata, T.; et al. Mutational signatures associated with tobacco smoking in human cancer. *Science* **2016**, *354*, 618–622. [CrossRef] [PubMed]
32. Gillison, M.L.; Akagi, K.; Xiao, W.; Jiang, B.; Pickard, R.K.L.; Li, J.; Swanson, B.J.; Agrawal, A.D.; Zucker, M.; Stache-Crain, B.; et al. Human papillomavirus and the landscape of secondary genetic alterations in oral cancers. *Genome Res.* **2019**, *29*, 1–17. [CrossRef]

33. Chang, J.; Tan, W.; Ling, Z.; Xi, R.; Shao, M.; Chen, M.; Luo, Y.; Zhao, Y.; Liu, Y.; Huang, X.; et al. Genomic analysis of oesophageal squamous-cell carcinoma identifies alcohol drinking-related mutation signature and genomic alterations. *Nat. Commun.* **2017**, *8*, 15290. [CrossRef] [PubMed]
34. Letouze, E.; Shinde, J.; Renault, V.; Couchy, G.; Blanc, J.F.; Tubacher, E.; Bayard, Q.; Bacq, D.; Meyer, V.; Semhoun, J.; et al. Mutational signatures reveal the dynamic interplay of risk factors and cellular processes during liver tumorigenesis. *Nat. Commun.* **2017**, *8*, 1315. [CrossRef]
35. Pickering, C.R.; Zhang, J.; Neskey, D.M.; Zhao, M.; Jasser, S.A.; Wang, J.; Ward, A.; Tsai, C.J.; Ortega Alves, M.V.; Zhou, J.H.; et al. Squamous cell carcinoma of the oral tongue in young non-smokers is genomically similar to tumors in older smokers. *Clin. Cancer Res.* **2014**, *20*, 3842–3848. [CrossRef] [PubMed]
36. Edge, S.; Byrd, D.R.; Compton, C.C.; Fritz, A.G.; Greene, F.; Trotti, A. (Eds.) *AJCC Cancer Staging Manual*, 7th ed.; Springer: New York, NY, USA, 2010.
37. Tamborero, D.; Gonzalez-Perez, A.; Lopez-Bigas, N. OncodriveCLUST: Exploiting the positional clustering of somatic mutations to identify cancer genes. *Bioinformatics* **2013**, *29*, 2238–2244. [CrossRef]
38. Lawrence, M.S.; Stojanov, P.; Polak, P.; Kryukov, G.V.; Cibulskis, K.; Sivachenko, A.; Carter, S.L.; Stewart, C.; Mermel, C.H.; Roberts, S.A.; et al. Mutational heterogeneity in cancer and the search for new cancer-associated genes. *Nature* **2013**, *499*, 214–218. [CrossRef] [PubMed]
39. DePristo, M.A.; Banks, E.; Poplin, R.; Garimella, K.V.; Maguire, J.R.; Hartl, C.; Philippakis, A.A.; del Angel, G.; Rivas, M.A.; Hanna, M.; et al. A framework for variation discovery and genotyping using next-generation DNA sequencing data. *Nat. Genet.* **2011**, *43*, 491–498. [CrossRef]
40. Van der Auwera, G.A.; Carneiro, M.O.; Hartl, C.; Poplin, R.; Del Angel, G.; Levy-Moonshine, A.; Jordan, T.; Shakir, K.; Roazen, D.; Thibault, J.; et al. From FastQ data to high confidence variant calls: The Genome Analysis Toolkit best practices pipeline. *Curr. Protoc. Bioinform.* **2013**, *43*, 11.10.1–11.10.33.
41. Cingolani, P.; Platts, A.; Wang le, L.; Coon, M.; Nguyen, T.; Wang, L.; Land, S.J.; Lu, X.; Ruden, D.M. A program for annotating and predicting the effects of single nucleotide polymorphisms, SnpEff: SNPs in the genome of Drosophila melanogaster strain w1118; iso-2; iso-3. *Fly Austin* **2012**, *6*, 80–92. [CrossRef]
42. Guo, Y.; Li, J.; Li, C.I.; Long, J.; Samuels, D.C.; Shyr, Y. The effect of strand bias in Illumina short-read sequencing data. *BMC Genom.* **2012**, *13*, 666. [CrossRef]
43. Mouradov, D.; Sloggett, C.; Jorissen, R.N.; Love, C.G.; Li, S.; Burgess, A.W.; Arango, D.; Strausberg, R.L.; Buchanan, D.; Wormald, S.; et al. Colorectal cancer cell lines are representative models of the main molecular subtypes of primary cancer. *Cancer Res.* **2014**, *74*, 3238–3247. [CrossRef] [PubMed]
44. Adzhubei, I.; Jordan, D.M.; Sunyaev, S.R. Predicting functional effect of human missense mutations using PolyPhen-2. *Curr. Protoc. Hum. Genet.* **2013**, *76*, 7–20. [CrossRef] [PubMed]
45. Plagnol, V.; Curtis, J.; Epstein, M.; Mok, K.Y.; Stebbings, E.; Grigoriadou, S.; Wood, N.W.; Hambleton, S.; Burns, S.O.; Thrasher, A.J.; et al. A robust model for read count data in exome sequencing experiments and implications for copy number variant calling. *Bioinformatic* **2012**, *28*, 2747–2754. [CrossRef]
46. Roca, I.; Gonzalez-Castro, L.; Fernandez, H.; Couce, M.L.; Fernandez-Marmiesse, A. Free-access copy-number variant detection tools for targeted next-generation sequencing data. *Mutat. Res.* **2019**, *779*, 114–125. [CrossRef]
47. Rajagopalan, R.; Murrell, J.R.; Luo, M.; Conlin, L.K. A highly sensitive and specific workflow for detecting rare copy-number variants from exome sequencing data. *Genome Med.* **2020**, *12*, 14. [CrossRef]
48. Derrien, T.; Estelle, J.; Marco Sola, S.; Knowles, D.G.; Raineri, E.; Guigo, R.; Ribeca, P. Fast computation and applications of genome mappability. *PLoS ONE* **2012**, *7*, e30377. [CrossRef] [PubMed]
49. R Core Team. *R: A Language and Environment for Statistical Computing*; R Foundation for Statistical Computing: Vienna, Austria, 2013.
50. Zeileis, A.; Kleiber, C.; Jackman, S. Regression Models for Count Data in R. *J. Stat. Softw.* **2008**, *27*, 25. [CrossRef]
51. DrinkWise Australia. Australian Drinking Habits: 2007 vs. 2017. Available online: https://drinkwise.org.au/our-work/australian-drinking-habits-2007-vs-2017 (accessed on 17 September 2020).
52. Belobrov, S.; Cornall, A.M.; Young, R.J.; Koo, K.; Angel, C.; Wiesenfeld, D.; Rischin, D.; Garland, S.M.; McCullough, M. The role of human papillomavirus in p16-positive oral cancers. *J. Oral Pathol. Med.* **2018**, *47*, 18–24. [CrossRef]
53. Kreimer, A.R.; Clifford, G.M.; Boyle, P.; Franceschi, S. Human papillomavirus types in head and neck squamous cell carcinomas worldwide: A systematic review. *Cancer Epidemiol. Biomark. Prev.* **2005**, *14*, 467–475. [CrossRef]
54. Scheffner, M.; Werness, B.A.; Huibregtse, J.M.; Levine, A.J.; Howley, P.M. The E6 oncoprotein encoded by human papillomavirus types 16 and 18 promotes the degradation of p53. *Cell* **1990**, *63*, 1129–1136. [CrossRef]
55. Tam, K.W.; Zhang, W.; Soh, J.; Stastny, V.; Chen, M.; Sun, H.; Thu, K.; Rios, J.J.; Yang, C.; Marconett, C.N.; et al. CDKN2A/p16 inactivation mechanisms and their relationship with smoke exposure and molecular features in non-small-cell lung cancer. *J. Thorac. Oncol.* **2013**, *8*, 1378–1388. [CrossRef]
56. Sivarajah, S.; Kostiuk, M.; Lindsay, C.; Puttagunta, L.; O'Connell, D.A.; Harris, J.; Seikaly, H.; Biron, V.L. EGFR as a biomarker of smoking status and survival in oropharyngeal squamous cell carcinoma. *J. Otolaryngol. Head Neck Surg.* **2019**, *48*, 1. [CrossRef] [PubMed]

57. Rudin, C.M.; Avila-Tang, E.; Harris, C.C.; Herman, J.G.; Hirsch, F.R.; Pao, W.; Schwartz, A.G.; Vahakangas, K.H.; Samet, J.M. Lung cancer in never smokers: Molecular profiles and therapeutic implications. *Clin. Cancer Res.* **2009**, *15*, 5646–5661. [CrossRef] [PubMed]
58. Sandulache, V.C.; Michikawa, C.; Kataria, P.; Gleber-Netto, F.O.; Bell, D.; Trivedi, S.; Rao, X.; Wang, J.; Zhao, M.; Jasser, S.; et al. High-Risk TP53 Mutations Are Associated with Extranodal Extension in Oral Cavity Squamous Cell Carcinoma. *Clin. Cancer Res.* **2018**, *24*, 1727–1733. [CrossRef] [PubMed]
59. Chen, W.S.; Bindra, R.S.; Mo, A.; Hayman, T.; Husain, Z.; Contessa, J.N.; Gaffney, S.G.; Townsend, J.P.; Yu, J.B. CDKN2A Copy Number Loss Is an Independent Prognostic Factor in HPV-Negative Head and Neck Squamous Cell Carcinoma. *Front. Oncol.* **2018**, *8*, 95. [CrossRef]
60. Michikawa, C.; Uzawa, N.; Sato, H.; Ohyama, Y.; Okada, N.; Amagasa, T. Epidermal growth factor receptor gene copy number aberration at the primary tumour is significantly associated with extracapsular spread in oral cancer. *Br. J. Cancer* **2011**, *104*, 850–855. [CrossRef]
61. Bissinger, O.; Kolk, A.; Drecoll, E.; Straub, M.; Lutz, C.; Wolff, K.D.; Gotz, C. EGFR and Cortactin: Markers for potential double target therapy in oral squamous cell carcinoma. *Exp. Ther. Med.* **2017**, *14*, 4620–4626.
62. Chen, I.H.; Chang, J.T.; Liao, C.T.; Wang, H.M.; Hsieh, L.L.; Cheng, A.J. Prognostic significance of EGFR and Her-2 in oral cavity cancer in betel quid prevalent area cancer prognosis. *Br. J. Cancer* **2003**, *89*, 681–686. [CrossRef]
63. Huang, S.F.; Cheng, S.D.; Chien, H.T.; Liao, C.T.; Chen, I.H.; Wang, H.M.; Chuang, W.Y.; Wang, C.Y.; Hsieh, L.L. Relationship between epidermal growth factor receptor gene copy number and protein expression in oral cavity squamous cell carcinoma. *Oral Oncol.* **2012**, *48*, 67–72. [CrossRef]
64. Chau, N.G.; Perez-Ordonez, B.; Zhang, K.; Pham, N.A.; Ho, J.; Zhang, T.; Ludkovski, O.; Wang, L.; Chen, E.X.; Tsao, M.S.; et al. The association between EGFR variant III, HPV, p16, c-MET, EGFR gene copy number and response to EGFR inhibitors in patients with recurrent or metastatic squamous cell carcinoma of the head and neck. *Head Neck Oncol.* **2011**, *3*, 11. [CrossRef]
65. Beaty, B.T.; Moon, D.H.; Shen, C.J.; Amdur, R.J.; Weiss, J.; Grilley-Olson, J.; Patel, S.; Zanation, A.; Hackman, T.G.; Thorp, B.; et al. PIK3CA Mutation in HPV-Associated OPSCC Patients Receiving Deintensified Chemoradiation. *J. Natl. Cancer Inst.* **2020**, *112*, 855–858. [CrossRef] [PubMed]

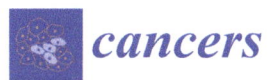

Editorial

Treatments of Squamous Cell Cancer

Darido Charbel [1,2]

1. The Peter MacCallum Cancer Centre, 305 Grattan St, Melbourne 3000, VIC, Australia; Charbel.Darido@petermac.org
2. Sir Peter MacCallum Department of Oncology, The University of Melbourne, Parkville 3010, VIC, Australia

Received: 29 September 2020; Accepted: 30 October 2020; Published: 2 November 2020

It is now clear that the most common solid cancer is squamous cell cancer (SCC) [1]. This malignant tumour originates mainly from epithelial cells that cover the skin, the surfaces of the respiratory and digestive tracts, and the linings of the hollow organs of the body that interface with the external environment. These epithelia are constantly challenged within diverse anatomical locations and share a common genetic mutational landscape [2]. Among the etiological factors of SCC, UV irradiation, exposure to carcinogen such as tobacco smoking and betel quid chewing, frequent alcohol use, genetic predisposition, immunosuppression, and the diverse commensal microbiome are highly cited. Treatments of SCC that consider the disease molecular drivers and its microenvironment have been embraced to overcome SCC heterogeneity [3].

Current conventional treatment regimens for SCC, including surgery, radiation, chemotherapy, targeted therapy and immunotherapy, are non-selective and are administered regardless of biomarkers [4]. Therapy resistance and/or cancer recurrence subsequently emerges leading to SCC patient mortality. Over the last decade, the SCC field has witnessed an unprecedented investment in the development, characterisation and translation of novel biomarkers to have real clinical value [5]. The enduring challenge ahead involves understanding how best to pair these biomarkers with preventative and therapeutic approaches to extract the maximum benefit for SCC patients. Central to this ambition is the knowledge of how to tailor SCC therapies to specific risk factors and molecular drivers while enhancing the immune response to eradicate the disease.

In this Special Issue, Dr Darido brings together experts in the field of SCC to provide an overview of the current treatment advances. As we develop a better understanding of the limitations of current therapies, we expect to highlight new diagnostic, prognostic/predictive and therapy response/resistance biomarkers for interventional modalities in emerging immuno-oncology therapeutic areas, and areas of unmet clinical need. Future prospects enabling improved therapies will provide an exciting therapeutic roadmap for the control of SCC and will ultimately contribute to alleviating the huge burden of SCC in patients.

Funding: This research received no external funding.

Conflicts of Interest: The author declares no conflict of interest.

References

1. Dotto, G.P.; Rustgi, A.K. Squamous Cell Cancers: A Unified Perspective on Biology and Genetics. *Cancer Cell* **2016**, *29*, 622–637. [CrossRef] [PubMed]
2. Sanchez-Danes, A.; Blanpain, C. Deciphering the cells of origin of squamous cell carcinomas. *Nat. Rev. Cancer* **2018**, *18*, 549–561. [CrossRef] [PubMed]
3. Murciano-Goroff, Y.R.; Warner, A.B.; Wolchok, J.D. The future of cancer immunotherapy: microenvironment-targeting combinations. *Cell Res.* **2020**, *30*, 507–519. [CrossRef] [PubMed]

4. Tan, F.H.; Bai, Y.; Saintigny, P.; Darido, C. mTOR Signalling in Head and Neck Cancer: Heads Up. *Cells* **2019**, *8*, 333. [CrossRef] [PubMed]
5. Siravegna, G.; Marsoni, S.; Siena, S.; Bardelli, A. Integrating liquid biopsies into the management of cancer. *Nat. Rev. Clin. Oncol.* **2017**, *14*, 531–548. [CrossRef] [PubMed]

Publisher's Note: MDPI stays neutral with regard to jurisdictional claims in published maps and institutional affiliations.

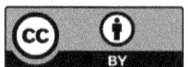 © 2020 by the author. Licensee MDPI, Basel, Switzerland. This article is an open access article distributed under the terms and conditions of the Creative Commons Attribution (CC BY) license (http://creativecommons.org/licenses/by/4.0/).

MDPI
St. Alban-Anlage 66
4052 Basel
Switzerland
Tel. +41 61 683 77 34
Fax +41 61 302 89 18
www.mdpi.com

Cancers Editorial Office
E-mail: cancers@mdpi.com
www.mdpi.com/journal/cancers

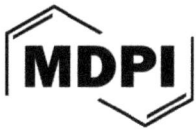